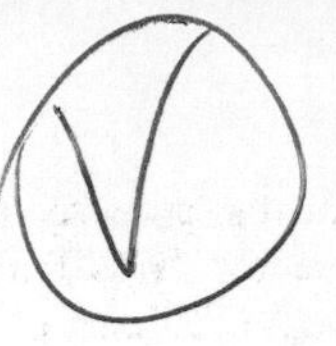

MRCP 1

Multiple True/False

Revision Book

Philip A Kalra MA MB BChir FRCP MD

Consultant Nephrologist and Honorary Lecturer
Hope Hospital, Salford Royal Hospitals Trust and
The University of Manchester

PAS
Dedicat

Egerton Court
Parkgate Estate
Knutsford
Cheshire WA16 8DX

Telephone: 01565 752000

First published 2002
Reprinted 2002

ISBN 1 901198 95 2

A catalogue record for this book is available from the British Library.

Typeset by Breeze Ltd, Manchester.
Printed by Bell and Bain Ltd, Glasgow.

CONTENTS

MRCP (UK) PART 1 EXAMINATION PAPER 1

The MRCP (UK) Part 1 Examination Paper 1 will contain 60 multiple true-false questions, including approximately 14 MCQs on all aspects of clinical science (molecular and membrane biology, anatomy, physiology, biochemistry, metabolism, immunology, genetics, elementary statistics, epidemiology, evidence-based medicine, microbiology and pharmacology) and some 46 questions which will test a candidate's knowledge of a wide range of common and important disorders in General Medicine, as set out in the published syllabus.

The composition of Paper 1 will be as follows:

Clinical science	14
Cardiology	4
Clinical haematology	4
Clinical pharmacology, therapeutics and toxicology	6
Dermatology	1
Endocrinology	4
Gastroenterology	4
Infectious diseases and tropical medicine	4
Nephrology	4
Neurology	4
Psychiatry	4
Respiratory medicine	4
Rheumatology	4
Miscellaneous (e.g. ophthalmology, sexually transmitted diseases)	1

PREFACE

It is recognised that Multiple Choice Questions (MCQs) are the most reliable, reproducible and internally consistent method we have of testing recall of factual knowledge, and they are also able to assess reasoning ability and an understanding of principles and concepts. Although major changes have recently occurred in the structure of the MRCP part 1, the multiple True/False style (MCQ) remains the cornerstone of the examination. Hence, within Paper 1 the candidate will be faced with 60 such questions to be completed within 2.5 hours; gone, thankfully, is the negative marking format, but now the pass mark will be set by a criterion-referenced system. In order to pass the overall Part 1 examination candidates will have to achieve a pass in both Paper 1 and 2 (the latter composed of 100 'Best answer from 5' questions).

Pastest have carefully observed the question content of the Royal College examinations over the last two decades, and this book attempts to reproduce the format, content and style of Paper 1 of the new MRCP part 1 examination. The proportion of questions in individual subjects within Paper 1 is similar to that composing the old-style Part 1 exam (see page opposite), and so, as before, there is an emphasis on clinical science. This book reflects this structure, with appropriate numbers of questions for each individual specialty within the Medical syllabus. One exception is Clinical Pharmacology and Toxicology, in which the variety and number of potential topics is quite diverse; this section accordingly carries a greater proportion of questions, relative to the exam, than would be expected. This book contains over 750 carefully evaluated MCQs, and this includes three complete and balanced Practice exams in order to aid your revision.

My thanks are due to many colleagues from the North West regional hospitals, in particular to Dr Malcolm Littley, for their help in producing the questions for this book, and especially to Kirsten Baxter and the team at Pastest who have expedited the production process in order to achieve a timely and quality publication.

Philip A Kalra
May 2002

CARDIOLOGY

Basic cardiology and the ECG

1. In the heart

- ❑ A the pulmonary valve is normally bicuspid
- ❑ B the right bundle branch of His divides into anterior and posterior hemibundles
- ❑ C the coronary sinus opens into the right atrium
- ❑ D blood leaving the coronary sinus is less de-oxygenated than the atrial blood into which it drains
- ❑ E the S-A node lies in the anterior wall of the left atrium

2. The following statements about the arterial pulse are correct:

- ❑ A pulsus paradoxus is diagnostic of cardiac tamponade
- ❑ B a bisferiens pulse suggests combined aortic stenosis and regurgitation
- ❑ C pulsus alternans is a sign of impaired left ventricular function
- ❑ D a slow rising carotid pulse is characteristic of severe mitral stenosis
- ❑ E the femoral pulses are diminished but not delayed in coarctation of the aorta

3. During the normal cardiac cycle

- ❑ A initial myocardial depolarisation occurs at a site near to the junction of the right atrium and inferior vena cava
- ❑ B there is no time when all cardiac chambers are simultaneously in diastole
- ❑ C the dicrotic notch of the aortic pressure trace coincides with the second heart sound
- ❑ D a third heart sound is never heard
- ❑ E the majority of coronary artery flow occurs during ventricular diastole

4. The right coronary artery

- ❑ A originates from the right coronary sinus and lies in the right atrio-ventricular groove
- ❑ B typically supplies the inferior aspect of the left ventricle
- ❑ C typically gives rise to the artery to the A-V node
- ❑ D gives rise to the posterior descending coronary artery in the majority of patients
- ❑ E occlusion has occurred in the majority of patients with right ventricular infarction and failure

5. Atrial natriuretic peptide

- ❑ A is secreted by the left atrium
- ❑ B receptors are found in the kidney
- ❑ C stimulates renal sodium reabsorption
- ❑ D consists of 28 amino acids
- ❑ E secretion is inhibited in congestive cardiac failure

6. The following statements are correct for the normal adult resting electro-cardiogram:

- ❑ A the mean frontal plane QRS axis is between 0° and +90°
- ❑ B the mean frontal plane T wave axis may not differ from the mean frontal plane QRS axis by more than 45°
- ❑ C the P wave should not exceed a height of 0.25 mV or a duration of 0.12 seconds
- ❑ D in the precordial leads at least one R wave should exceed a height of 8 mm (0.8 mV) but no R wave should be greater than 27 mm (2.7 mV)
- ❑ E the sum of the tallest R wave in the left precordial leads and the deepest S wave in the right precordial leads must not exceed 30 mm

7. ST depression on ECG is a feature of

- ❑ A digitalis toxicity
- ❑ B hypertension
- ❑ C patients with cardiac syndrome X on exertion
- ❑ D chronic pericarditis
- ❑ E hypokalaemia

8. On the resting adult electrocardiogram, T wave inversion

- ❑ A in V1 is always abnormal
- ❑ B in V2 is always abnormal
- ❑ C in V5 is always abnormal
- ❑ D may be seen in subendocardial ischaemia
- ❑ E may be generalised in pericarditis

Arrhythmias and conduction disorders

9. The following statements are correct for heart block:

- ❑ A the Wenckebach phenomenon may occur in healthy individuals
- ❑ B after an acute anterior myocardial infarction, development of bifascicular block has a poor prognosis
- ❑ C in asymptomatic individuals, the chance finding of slight lengthening of the PR interval is of no significance
- ❑ D patients with recurrent symptomatic episodes of complete heart block should be given a trial of oral isoprenaline before consideration for permanent pacemaker implantation
- ❑ E complete heart block developing during the first day after an inferior myocardial infarction will usually require permanent pacing because the artery to the atrioventricular node is involved in the disease territory

10. Characteristic findings in complete atrio-ventricular (heart) block include

- ❑ A variable intensity of the second heart sound
- ❑ B increased ventricular rate after atropine
- ❑ C collapsing brachial pulse
- ❑ D regular giant 'a' waves in the jugular venous pulse
- ❑ E beat-to-beat variation in the blood pressure

11. The following are appropriate pacing modes for patients with heart block:

- ❑ A DDD pacing for permanent atrial fibrillation with prolonged symptomatic pauses
- ❑ B DDD pacing for complete heart block associated with sinus node disease
- ❑ C AAIR pacing in patients with sinus node disease in the absence of AV block
- ❑ D VVI pacing for atrial fibrillation with persistent bradycardia
- ❑ E DDD pacing for complete heart block in the absence of sinus node disease

12. Features of cardiac syncope include

- ❑ A transient unconsciousness with rapid return to consciousness
- ❑ B preceding aura
- ❑ C distinction from epilepsy of tonic/clonic phases
- ❑ D tachyarrhythmias
- ❑ E occurrence in the erect or supine position

13. Right bundle branch block

- ❑ A is associated with a deep S wave in V6
- ❑ B may occur in normal individuals
- ❑ C is found in 30% of cases of atrial septal defect
- ❑ D is an indication for temporary pacing in patients undergoing general anaesthesia
- ❑ E may occur in patients with pulmonary embolus

14. Causes of atrial fibrillation include

- ❑ A hyperthyroidism
- ❑ B recent myocardial infarction
- ❑ C chronic hypertension
- ❑ D cardiac surgery
- ❑ E subdural haematoma

15. The following statements about atrial flutter are correct:

- ❑ A the ventricular rate is characteristically about 150/min
- ❑ B an irregular pulse is a recognised finding
- ❑ C DC counter shock is a treatment of choice
- ❑ D quinidine alone is a recognised treatment
- ❑ E carotid sinus pressure is of value in diagnosis

16. Wolff-Parkinson-White syndrome

- ❑ A is due to an anomalous pathway known as the bundle of Kent situated along the A–V ring
- ❑ B is associated with an increased incidence of atrial fibrillation
- ❑ C is treated with radiofrequency ablation of the atrioventricular node
- ❑ D may be associated with mitral leaflet prolapse
- ❑ E may be treated with prophylactic digoxin to prevent fast atrial fibrillation

17. The following statements are correct for electromechanical dissociation:

- ❑ A the electrocardiogram shows no cardiac activity
- ❑ B it responds to DC cardioversion
- ❑ C it has a better prognosis than ventricular fibrillation
- ❑ D when it occurs a week after acute myocardial infarction it is characteristically the result of cardiac rupture
- ❑ E it may respond to adrenaline injected down an endotracheal tube if intravenous access is not available

Valvular disease and heart sounds

18. A cardiac murmur is likely to be innocent (i.e. not associated with demonstrable structural abnormality) if

- ❑ A it is diastolic
- ❑ B the only finding is a soft ejection systolic murmur at the left sternal edge in a healthy young child
- ❑ C it is associated with a palpable thrill
- ❑ D it is systolic with an ejection click
- ❑ E it is continuous, and disappears on neck vein compression or when lying down

19. A third heart sound in a 45-year-old man

- ❑ A is a sign of heart disease
- ❑ B excludes significant A-V valve stenosis
- ❑ C could be due to tricuspid regurgitation
- ❑ D is a feature of constrictive pericarditis
- ❑ E could indicate hypertensive heart disease

20. Isolated calcific aortic stenosis in the elderly

- ❑ A is rheumatic in origin in the majority of cases
- ❑ B may present as congestive cardiac failure
- ❑ C is associated characteristically with a systolic ejection click
- ❑ D tends to soften and delay the aortic component of the second sound
- ❑ E is not haemodynamically important in the absence of a thrill

21. In aortic regurgitation

- ❑ A the Austin-Flint murmur is associated with a mitral opening snap
- ❑ B an aortic ejection systolic murmur indicates co-existing aortic stenosis
- ❑ C increasing severity of regurgitation prolongs the murmur
- ❑ D increasing severity of regurgitation lowers diastolic blood pressure
- ❑ E antibiotic prophylaxis is not required

22. A rumbling apical diastolic murmur is a recognised finding in

- ❑ A systemic arterial hypertension
- ❑ B thyrotoxicosis
- ❑ C mitral regurgitation
- ❑ D complete heart block
- ❑ E ventricular septal defect

23. In a patient with mitral stenosis in sinus rhythm, the following findings would indicate a severe lesion:

- ❑ A long mid-diastolic murmur
- ❑ B late, loud, opening snap
- ❑ C soft first heart sound
- ❑ D Graham-Steel murmur
- ❑ E third heart sound

24. Characteristic features of mitral valve prolapse syndrome include

❏ A early systolic murmur at apex
❏ B mid-systolic click
❏ C a liability to infective endocarditis
❏ D a poor prognosis
❏ E a higher incidence in males

25. Recognised features of mitral regurgitation include

❏ A loud first heart sound
❏ B mid-systolic click followed by late systolic murmur
❏ C third heart sound
❏ D pansystolic murmur and apical thrill with ECG evidence of a recent posterior infarct
❏ E reversed splitting of the second sound

26. The following statements concerning pulmonary stenosis are correct:

❏ A it is the commonest cardiovascular abnormality in Turner's syndrome
❏ B the chest X-ray typically shows plethoric lung fields
❏ C there is a recognised association with carcinoid syndrome
❏ D an ejection click indicates that the stenosis is likely to be subvalvular
❏ E the pulmonary component of the second sound is accentuated when the stenosis is severe

27. In ostium secundum atrial septal defect

❏ A pregnancy is typically poorly tolerated
❏ B a mid-diastolic murmur suggests a large shunt
❏ C there is reversed splitting of the second heart sound
❏ D atrial arrhythmias are an important feature
❏ E the electrocardiograph shows left axis deviation

28. Ventricular septal defects

- ❑ A do not produce right atrial volume overload unless a Gerbode defect is present
- ❑ B may be complicated by infective endocarditis no matter how small the defect
- ❑ C do not produce the Eisenmenger syndrome until adult life
- ❑ D usually affect the muscular part of the septum
- ❑ E are characterised by a systolic murmur at the sternal edge and right bundle branch block on the electrocardiogram

29. The following statements about infective endocarditis are correct:

- ❑ A the most frequent manifestation of renal involvement is a nephrotic syndrome
- ❑ B a common organism responsible for acute endocarditis is *Streptococcus faecalis*
- ❑ C purpuric lesions are usually due to thrombocytopenia
- ❑ D anti-nuclear factor is found in about 50% of cases
- ❑ E the prognosis is worse with prolonged duration of symptoms

30. The following are indications for surgery in infective endocarditis:

- ❑ A persistence of vegetations on echocardiography after one week of antibiotic therapy
- ❑ B lengthening of the PR interval on ECG
- ❑ C the development of pulmonary oedema in a patient with associated aortic regurgitation
- ❑ D fungal endocarditis
- ❑ E recurrent embolisation in the presence of a mobile vegetation on echocardiography

Disorders of heart muscle

31. The following statements concerning exercise testing in heart disease are correct:

- ❑ A a normal exercise test excludes significant ischaemic heart disease
- ❑ B exercise testing is a useful way of assessing the severity of aortic stenosis in adults
- ❑ C exercise testing may reveal significant arrhythmias
- ❑ D digoxin therapy may cause difficulty in interpreting the ECG changes occurring with exercise
- ❑ E a fall in systolic blood pressure by 20 mmHg or more during exercise suggests that severe coronary artery disease may be present

32. The risk of atheromatous coronary disease is increased

- ❑ A in WHO type 1 hyperlipidaemia
- ❑ B when HDL cholesterol >2.0 mmol/l
- ❑ C when proteinuria complicates type 2 diabetes
- ❑ D in heterozygous familial hypercholesterolaemia
- ❑ E when LDL cholesterol >4.5 mmol/l

33. The following statements about angina pectoris are correct:

- ❑ A it may occur with normal coronary arteries
- ❑ B it is associated with abnormal resting ECG between attacks in about 90% of cases
- ❑ C it is typically worse later in the day
- ❑ D ST segment elevation on ECG is usual during an attack
- ❑ E it may be aggravated by lying down

34. In the management of acute myocardial infarction, intravenous streptokinase

- ❑ A reduces mortality by 50% if given within 12 hours
- ❑ B is more effective than alteplase for anterior infarcts
- ❑ C shortens the partial thromboplastin time
- ❑ D efficacy is enhanced by recent streptococcal infection
- ❑ E is contraindicated by systolic BP >200 mmHg

35. Following myocardial infarction

- ❑ A persistent ST elevation with Q wave formation is associated with the development of a left ventricular aneurysm
- ❑ B the development of frequent ventricular ectopic beats (>10/hr) is associated with a six month mortality of about 5% and should therefore be treated with flecainide
- ❑ C a pansystolic murmur associated with an inferior myocardial infarction is most commonly associated with a ventricular septal defect
- ❑ D left ventricular function is a more important prognostic indicator than the presence of ST depression on exercise testing
- ❑ E patients with a Group 2 HGV/PSV licence are not permitted to return to work unless they are able to complete three stages of the standard Bruce protocol off all medication without symptoms or significant ST depression

36. The following statements are correct:

- ❑ A coronary angioplasty is associated with a restenosis rate of 30–40%
- ❑ B coronary artery bypass grafting improves survival in patients with single vessel coronary disease
- ❑ C use of the internal mammary artery for bypass grafting should be limited to patients in whom vein grafts are not available
- ❑ D coronary artery bypass grafting (CABG) in uncomplicated cases is associated with an operative mortality of about 5%
- ❑ E aortic valve replacement should not be performed in patients with aortic stenosis and impaired left ventricular function because of an unacceptably high operative mortality

37. Recognised features of congestive (dilated) cardiomyopathy include

- ❑ A an increased risk of systemic embolism
- ❑ B pansystolic murmurs
- ❑ C asymmetrical hypertrophy of the intraventricular septum
- ❑ D a history of alcoholism
- ❑ E a family history of sudden death

38. In dilated cardiomyopathy

- ❑ A involvement of both left and right ventricles is common
- ❑ B histological evidence of an acute myocarditis is found in about 90% of cases
- ❑ C anticoagulation is indicated in patients with severe LV dilatation in the absence of atrial fibrillation
- ❑ D due to haemochromatosis, diabetes mellitus is an uncommon finding
- ❑ E a family history of cardiomyopathy may be found in up to 20% of cases

39. In left ventricular failure

- ❑ A alveolar PCO_2 is increased
- ❑ B carbon monoxide diffusion capacity is reduced
- ❑ C pulmonary venous pressure is raised
- ❑ D left ventricular end-diastolic pressure is reduced
- ❑ E basal crepitations are heard before chest X-ray changes are seen

40. In refractory heart failure

- ❑ A hyponatraemia is of prognostic significance
- ❑ B enalapril acts primarily by reducing venous return
- ❑ C antacids are a potential hazard
- ❑ D splenomegaly is a recognised finding
- ❑ E blood urea levels rise in part due to overproduction of urea

41. In hypertrophic cardiomyopathy

- ❑ A atrial fibrillation indicates a poor prognosis
- ❑ B the characteristic murmur is typically loudest in the aortic area
- ❑ C a diastolic murmur is present in the majority of cases
- ❑ D GTN reduces outflow obstruction
- ❑ E there are characteristic echocardiographic findings

Miscellaneous cardiology

42. Coarctation of the thoracic aorta

- ❑ A is a predominantly female disease
- ❑ B occurs characteristically proximal to the origin of the left subclavian artery
- ❑ C can give a continuous murmur
- ❑ D is associated with bicuspid aortic valves
- ❑ E has a good prognosis untreated after the age of 20

43. The following conditions are recognised as predisposing to dissecting aneurysms of the aorta:

- ❑ A syphilitic aortitis
- ❑ B rheumatic aortic valve disease
- ❑ C Marfan's syndrome
- ❑ D hypertension
- ❑ E pregnancy

44. The following statements about abdominal aortic aneurysms are correct:

- ❑ A they typically arise above the renal arteries
- ❑ B they are a recognised cause of ureteric obstruction
- ❑ C cross-sectional ultrasound is the best way to detect and size the aneurysm
- ❑ D the patient's prognosis is related to the size of the aneurysm
- ❑ E a majority of cases present with rupture

45. The following statements are correct for pulmonary embolism:

- ❑ A a clinical picture similar to primary pulmonary hypertension is recognised as resulting from recurrent small pulmonary emboli
- ❑ B measurement of arterial gases whilst breathing air after pulmonary embolism typically shows a raised PCO_2 and reduced PO_2
- ❑ C after pulmonary embolism, the right atrial pressure may exceed left atrial pressure
- ❑ D pulmonary emboli typically originate from leg or pelvic venous thrombi
- ❑ E demonstration of the presence of pulmonary emboli by ventilation/perfusion lung scanning is easy and entirely safe

46. The following are typical findings in acute rheumatic fever:

❑ A apical rumbling presystolic murmur
❑ B tender subcutaneous nodules
❑ C cardiac conduction defects
❑ D nail bed changes
❑ E urticaria

47. Acute pericarditis is a recognised complication of

❑ A polyarteritis nodosa
❑ B gonorrhoea
❑ C thyrotoxicosis
❑ D amoebiasis
❑ E congestive cardiac failure

48. Post myocardial infarction pericarditis (Dressler's syndrome)

❑ A occurs in 25% of all myocardial infarctions
❑ B occurs only a month or more after myocardial infarction
❑ C is usually associated with pain and fever
❑ D responds to treatment with non-steroidal anti-inflammatory drugs
❑ E is frequently associated with the subsequent development of constrictive pericarditis

49. The following are characteristic findings in constrictive pericarditis:

❑ A atrial fibrillation
❑ B normal heart size
❑ C acute pulmonary oedema
❑ D pulsus alternans
❑ E third heart sound

50. Left atrial myxoma is associated with

❑ A signs suggesting mitral stenosis
❑ B syncope
❑ C acute pulmonary oedema
❑ D cerebrovascular accident
❑ E increased erythrocyte sedimentation rate

CLINICAL PHARMACOLOGY AND TOXICOLOGY

Drug pharmokinetics, pharmacodynamics and interactions

1. Regarding drug absorption from the gastro-intestinal tract

❑ A acidic drugs are mostly absorbed from the stomach by passive transport
❑ B water-soluble, polar drugs are absorbed from the small intestine by active transport
❑ C active transport absorptive processes in the small intestine are saturable
❑ D a delay in gastric emptying decreases the amount of drug absorbed
❑ E coeliac disease may result in either an increase or a decrease in drug bioavailability, depending on the compound

2. A drug with a high first-pass effect

❑ A is largely excreted unchanged in the urine
❑ B is poorly absorbed
❑ C is extensively metabolised in the liver and/or gut wall
❑ D will have a high extraction ratio
❑ E will have its extraction ratio decreased if the patient has severe hepatic cirrhosis

3. The bioavailability of the following drugs is increased in the presence of hepatic cirrhosis:

❑ A digoxin
❑ B propranolol
❑ C metoclopramide
❑ D gentamicin
❑ E imipramine

4. Enterohepatic recirculation makes an important contribution to the bioavailability of the following drugs:

- ❑ A ethinyloestradiol
- ❑ B diazepam
- ❑ C warfarin
- ❑ D phenytoin
- ❑ E lithium

5. The blood-brain barrier is rapidly permeable to

- ❑ A highly polar water-soluble drugs
- ❑ B strong acids
- ❑ C weak bases
- ❑ D adrenaline
- ❑ E amphetamine

6. The following drugs are subject to polymorphic metabolism:

- ❑ A lignocaine
- ❑ B metoprolol
- ❑ C hydralazine
- ❑ D 6-mercaptopurine
- ❑ E gentamicin

7. Slow acetylators are more prone to the following adverse drug effect:

- ❑ A hypertensive crisis with hydralazine
- ❑ B hepatitis with isoniazid
- ❑ C nausea and vomiting with sulphasalazine
- ❑ D peripheral neuropathy with isoniazid
- ❑ E systemic lupus syndrome with hydralazine

8. Enzyme induction

- ❑ A with anticonvulsants may cause osteomalacia
- ❑ B contributes to tolerance to the effects of atenolol
- ❑ C can cause failure of the contraceptive pill
- ❑ D may occur as a result of smoking
- ❑ E lowers plasma bilirubin concentration

9. Competitive enzyme inhibitors include

- ❑ A metyrapone
- ❑ B finasteride
- ❑ C enalaprilat
- ❑ D pralidoxime
- ❑ E pyridostigmine

10. Sympathomimetic amine actions at the α-receptor include

- ❑ A decrease in gut motility
- ❑ B relaxation of the pregnant uterus
- ❑ C decreased bronchial secretions
- ❑ D stimulation of gluconeogenesis
- ❑ E contraction of ciliary muscle of the iris

11. The following drugs act as α-receptor antagonists:

- ❑ A phenoxybenzamine
- ❑ B doxazosin
- ❑ C lignocaine
- ❑ D phenytoin
- ❑ E chlorpromazine

12. Regarding β-adrenoceptor antagonists

- ❑ A drugs with intrinsic sympathomimetic activity are less likely to cause bradycardia
- ❑ B atenolol is a cardio-specific drug
- ❑ C propranolol causes prolongation of the Q-T interval
- ❑ D celiprolol increases total peripheral resistance
- ❑ E esmolol can be administered intravenously to treat patients with supraventricular arrhythmias

13. The following drug combinations are usually undesirable:

- ❑ A digoxin and amiodarone
- ❑ B metoclopramide and chlorpromazine
- ❑ C cholestyramine and prednisolone
- ❑ D levodopa and nifedipine
- ❑ E ranitidine and metronidazole

14. Warfarin metabolism can be inhibited by

- ❑ A zafirlukast
- ❑ B terfenadine
- ❑ C omeprazole
- ❑ D fluvoxamine
- ❑ E bezafibrate

15. Aspirin potentiates the therapeutic action of the following:

- ❑ A warfarin
- ❑ B probenecid
- ❑ C indomethacin
- ❑ D diazepam
- ❑ E tetracyclines

16. An increase in plasma digoxin levels would be expected on introduction of

- ❑ A amiodarone
- ❑ B nifedipine
- ❑ C quinidine
- ❑ D cholestyramine
- ❑ E rifampicin

17. The risk of pregnancy despite combined contraceptive steroid usage is increased by concurrent treatment with

- ❑ A diazepam
- ❑ B isoniazid
- ❑ C carbamazepine
- ❑ D phenytoin
- ❑ E rifampicin

18. Cigarette smoking accelerates the metabolism of

- ❑ A theophylline
- ❑ B phenytoin
- ❑ C alcohol
- ❑ D dextropropoxyphene
- ❑ E amitriptyline

19. Chronic alcohol intake increases the metabolism of

- ❑ A alcohol
- ❑ B ciprofloxacin
- ❑ C cimetidine
- ❑ D atenolol
- ❑ E paracetamol

Prescribing in specific clinical situations

20. The following drugs are excreted in breast milk in sufficient quantities to cause harm to the infant:

- ❑ A cyclosporin
- ❑ B phenindione
- ❑ C tetracycline
- ❑ D digoxin
- ❑ E mefloquine

21. The following drugs may have a causative association with the following renal diseases:

- ❑ A tetracycline and uraemia
- ❑ B penicillamine and papillary necrosis
- ❑ C allopurinol and uric acid nephropathy
- ❑ D gold and heavy proteinuria
- ❑ E procainamide and glomerulonephritis

22. The following drugs should be avoided in renal failure:

- ❑ A ampicillin
- ❑ B oxytetracycline
- ❑ C aluminium hydroxide
- ❑ D ferrous sulphate
- ❑ E nitrofurantoin

23. In chronic liver disease the following should be avoided:

- ❑ A digoxin
- ❑ B pethidine
- ❑ C paracetamol
- ❑ D isoniazid
- ❑ E imipramine

24. Patients with acute intermittent porphyria should avoid

- ❑ A alcohol
- ❑ B rifampicin
- ❑ C phenytoin
- ❑ D aspirin
- ❑ E oral contraceptives

Drugs in cardiology

25. Amiodarone

- ❑ A has a short half-life
- ❑ B has anti-anginal effects
- ❑ C causes hyperthyroidism more commonly than hypothyroidism
- ❑ D can precipitate digoxin toxicity by inhibiting its metabolism
- ❑ E blocks potassium channels

26. Adenosine

- ❑ A stimulates adenosine (A2) receptors
- ❑ B is more likely to terminate junctional tachycardias than arrhythmias arising within the atria
- ❑ C will slow heart rate in patients with ventricular tachycardia
- ❑ D can cause bronchospasm
- ❑ E is recommended as an essential drug to be carried by General Practitioners

27. Significant negative inotropic action is a feature of

- ❑ A diltiazem
- ❑ B lisinopril
- ❑ C propafenone
- ❑ D bisoprolol
- ❑ E thyroxine

28. Regarding calcium channel blockers

❑ A there is a good correlation between serum levels and clinical effects
❑ B dihydropyridines may worsen angina
❑ C they improve survival after myocardial infarction
❑ D they have been shown to reduce left ventricular mass in hypertensive patients with left ventricular hypertrophy
❑ E both diltiazem and verapamil permit an increase in heart rate with exercise

29. The following are true statements concerning calcium channel blocking drugs:

❑ A diltiazem has no anti-arrhythmic properties
❑ B they dilate arteries more than veins
❑ C nifedipine increases pulse rate
❑ D verapamil is the most likely to cause constipation
❑ E verapamil is the least likely to produce heart failure

30. The following adverse effects are associated with the use of enalapril:

❑ A angioneurotic oedema
❑ B cough in around 10% of patients
❑ C retroperitoneal fibrosis
❑ D acute renal failure
❑ E hypercholesterolaemia

31. The following drugs may reduce mortality in patients with heart failure:

❑ A enalapril
❑ B frusemide
❑ C digoxin
❑ D carvedilol
❑ E verapamil

32. Nicorandil

- ❑ A causes dilatation of the arteries and veins
- ❑ B has been shown to have an additive effect when used in combination with other anti-anginals
- ❑ C reduces cardiac output in patients with cardiac failure
- ❑ D tolerance occurs and is equivalent to that seen with nitrates
- ❑ E increases efflux of potassium ions and inhibits entry of calcium ions

33. Regarding the use of moxonidine in hypertension

- ❑ A it acts as an imidazoline (I1) receptor antagonist
- ❑ B its antihypertensive effects diminish with time
- ❑ C its efficacy is comparable to other first-line agents used for the treatment of hypertension
- ❑ D it improves insulin responsiveness in insulin-resistant patients
- ❑ E sedation is an adverse effect

34. Minoxidil

- ❑ A causes arteriolar vasodilation
- ❑ B accumulates dangerously in renal failure
- ❑ C must not be used with a loop diuretic
- ❑ D increases growth of body hair
- ❑ E causes flattening or inversion of the T-wave on the ECG

35. Alteplase (recombinant tissue plasminogen activator)

- ❑ A has high affinity for free plasminogen
- ❑ B is associated with a higher rate of intracerebral haemorrhage than streptokinase
- ❑ C commonly causes anaphylaxis
- ❑ D has a longer half-life than streptokinase
- ❑ E reduces mortality of patients with acute ischaemic stroke

36. The following drugs affect platelet function:

- ❑ A aspirin
- ❑ B hirudin
- ❑ C ticlopidine
- ❑ D abciximab
- ❑ E warfarin

37. Drugs which lower serum LDL cholesterol concentration include

❑ A simvastatin
❑ B cholestyramine
❑ C propranolol
❑ D fenofibrate
❑ E omega-3 marine oil

38. Simvastatin

❑ A has been shown to reduce mortality in hypercholesterolaemic patients with known ischaemic heart disease
❑ B acts by increasing the faecal loss of cholesterol
❑ C can be used safely in patients with acute porphyria
❑ D causes rhabdomyolysis, the risk of which is increased by concomitant administration of mibefradil
❑ E is more effective than ciprofibrate in raising HDL cholesterol

Drugs in endocrinology

39. Glibenclamide

❑ A has no biologically active metabolites
❑ B has a shorter half life than chlorpropamide
❑ C stimulates gluconeogenesis
❑ D does not cross the placenta
❑ E is safe in renal impairment

40. Regarding the use of anti-thyroid drugs, the following statements are correct:

❑ A propylthiouracil inhibits the peripheral conversion of T4 to T3
❑ B beta-blockers reduce the basal metabolic rate
❑ C carbimazole produces an improvement in two days
❑ D iodide can cause a goitre in euthyroid patients
❑ E radioactive iodine (I^{131}) predominantly emits γ rays

41. Regarding radioiodine therapy

- ❑ A breast-feeding should be avoided for eight weeks after treatment
- ❑ B it can be used in patients with hyperthyroidism caused by thyroiditis
- ❑ C it improves Graves' ophthalmopathy
- ❑ D it can be used to treat both thyroid cancer and its bony metastases simultaneously
- ❑ E it induces euthyroidism in hyperthyroid patients within one week

Drugs in neurology

42. In the treatment of status epilepticus

- ❑ A it has been shown that the response to first-line therapy is greater the sooner treatment is started
- ❑ B intravenous diazepam is more effective than lorazepam in controlling seizures
- ❑ C lorazepam has a longer duration of anti-seizure effect than diazepam
- ❑ D out of hospital, the preferred route of administration of diazepam is intramuscular
- ❑ E intravenous phenytoin causes cardiac arrhythmias in 50% of patients

43. Rare adverse effects of phenytoin include

- ❑ A memory impairment
- ❑ B aplastic anaemia
- ❑ C ataxia
- ❑ D skin rash
- ❑ E selective IgA deficiency

44. In the treatment of migraine

- ❑ A attacks can be prevented by sodium valproate
- ❑ B sumatriptan works by inhibiting release of calcitonin gene-related peptide (CGRP)
- ❑ C ergot alkaloids cause systemic vasodilatation
- ❑ D sumatriptan prevents the aura associated with migraine
- ❑ E sumatriptan use is contraindicated in patients with coronary artery disease

45. Donepezil

- ❑ A inhibits the action of acetylcholine in the central nervous system
- ❑ B has been shown to improve quality of life in patients with Alzheimer's disease
- ❑ C may cause hallucinations
- ❑ D has predictable beneficial effects in patients with Alzheimer's disease
- ❑ E causes constipation

46. In patients with the Guillain-Barré syndrome

- ❑ A suxamethonium can lead to hyperkalaemia
- ❑ B intravenous immunoglobulin should be used to hasten recovery
- ❑ C intravenous immunoglobulin is as effective as plasma exchange
- ❑ D corticosteroids have been shown to be of benefit
- ❑ E antibodies to ganglioside GM1 are useful for monitoring response to therapy

Drugs in psychiatry

47. Benzodiazepine anxiolytics

- ❑ A are mainly metabolised to sulphate conjugates
- ❑ B have no active metabolites
- ❑ C differ significantly in their duration of action
- ❑ D differ significantly in their sedative effect relative to anxiolytic activity
- ❑ E increase body sway

48. Tricyclic antidepressants

- ❑ A are contraindicated in patients with glaucoma
- ❑ B may cause dry mouth
- ❑ C produce prolonged PR and QT intervals on the ECG
- ❑ D are safe in patients anticoagulated with warfarin
- ❑ E are contraindicated in patients with ischaemic heart disease

49. Phenothiazines may cause

- ❑ A agranulocytosis
- ❑ B photosensitivity
- ❑ C increased lacrimation
- ❑ D priapism
- ❑ E cholestatic jaundice

50. Recognised side-effects of lithium carbonate include

- ❑ A polyuria
- ❑ B hypopituitarism
- ❑ C diarrhoea
- ❑ D intention tremor
- ❑ E hypothyroidism

Drugs in haematology

51. Regarding cytotoxic chemotherapeutic agents

- ❑ A they all act on the proliferative phase of the cell cycle
- ❑ B tumour cells are killed by a process of apoptosis
- ❑ C combination therapy may reduce unwanted adverse effects
- ❑ D a given dose will kill a given percentage of tumour cells rather than a given number
- ❑ E they affect normal as well as malignant cells

52. Correct descriptions of chemotherapeutic agents include

- ❑ A cyclophosphamide: alkylating agent
- ❑ B methotrexate: folic acid antagonist
- ❑ C azathioprine: vinca alkaloid
- ❑ D vinblastine: pyrimidine analogue
- ❑ E cytosine arabinoside: purine analogue

53. Methotrexate

- ❑ A should not be used in children
- ❑ B may have a steroid-sparing effect in patients with severe asthma
- ❑ C can cause mucositis within a few hours of administration
- ❑ D toxicity may develop in patients treated with naproxen
- ❑ E concentrations in plasma can allow prediction of therapeutic effect

Drugs in anaesthetics

54. Lignocaine

- ❑ A prevents the generation of nerve impulses
- ❑ B prevents the conduction of nerve impulses
- ❑ C may lead to methaemoglobinaemia
- ❑ D can only be used parenterally
- ❑ E can be used for the treatment of both atrial and ventricular arrhythmias

55. The following are known effects of halothane:

- ❑ A increased blood pressure
- ❑ B hepatitis
- ❑ C increased tendency to arrhythmias
- ❑ D increased sensitivity to catecholamines
- ❑ E increased cardiac output

Miscellaneous drugs

56. Inhaled corticosteroids used in the treatment of asthma can cause the following adverse effects:

- ❑ A diabetes mellitus
- ❑ B cataracts
- ❑ C glaucoma
- ❑ D osteoporosis
- ❑ E skin bruising

57. Terfenadine

- ❑ A is a pro-drug
- ❑ B metabolism can be inhibited by ketoconazole
- ❑ C can usually be detected in plasma of healthy individuals on no other drugs
- ❑ D inhibits cardiac sodium channels
- ❑ E causes atrial fibrillation

58. Morphine

- ❑ A is mainly excreted unchanged by the kidneys
- ❑ B produces mydriasis
- ❑ C decreases intestinal smooth muscle tone
- ❑ D decreases peripheral venous capacitance
- ❑ E is antagonised by naloxone

59. The following are causally related:

- ❑ A melphalan and pulmonary fibrosis
- ❑ B hydrochlorothiazide and pulmonary oedema
- ❑ C barbiturates and hyperventilation
- ❑ D phenytoin and SLE
- ❑ E prostaglandin F2 alpha and bronchodilatation

60. The following antiviral therapies are of proven benefit:

- ❑ A amantadine for treatment of influenza A
- ❑ B intravenous acyclovir in chickenpox pneumonitis
- ❑ C zidovudine (AZT) in asymptomatic HIV infection with CD4 count >500 x 10^6/l
- ❑ D interferon in chronic hepatitis C
- ❑ E ribavirin in Lassa fever

61. The following drugs are useful in the treatment of generalised pruritus:

- ❑ A cholestyramine
- ❑ B hydroxyzine
- ❑ C trimeprazine
- ❑ D codeine
- ❑ E carbamazepine

Antimicrobials

62. Aminoglycosides

- ❑ A should be given once daily in patients with endocarditis
- ❑ B are concentrated within the renal cortex
- ❑ C are effective against β-lactamase producing strains of *Staphylococcus aureus*
- ❑ D are effective against streptococci
- ❑ E have a reduced half-life in patients with Paget's disease of bone

63. Ciprofloxacin

- ❑ A inhibits DNA-dependent RNA polymerase
- ❑ B is highly active against *Streptococcus pneumoniae*
- ❑ C should be used with caution in epileptics
- ❑ D can cause tenosynovitis
- ❑ E increases plasma theophylline concentrations

64. Rifampicin

- ❑ A produces a clinically significant interaction with cyclosporin
- ❑ B can be used as chemoprophylaxis for meningococcal disease
- ❑ C is not effective against intracellular organisms
- ❑ D can cause a flu-like illness if administered less than twice weekly
- ❑ E can be used safely in patients who wear soft contact lenses

65. Tetracycline

- ❑ A should be administered with meals to ensure adequate absorption
- ❑ B dose should be reduced in patients with renal failure
- ❑ C can be used for the treatment of infections caused by *Enterococcus faecalis*
- ❑ D can be used safely in patients on the oral contraceptive pill
- ❑ E enhances the anticoagulant effect of warfarin

66. Regarding the use of co-trimoxazole (sulphamethoxazole and trimethoprim) in HIV-positive patients

❑ A it provides prophylaxis against both *Pneumocystis carinii* pneumonia and *Toxoplasma gondii* encephalitis
❑ B trimethoprim by itself is as effective as sulphamethoxazole in the treatment of *Pneumocystis carinii* pneumonia
❑ C co-trimoxazole is more effective than dapsone-trimethoprim in the treatment of *Pneumocystis carinii* pneumonia
❑ D both drugs inhibit dihydrofolate reductase in *Pneumocystis carinii*
❑ E rash is a common side-effect

67. The following antibiotics are correctly paired with their adverse effects:

❑ A fusidic acid: nephrotoxicity
❑ B vancomycin: 'red man' syndrome
❑ C cefotaxime: haemolysis
❑ D metronidazole: motor neuropathy
❑ E minocycline: hepatitis

68. Ketoconazole

❑ A blocks gonadal and adrenal steroid synthesis in humans
❑ B acts in a synergistic manner with amphotericin
❑ C causes renal failure
❑ D resistance is common
❑ E inhibits C-14 a-demethylase in fungal cells

Specific adverse effects

69. The following drugs cause hyperprolactinaemia:

❑ A risperidone
❑ B cimetidine
❑ C sodium valproate
❑ D ergotamine
❑ E fluvoxamine

70. The following drugs have been associated with impairment of glucose tolerance:

- ❑ A bendrofluazide
- ❑ B combined oestrogen/progestogen oral contraceptive pill
- ❑ C glipizide
- ❑ D prednisolone
- ❑ E spironolactone

71. QT interval prolongation on the surface electrocardiogram is seen with the following drugs:

- ❑ A gentamicin
- ❑ B sertindole
- ❑ C halofantrine
- ❑ D imipramine
- ❑ E astemizole

72. Thrombocytopenia is a recognised side-effect of

- ❑ A warfarin
- ❑ B heparin
- ❑ C gold
- ❑ D bendrofluazide
- ❑ E quinine

73. The following drugs can cause haemolysis in patients with glucose-6-phosphate dehydrogenase deficiency:

- ❑ A nitrofurantoin
- ❑ B nalidixic acid
- ❑ C ciprofloxacin
- ❑ D trimethoprim
- ❑ E primaquine

74. The following drugs can cause acute renal failure:

- ❑ A captopril
- ❑ B amoxycillin
- ❑ C sulphamethoxazole
- ❑ D mesalazine
- ❑ E atenolol

75. Parkinson-like extrapyramidal effects occur during treatment with

- ❑ A haloperidol
- ❑ B imipramine
- ❑ C prochlorperazine
- ❑ D phenytoin
- ❑ E trifluoperazine

76. The following drugs cause retinopathy:

- ❑ A glibenclamide
- ❑ B tamoxifen
- ❑ C thioridazine
- ❑ D tacrolimus
- ❑ E vigabatrin

77. Diarrhoea is commonly produced by treatment with

- ❑ A magnesium trisilicate
- ❑ B aluminium hydroxide
- ❑ C verapamil
- ❑ D colchicine
- ❑ E misoprostol

78. Abrupt discontinuation of the following drugs can result in a withdrawal syndrome:

- ❑ A paroxetine
- ❑ B amiodarone
- ❑ C indomethacin
- ❑ D diazepam
- ❑ E venlafaxine

79. Regarding drug-induced anaphylaxis

- ❑ A it is mediated by both IgE and IgA antibodies
- ❑ B it is more severe with parenteral compounds when compared to the same compound administered orally
- ❑ C prophylactic corticosteroids will prevent such a reaction
- ❑ D a history of prior sensitisation to the antigen may not be available
- ❑ E it is more common in patients with underlying atopy

Poisoning

80. Monitoring plasma concentrations is of value in the management of overdosage of

- ❑ A propranolol
- ❑ B lithium
- ❑ C amitriptyline
- ❑ D iron
- ❑ E digoxin

81. An adult has taken 50 aspirin tablets; after four hours

- ❑ A coma is to be expected
- ❑ B gastric lavage is of no value
- ❑ C alkaline diuresis is the treatment of choice
- ❑ D peritoneal dialysis could be of value therapeutically
- ❑ E hypoglycaemia may be present

82. In paracetamol poisoning

- ❑ A the earliest sign of hepatotoxicity is a raised alanine transaminase (ALT)
- ❑ B patients established on cimetidine are at increased risk
- ❑ C smokers are at decreased risk
- ❑ D N-acetylcysteine is effective because it can donate –SH groups
- ❑ E after recovery, future therapy with paracetamol is contraindicated

83. Hepatic damage following paracetamol overdosage is more likely to occur in the following patient groups:

- ❑ A chronic alcoholics
- ❑ B patients on cimetidine
- ❑ C patients on phenytoin
- ❑ D patients on sodium valproate
- ❑ E children

84. Severe poisoning with iron is characterised by

- ❑ A a total white cell count of less than 4×10^9/l
- ❑ B a blood glucose greater than 8.3 mmol/l
- ❑ C a normal plain abdominal X-ray
- ❑ D hypotension
- ❑ E the appearance of black stools

85. Digoxin toxicity may be

- ❑ A potentiated by hypokalaemia
- ❑ B potentiated by hyponatraemia
- ❑ C diagnosed by ST elevation on the ECG
- ❑ D treated with phenytoin
- ❑ E treated with an infusion of calcium chloride

86. Features of lithium poisoning include

- ❑ A constipation
- ❑ B inappropriate ADH secretion
- ❑ C cerebellar signs
- ❑ D hypokalaemia
- ❑ E coma

87. The following are features of atropine poisoning:

- ❑ A fever
- ❑ B bradycardia
- ❑ C profuse sweating
- ❑ D pin-point pupils
- ❑ E hallucinations

88. In theophylline overdosage

❑ A plasma theophylline concentrations are a poor guide to toxicity
❑ B convulsions indicate a bad prognosis
❑ C hypokalaemia can be profound
❑ D activated charcoal is ineffective
❑ E centrally induced nausea and vomiting are poorly responsive to anti-emetics

DERMATOLOGY

1. Alopecia areata

- ❑ A is a scarring process with permanent loss of follicles
- ❑ B is associated with autoimmune thyroid disease
- ❑ C is confined to scalp hairs
- ❑ D is a recognised association of Down's syndrome
- ❑ E may be associated with nail changes

2. Changes to the nail or adjacent tissue are seen

- ❑ A in dermatomyositis
- ❑ B in psoriasis
- ❑ C in epidermolysis bullosa
- ❑ D in pyoderma gangrenosum
- ❑ E following severe illness

3. Exfoliative dermatitis

- ❑ A may contribute to heart failure
- ❑ B gives hyperpyrexia
- ❑ C with pruritus indicates a lymphoma
- ❑ D can complicate psoriasis
- ❑ E may be responsible for lymphadenopathy

4. Bullae are a feature of

- ❑ A orf
- ❑ B pompholyx eczema
- ❑ C erythema nodosum
- ❑ D pemphigoid
- ❑ E erythema multiforme

5. The following are features of dermatitis herpetiformis:

- ❑ A a granular pattern of IgA antibodies at the dermo-epidermal junction of uninvolved skin
- ❑ B a rapid response to oral dapsone
- ❑ C gastrointestinal malabsorption
- ❑ D an increased incidence of malignancy
- ❑ E an association with HLA types B8, Dw3 and DRw3

6. Strawberry naevi (cavernous haemangiomata)

❑ A have a significant predisposition to malignant change
❑ B often enlarge during the first year of life
❑ C should be treated by surgical excision
❑ D are associated with mental retardation
❑ E if very large, may be associated with thrombocytopenia

7. Recognised causes of erythema nodosum include:

❑ A sarcoidosis
❑ B oral contraceptives
❑ C preceding mycoplasmal infection
❑ D diabetes mellitus
❑ E cryptogenic false-fibrosing alveolitis

8. Purpuric skin lesions are a feature of

❑ A vitamin A deficiency
❑ B T cell lymphoma
❑ C corticosteroid therapy
❑ D pemphigus
❑ E pityriasis rosea

9. The following conditions are more prevalent in immuno-compromised patients:

❑ A viral warts
❑ B Kaposi's sarcoma
❑ C squamous cell carcinomas
❑ D seborrhoeic dermatitis
❑ E scabies

10. The following drugs are recognised causes of the rashes mentioned:

❑ A captopril and lichenoid eruptions
❑ B minocycline and skin pigmentation
❑ C gold and exfoliative dermatitis
❑ D aspirin and urticaria
❑ E thiazides and photosensitivity

ENDOCRINOLOGY

Glycaemic control and diabetes

1. Actions of glucagon include

❑ A stimulation of hepatic glycogenolysis
❑ B inhibition of insulin secretion
❑ C stimulation of hepatic gluconeogenesis
❑ D inhibition of adenyl cyclase
❑ E a positive cardiac inotropic effect

2. A diagnosis of diabetes mellitus is confirmed by the presence of

❑ A generalised pruritus
❑ B fast venous plasma glucose 6.8 mmol/l
❑ C glycosuria
❑ D polyuria and polydipsia
❑ E venous plasma glucose 11.2 mmol/l, 2 hours after 75 g oral glucose

3. In insulin dependent diabetes (IDDM)

❑ A persistence of islet cell antibodies increases the likelihood of associated autoimmune disease
❑ B there is an increased incident of HLA B8 status
❑ C there is 90% concordance in identical twins
❑ D a history of recent mumps virus infection is common at presentation
❑ E retinopathy is usually present at diagnosis

4. In diabetic glomerulosclerosis

❑ A arteriosclerosis is generally thought to play an important initiating role
❑ B hypertension is usually the first clinical feature
❑ C absence of diabetic retinopathy is exceptional
❑ D nodular sclerosis (Kimmelstiel-Wilson lesion) is the commonest histological finding
❑ E renal amyloid may be a late complication

5. Insulin resistance is

- ❑ A associated with raised HDL-cholesterol
- ❑ B associated with hypertension
- ❑ C unaffected by physical training
- ❑ D characterised clinically by acanthosis nigricans
- ❑ E due to a reduced number of insulin receptors

6. The following are characteristically associated with hypoglycaemia:

- ❑ A adrenocortical insufficiency
- ❑ B retroperitoneal sarcoma
- ❑ C alcohol intoxication
- ❑ D multiple endocrine neoplasia Type IIa
- ❑ E von Gierke's disease

Thyroid/parathyroid disease

7. Total serum thyroxine levels are reduced by

- ❑ A pregnancy
- ❑ B phenytoin treatment
- ❑ C panhypopituitarism
- ❑ D combined oral contraceptives
- ❑ E salicylate

8. In a normal individual

- ❑ A 80% of circulating thyroxine is protein bound
- ❑ B most serum triiodothyronine is produced in the thyroid
- ❑ C thyroglobulin binds thyroxine in serum
- ❑ D thyroxine half life is >24 hours
- ❑ E thyrotropin (TSH) inhibits thyroid growth

9. The following are recognised features of hypothyroidism:

- ❑ A menorrhagia
- ❑ B ascites
- ❑ C cerebellar ataxia
- ❑ D clubbing
- ❑ E normochromic anaemia

10. In autoimmune thyroid eye disease

- ❑ A exophthalmos is due to retro-orbital fluid
- ❑ B there is exacerbation by cigarette smoking
- ❑ C diplopia is normally due to 3rd nerve palsy
- ❑ D high dose steroids are mandatory
- ❑ E improvement follows 131-Iodine treatment

11. Intact parathyroid hormone

- ❑ A levels are increased in the hypercalcaemia of sarcoidosis
- ❑ B concentration is low in primary hyperparathyroidism
- ❑ C can be measured by immunoradiometric assay
- ❑ D inhibits renal 1-alpha hydroxylase
- ❑ E consists of 52 amino acids

12. In primary hyperparathyroidism there is

- ❑ A an invariable increase in the level of parathyroid hormone in blood
- ❑ B an increase in tubular reabsorption of calcium in the presence of hypercalciuria
- ❑ C the possibility of hypocalcaemic tetany in a neonate whose mother has the condition
- ❑ D a single adenoma in about 40% of cases
- ❑ E a recognised association with systemic arterial hypertension

13. Features of primary hypoparathyroidism include

- ❑ A basal ganglia calcification
- ❑ B carpopedal spasm
- ❑ C serum phosphate 0.5 mmol/l
- ❑ D elevated serum alkaline phosphatase
- ❑ E delayed relaxation of tendon reflexes

Pituitary disorders

14. The close anatomical relations of the pituitary fossa include the

- ❑ A cavernous sinus
- ❑ B internal carotid artery
- ❑ C III cranial nerve
- ❑ D sphenoidal sinus
- ❑ E VIII cranial nerve

15. Non-secreting adenomas of the pituitary gland

- ❑ A are composed entirely of chromophobe cells
- ❑ B rarely cause expansion of the pituitary fossa
- ❑ C rarely give rise to pituitary failure
- ❑ D are a recognised association in patients with primary hyperparathyroidism due to hyperplasia of the parathyroid glands
- ❑ E may progress to involve the supraopticohypophysial tract thereby causing diabetes insipidus

16. Prolactin

- ❑ A has no established function in males
- ❑ B secretion occurs in response to stress
- ❑ C in excess can give amenorrhoea
- ❑ D is mainly controlled by a hypothalamic releasing hormone
- ❑ E secretion may be increased in primary hypothyroidism

17. Vasopressin (ADH)

- ❑ A is synthesised in the hypothalamus
- ❑ B is a steroid
- ❑ C increases permeability of the loop of Henle to water
- ❑ D is released in response to a fall in blood volume
- ❑ E relaxes smooth muscle

18. The following statements regarding diabetes insipidus are correct:

❑ A the condition is more often produced by hypothalamic than pituitary lesions
❑ B the treatment of choice in children is chlorpropamide
❑ C the treatment of choice in adults is DDAVP
❑ D the absence of nocturia is strong evidence against this diagnosis
❑ E the symptoms of nephrogenic diabetes insipidus can be improved by thiazide diuretics

19. Features of acromegaly include

❑ A carpal tunnel syndrome
❑ B elevated serum IGF-1 concentration
❑ C tunnel vision
❑ D increased risk of colonic carcinoma
❑ E frontal sinus destruction

20. In active acromegaly

❑ A treatment is not necessary for a small intrasellar tumour which is not expanding
❑ B external beam radiotherapy will normalise growth hormone (GH) levels in most cases within six months
❑ C transphenoidal surgical removal is the treatment of choice for large tumours causing visual field constriction
❑ D bromocriptine will normalise GH levels in over 90% of cases
❑ E somatostatin analogues can achieve clinical and biochemical remission

Adrenal disorders

21. The rate of aldosterone secretion

❑ A is controlled by the renin-angiotensin system
❑ B is increased by increased sodium concentrations in the extra-cellular fluid
❑ C increases when plasma potassium concentrations rise
❑ D is inversely related to plasma volume
❑ E is increased by stimulation of the sympathetic supply of the adrenal gland

22. In untreated 21 hydroxylase deficiency

❑ A female clitoromegaly is characteristic
❑ B pregnanetriol excretion is increased
❑ C plasma renin activity is suppressed
❑ D serum progesterone level is reduced
❑ E delayed puberty is common in affected males

23. Features of Cushing's disease include

❑ A hypertension
❑ B psychiatric symptoms
❑ C tall stature in children
❑ D hypertrichosis
❑ E macrocytic anaemia

24. In the investigation of Cushing's syndrome

❑ A 24 hour urine free cortisol collection is a first-line investigation
❑ B ACTH levels in the normal range suggest an adrenal tumour
❑ C a rise in ACTH levels following an injection of corticotrophin releasing hormone (CRH) suggests a pituitary tumour
❑ D MRI scanning of the pituitary is the best investigation to differentiate ectopic ACTH production from pituitary-dependent disease (Cushing's disease)
❑ E plasma cortisol is characteristically suppressed following high doses of dexamethasone (8 mg/day) in Cushing's syndrome due to ectopic ACTH production

25. In patients with phaeochromocytoma

❑ A a tumour secreting adrenaline only is more likely to arise from a site other than the adrenals
❑ B tumours in both adrenals occur in about 10% of cases
❑ C preparation for surgery should generally start with a beta blocker drug
❑ D hypercalcaemia is a recognised finding
❑ E there is an association with follicular carcinoma of the thyroid

Miscellaneous endocrinology

26. The following statements are true:

- ❑ A growth hormone deficiency in adults produces no effects
- ❑ B magnesium is excreted in both urine and faeces
- ❑ C steroid receptors are present at the cell surface
- ❑ D steroid receptors can bind to DNA
- ❑ E thyroid hormone receptors can bind to DNA

27. The following statements about endocrinopathies are correct:

- ❑ A hypoparathyroidism is associated with osteoporosis
- ❑ B hyperparathyroidism produces features of ligament calcification similar to ankylosing spondylitis
- ❑ C acute pseudogout is a feature of acromegaly
- ❑ D diabetes mellitus is associated with 'hypertrophic ankylosing hyperostosis' (Forestier's disease)
- ❑ E the soft tissue swelling of thyroid acropachy responds to treatment of the underlying thyrotoxicosis

28. Breast development in a five-year-old girl

- ❑ A may be due to an arrhenoblastoma of the ovary
- ❑ B frequently has no identifiable organic cause
- ❑ C is a common result of XXY chromosomal constitution
- ❑ D requires urgent laparotomy to examine the ovaries
- ❑ E may be a late result of maternal oestrogens transferred before birth

29. Causes of gynaecomastia include

- ❑ A prostatic carcinoma
- ❑ B normal puberty
- ❑ C hypothyroidism
- ❑ D diabetes mellitus
- ❑ E cimetidine

30. Testicular malfunction

❏ A resulting in infertility is usually accompanied by androgen deficiency
❏ B resulting in androgen deficiency is usually accompanied by infertility
❏ C is the commonest cause of impotence
❏ D in Klinefelter's syndrome will show a plasma testosterone response to human chorionic gonadotrophin
❏ E occurs in hyperprolactinaemia

31. Polycystic ovary syndrome

❏ A occurs in 20% of young women
❏ B causes anovulatory infertility
❏ C leads to elevated serum FSH levels
❏ D is associated with hyperprolactinaemia
❏ E is common in ballet dancers

32. At the female menopause

❏ A the patient has her greatest bone mass
❏ B oestrogen secretion causes hot flushes
❏ C myocardial infarction is common
❏ D bowel transit time increases
❏ E serum FSH is higher than serum LH

33. The following are true statements concerning carninoid tumours and the carcinoid syndrome:

❏ A the commonest primary site is the jejunum
❏ B with a small bowel primary tumour, the development of the carcinoid syndrome implies liver metastases
❏ C left-sided cardiac lesions do not occur
❏ D high volume secretory diarrhoea may occur
❏ E tumours are most commonly incidental findings

GASTROENTEROLOGY

Disorders of the upper GI tract

1. Characteristic features of diffuse oesophageal spasm are

- ❑ A central chest pain relieved by glyceryl trinitrate
- ❑ B effort-related pain
- ❑ C the presence of a corkscrew oesophagus on barium swallow
- ❑ D the absence of simultaneous contractions on manometry
- ❑ E a low incidence below the age of 50 years

2. Significant elevation of plasma gastrin level is found

- ❑ A after massive small bowel resection
- ❑ B in patients treated with omeprazole
- ❑ C in chronic renal failure
- ❑ D in duodenal ulcer
- ❑ E in multiple endocrine neoplasia type IIB

3. The following factors influence the rate of gastric emptying of liquids:

- ❑ A the volume of the ingested liquid
- ❑ B smoking
- ❑ C the frequency of the migrating motor complex
- ❑ D the concomitant ingestion of food
- ❑ E the presence of disaccharides in the liquid

4. *Helicobacter pylori*

- ❑ A are found in normal asymptomatic people
- ❑ B respond poorly to H_2 antagonists
- ❑ C are found in ectopic gastric tissue in the duodenum
- ❑ D are eliminated by bismuth therapy
- ❑ E cause acute gastritis

5. In the upper gastrointestinal tract

- ❑ A ranitidine competitively blocks histamine H_1 receptors
- ❑ B cisapride has anticholinergic actions
- ❑ C omeprazole lowers intragastric pH
- ❑ D domperidone stimulates dopamine D2 receptors
- ❑ E sucralfate is a potent acid neutralising agent

6. In acute pancreatitis

- ❑ A urgent ultrasound is required if the patient is jaundiced
- ❑ B emergency ERCP is needed to confirm the diagnosis
- ❑ C pancreatic pseudo-cyst is a likely cause of persistent hyperamylasaemia
- ❑ D progression to chronic pancreatitis is common
- ❑ E hypercalcaemia may follow the acute presentation

7. In chronic pancreatitis

- ❑ A plasma amylase is often raised even when patients are asymptomatic
- ❑ B after 50% gland destruction, diabetes is inevitable
- ❑ C histology is important in order to make a diagnosis
- ❑ D sub-total pancreatectomy provides excellent pain relief at the expense of exocrine insufficiency
- ❑ E the commonest known aetiological agent in Western societies is alcohol

Small bowel disorders

8. In acute gastroenteritis

- ❑ A patients with an ileostomy are at increased risk from dehydration
- ❑ B re-feeding should commence as soon as the appetite returns
- ❑ C oral rehydration therapy (ORT) improves the diarrhoea
- ❑ D antibiotics are contraindicated with Campylobacter infection
- ❑ E commercial ORT is inadequate for children less than 2 years of age

9. In coeliac disease

- ❑ A there is a biphasic peak of presentation
- ❑ B gluten withdrawal includes abstinence from oats and maize
- ❑ C patients with well controlled diet may have a normal jejunal biopsy
- ❑ D when the diagnosis has been made in infancy, a gluten-free diet can often be withdrawn at puberty
- ❑ E hyposplenism is a recognised feature

10. Concerning bacterial overgrowth of the gastrointestinal tract

- ❑ A it is rarely seen in the elderly
- ❑ B it is more common after partial gastrectomy
- ❑ C it does not occur in patients with an ileostomy
- ❑ D the most cost-effective investigation is breath hydrogen analysis
- ❑ E breath tests cannot easily distinguish bacterial overgrowth from rapid intestinal transit

11. Malabsorption of fat due to bile acid deficiency occurs in

- ❑ A Crohn's disease
- ❑ B radiation enteritis
- ❑ C cystic fibrosis
- ❑ D coeliac disease
- ❑ E giardiasis

Inflammatory bowel disease and large bowel disorders

12. Crohn's disease

- ❑ A presents with fistulae into other organs
- ❑ B is effectively treated with elemental diet alone
- ❑ C commonly involves the stomach
- ❑ D involving the small bowel can be treated with 5-amino salicylic acid
- ❑ E is more closely associated with sclerosing cholangitis than ulcerative colitis

13. In ulcerative colitis

- ❑ A the rectum is involved in more than 90% of cases
- ❑ B 5-ASA analogues are more effective at preventing relapses than sulphasalazine
- ❑ C distal proctitis responds poorly to systemic steroids
- ❑ D sulphasalazine induces a reversible reduction in sperm count sufficient to cause male infertility
- ❑ E ileo-anal anastomosis gives equally good results as in Crohn's disease

14. *Clostridium difficile*

- ❑ A is present in the normal colonic flora of 15–20% of adults
- ❑ B colitis is more likely the longer the preceding antibiotic treatment
- ❑ C occasionally produces fulminant colitis requiring urgent colectomy
- ❑ D produces diagnostic histological changes
- ❑ E colitis is best treated with i.v. metronidazole

15. The following are true of colonic gas:

- ❑ A it contains methane in over 90% of cases
- ❑ B the hydrogen component is decreased by fasting
- ❑ C flatus is largely produced by the hydrolysis of complex carbohydrate by brush border enzymes
- ❑ D production is related to the amount of air swallowed
- ❑ E production is usually increased in subjects with lactase deficiency

16. Concerning colonic polyps

- ❑ A only adenomas have malignant potential
- ❑ B colonoscopy is the preferred investigation
- ❑ C polyps >2 cm are more likely to be malignant
- ❑ D small polyps (<2 mm) do not require removal
- ❑ E red meat and low fibre have been aetiologically linked

17. Intestinal pseudo-obstruction may be a manifestation of

❑ A amyloidosis
❑ B squamous cell carcinoma of the lung
❑ C lead poisoning
❑ D Parkinson's disease
❑ E sarcoidosis

18. Irritable bowel syndrome

❑ A may follow an episode of infective diarrhoea
❑ B is a diagnosis which can only be safely made following a normal colonoscopy or barium enema
❑ C is commonly found to have been present in early adult life in patients presenting with diverticular disease in middle age
❑ D rarely presents over the age of 60
❑ E spares the upper GI tract

Liver disease

19. Drug-induced acute hepatitis may occur following treatment with

❑ A tetracycline
❑ B indomethacin
❑ C vitamin A
❑ D rifampicin
❑ E carbamazepine

20. Hepatitis C

❑ A is an RNA virus
❑ B is more likely to produce jaundice than hepatitis B
❑ C is associated with hepatocellular carcinoma
❑ D infection may be complicated by hepatitis D
❑ E is more likely to result in cirrhosis than hepatitis B

21. The following are true of infectious hepatitis:

- ❑ A hepatitis C is food/water borne
- ❑ B patients are maximally infectious prior to the onset of jaundice
- ❑ C vaccine to hepatitis B may reduce the incidence of hepatoma
- ❑ D alkaline phosphatase is rarely more than double the upper limit of the reference range
- ❑ E hepatitis D is now the commonest blood borne hepatitis in the UK

22. The following are true in liver failure:

- ❑ A a bleeding diathesis is more likely in cirrhosis than after a paracetamol overdose
- ❑ B neomycin is superior to metronidazole
- ❑ C lactulose reduces gut pH
- ❑ D it may be precipitated by constipation
- ❑ E deep coma is associated with opiate analgesia

23. Hepatic encephalopathy may be precipitated by

- ❑ A metabolic alkalosis
- ❑ B therapeutic paracentesis
- ❑ C treatment with omeprazole
- ❑ D intravenous normal saline
- ❑ E intravenous salt poor albumin

24. Cholestatic jaundice occurs with

- ❑ A pregnancy
- ❑ B erythromycin stearate
- ❑ C verapamil
- ❑ D prochlorperazine
- ❑ E amitriptyline

25. The following are true statements concerning haemochromatosis:

- ❑ A there is an association with B8 and Dw3 HLA antigens
- ❑ B it is the commonest cause of hepatoma in Britain
- ❑ C it can lead to pituitary failure
- ❑ D asymptomatic relatives should be screened for a raised plasma ferritin
- ❑ E a plasma ferritin value more than five times the upper reference range limit is diagnostic

26. Hepatocellular carcinoma

- ❑ A is more common in women
- ❑ B is usually associated with chronic hepatitis B
- ❑ C may present as an acute abdomen
- ❑ D needs a liver biopsy to confirm the diagnosis
- ❑ E rarely produces hepatomegaly

Miscellaneous gastroenterology

27. The following are true statements concerning artificial nutrition:

- ❑ A a low serum albumin indicates malnutrition
- ❑ B parenteral nutrition is more effective than enteral nutrition
- ❑ C the main complication of TPN is catheter occlusion
- ❑ D all enteral feeds are gluten-free
- ❑ E the major cause of weight loss in cancer patients is poor nutritional intake

28. In the investigation of acute gastrointestinal bleeding

- ❑ A a low haemoglobin with a normal MCV indicates recent haemorrhage
- ❑ B a raised blood urea indicates proximal bleeding
- ❑ C in patients over 60, angiodysplasia of the colon is an important cause
- ❑ D angiography is helpful if endoscopy is negative
- ❑ E persistent early morning vomiting suggests alcoholic gastritis

29. Gallstones are associated with

- ❑ A Gilbert's syndrome
- ❑ B Crohn's disease
- ❑ C familial hypercholesterolaemia
- ❑ D hereditary spherocytosis
- ❑ E cystic fibrosis

30. The carcinoid syndrome

- ❑ A frequently responds to octreotide
- ❑ B usually causes mitral valve dysfunction
- ❑ C is invariably fatal within 5 years
- ❑ D causes pallor and sweating
- ❑ E is diagnosed with fasting blood specimens

31. Ascites is a feature of

- ❑ A syndrome of inappropriate antidiuretic hormone secretion
- ❑ B mesothelioma
- ❑ C acute pericarditis
- ❑ D marasmus
- ❑ E hepatocellular carcinoma

GENETICS

Chromosomes

1. The following are true:

- ❑ A Klinefelter's syndrome is the result of non-disjunction in either of the parents
- ❑ B patients with the karyotype 45,XO have an increased risk of coarctation of aorta
- ❑ C a Barr body is an inactivated X chromosome
- ❑ D patients with the karyotype 47,XYY generally lead normal lives
- ❑ E the fragile-X syndrome is found predominantly in females

2. HLA molecules

- ❑ A are encoded for by genes on chromosome 6
- ❑ B are constitutively expressed only on leucocytes
- ❑ C form part of the T cell receptor
- ❑ D present antigen
- ❑ E are associated with beta-2 microglobulin

Mendelian inheritance

3. The following are true:

- ❑ A Gaucher's disease is more common in Ashkenazi Jews
- ❑ B Erb's muscular dystrophy is X-linked
- ❑ C ataxia telangiectasia is commoner in men
- ❑ D defective LDL receptors associated with familial hypercholesterolaemia are inherited in an autosomal dominant fashion
- ❑ E nephrogenic diabetes insipidus is inherited as an autosomal recessive trait

4. The following conditions have an autosomal dominant inheritance:

- ❑ A familial Mediterranean fever
- ❑ B neurofibromatosis
- ❑ C Friedreich's ataxia
- ❑ D dystrophia myotonica
- ❑ E haemochromatosis

5. The following are autosomal recessively inherited conditions:

- ❑ A Alport's syndrome
- ❑ B cystinosis
- ❑ C cystinuria
- ❑ D nephrogenic diabetes insipidus
- ❑ E primary hyperoxaluria

6. An X chromosome containing an abnormal gene is found in the following:

- ❑ A haemophilia B
- ❑ B Duchenne muscular dystrophy
- ❑ C congenital pyloric stenosis
- ❑ D nephrogenic diabetes insipidus
- ❑ E ataxia telangiectasia

Genetic disorders

7. The following are recognised findings in osteogenesis imperfecta:

- ❑ A blue sclerae
- ❑ B otosclerosis
- ❑ C pathological fracture
- ❑ D low alkaline phosphatase
- ❑ E partial remission in the female reproductive years

8. The following statements are true of Huntington's disease (chorea):

- ❑ A the gene is localised on the short arm of chromosome 5
- ❑ B it is associated with cortical dementia
- ❑ C prominent rigidity with little chorea is associated with a juvenile onset
- ❑ D the prominent abnormality on CT imaging is atrophy of the caudate nucleus
- ❑ E L-dopa medication typically improves chorea

9. Neurofibromatosis is associated with

❑ A phaeochromocytoma
❑ B retinal phacoma
❑ C acoustic neuroma
❑ D meningioma
❑ E plexiform neuroma

10. Klinefelter's syndrome leads to

❑ A infertility
❑ B gynaecomastia
❑ C mental retardation
❑ D high serum gonadotrophins
❑ E premature balding

11. Cystic fibrosis

❑ A affects 1 in every 1000 infants
❑ B is due to a specific mutation of the cystic fibrosis transmembrane
❑ C cystic fibrosis conductance regulator gene therapy is delivered by a viral vector
❑ D is due to defective Na^+:K^+ transport
❑ E gene therapy need only be given once

12. Recognised features of Wilson's disease include

❑ A retinitis pigmentosa
❑ B low urinary copper
❑ C liver disease resembling chronic active hepatitis
❑ D reduced plasma caeruloplasmin
❑ E osteomalacia

13. Alport's syndrome

❑ A is autosomal recessive
❑ B is due to a mutation of the Goodpasture antigen
❑ C results in basement membrane changes in the eye
❑ D can recur in renal transplants
❑ E is associated with tracheobronchial leiomyomatosis

14. In Turner's syndrome

- ❑ A 45 XO karyotype is universal
- ❑ B tall stature in prepuberty is characteristic
- ❑ C there is poor breast development
- ❑ D serum FSH is high in the adult
- ❑ E uterine agenesis is characteristic

Molecular genetics

15. In genetic technology

- ❑ A a codon consists of three nucleotides
- ❑ B introns are transcribed into messenger RNA
- ❑ C endonucleases polymerise DNA fragments
- ❑ D thymidine is not found in messenger RNA
- ❑ E transcription can be measured by Northern blotting

16. The following are true:

- ❑ A restriction fragment length polymorphisms allow a defective gene to be detected only if the gene is known
- ❑ B oligonucleotide probes can be used to detect a condition caused by a deleted gene
- ❑ C Down's syndrome may be caused by a translocation
- ❑ D Gaucher's disease may be diagnosed prenatally
- ❑ E inherited factor eight deficiency may be diagnosed using a chorionic villus sample

Miscellaneous genetics

17. The following are true:

❑ A measuring maternal serum alpha fetoprotein (AFP) is useful in assessing the risk of the fetus having Down's syndrome
❑ B over 50% of spontaneous first trimester abortions are the result of fetal chromosomal abnormalities
❑ C fetal blood samples are necessary if a pre-natal diagnosis of haemophilia A is to be made
❑ D chorionic villus sampling allows fetal cystic fibrosis to be diagnosed in the first trimester
❑ E amniocentesis allows all fetal chromosomal abnormalities to be identified

18. The following are more common in men than in women:

❑ A agammaglobulinaemia
❑ B Lesch-Nyhan syndrome
❑ C mixed connective tissue disease
❑ D insulin-dependent diabetes mellitus
❑ E favism

GENITOURINARY MEDICINE AND HIV/AIDS

HIV/AIDS

1. Characteristic features of HIV seroconversion illness include

❑ A oral ulceration
❑ B petechial rash
❑ C positive HIV P24 antigen
❑ D aseptic meningitis
❑ E an association with good prognosis

2. In the HIV sero-positive patient

❑ A diarrhoea in the immunocompromised is most often caused by protozoal infection
❑ B *Pneumocystis carinii* is a zoonosis
❑ C *P. carinii* may appear as lobar consolidation on a chest radiograph
❑ D tuberculosis can increase the load and spread of HIV
❑ E central nervous system infection is a common early feature of disease

3. The following haematological disorders are seen in association with infection by HIV:

❑ A atypical lymphocytes in the peripheral blood
❑ B immune thrombocytopenic purpura (ITP)
❑ C megaloblastic erythroblasts in the bone marrow in the absence of vitamin B12/folate deficiency
❑ D positive lupus anticoagulant screen
❑ E monocytopenia

4. Amongst the complications of HIV and AIDS

- ❑ A focal skin Kaposi sarcoma responds best to intralesional alpha-interferon
- ❑ B large cell lymphomas are associated with Epstein–Barr virus (EBV)
- ❑ C opportunistic infection of peripheral nerve and muscle is uncommon
- ❑ D retinal microvascular cotton wool spots always require urgent treatment
- ❑ E abdominal pain may be due to sclerosing cholangitis

5. In HIV-positive patients, prophylactic agents are of proven benefit in reducing the incidence of the following opportunistic infections:

- ❑ A cytomegalovirus (CMV) retinitis
- ❑ B *Pneumocystis carinii* pneumonia (PCP)
- ❑ C *Mycobacterium avium* complex bacteraemia (MACBAC)
- ❑ D toxoplasma encephalitis
- ❑ E cryptosporidial diarrhoea

6. In AIDS

- ❑ A CNS lymphoma is common
- ❑ B herpes simplex and herpes zoster are common
- ❑ C cerebral atrophy occurs
- ❑ D peripheral neuropathy occurs in about 20%
- ❑ E myopathy may be induced by zidovudine

7. The findings of an intracranial space-occupying lesion in a patient with HIV infection may indicate

- ❑ A *Toxoplasma gondii*
- ❑ B *Mycobacterium tuberculosis*
- ❑ C *Mycobacterium avium-intracellulare*
- ❑ D *Cryptococcus neoformans*
- ❑ E Progressive multifocal leuco-encephalopathy

8. HIV patients are particularly susceptible to the following enteric pathogens:

- ❑ A microsporidia
- ❑ B *Isospora belli*
- ❑ C *Helicobacter pylori*
- ❑ D *Hymenolepis nana*
- ❑ E *Entamoeba hartmanni*

Genito-urinary infections

9. In syphilis

- ❑ A the majority of patients with secondary syphilis have mucosal ulcers
- ❑ B accelerated progression may occur in HIV-positive patients
- ❑ C the TPHA test usually becomes negative after treatment
- ❑ D phenoxy methyl penicillin is the treatment of choice
- ❑ E condylomata acuminata occurs in the perianal region

10. *Neisseria gonorrhoeae* may cause

- ❑ A a pustular rash
- ❑ B tenosynovitis
- ❑ C meningitis
- ❑ D perihepatitis
- ❑ E proctitis

11. Non-gonococcal urethritis may result from

- ❑ A *Mycoplasma hominis*
- ❑ B *Mycoplasma genitalium*
- ❑ C *Chlamydia trachomatis*
- ❑ D bifidobacteria
- ❑ E *Ureaplasma urealyticum*

12. The following organisms cause the following diseases:

- ❑ A *Calymmatobacterium granulomatosis* – lymphogranuloma venereum
- ❑ B *Haemophilus ducreyi* – granuloma inguinale
- ❑ C *Chlamydia trachomatis* – chancroid
- ❑ D *Treponema pallidum* – condylomata acuminata
- ❑ E *Pediculosis corporis* – pubic louse (crabs)

HAEMATOLOGY

Anaemias

1. A normochromic-normocytic anaemia can be seen in the following circumstances:

- ❑ A hypopituitarism
- ❑ B sideroblastic anaemia
- ❑ C acute blood loss
- ❑ D aplastic anaemia
- ❑ E long-term phenytoin administration

2. Macrocytosis of red cells is a recognised finding in

- ❑ A coeliac disease
- ❑ B ulcerative colitis
- ❑ C alcoholism
- ❑ D aplastic anaemia

3. Iron deficiency

- ❑ A is associated with a reduction in the serum transferrin concentration
- ❑ B results in defective globin synthesis
- ❑ C can result in gastrointestinal malabsorption
- ❑ D is seen in patients with paroxysmal nocturnal haemoglobinuria
- ❑ E is associated with glossitis

4. Oral iron treatment

- ❑ A imparts a characteristic slate grey colour to the stools
- ❑ B increases the risk of fits in patients with epilepsy
- ❑ C results in a slower haemoglobin recovery than intramuscular iron
- ❑ D may cause dose-related abdominal side effects
- ❑ E may be purchased from pharmacies without a prescription

5. A low serum folate is a common finding in

- ❑ A tropical sprue
- ❑ B pernicious anaemia
- ❑ C megaloblastic anaemia of pregnancy
- ❑ D myxoedema
- ❑ E cirrhosis of the liver

6. With regard to vitamin B12

- ❑ A deficiency causes malabsorption
- ❑ B intramuscular administration of more than 1 mg/week results in haemolysis
- ❑ C serum levels are increased in polycythaemia rubra vera
- ❑ D the presence of intrinsic factor antibodies provides strong supportive evidence for the diagnosis of pernicious anaemia
- ❑ E hydroxocobalamin is derived from liver extract

7. A falling haemoglobin with a 20% reticulocyte count may be due to

- ❑ A menorrhagia
- ❑ B congenital spherocytosis
- ❑ C sideroblastic anaemia
- ❑ D lead
- ❑ E methyl dopa

8. In Addisonian pernicious anaemia (PA)

- ❑ A the serum folate is often raised in association with a low red cell folate
- ❑ B antibodies to intrinsic factor are found in the serum of 90% of patients
- ❑ C a response to treatment with corticosteroids is common
- ❑ D is associated with a higher than normal incidence of carcinoma of the stomach
- ❑ E infertility is a rare presentation

Haemoglobinopathies

9. Features of sickle cell anaemia in adults include

- ❑ A leg ulcers
- ❑ B aseptic bone necrosis
- ❑ C dysphagia
- ❑ D priapism
- ❑ E nocturia

10. Complications seen in patients suffering from sickle cell disease include

- ❑ A priapism
- ❑ B pneumothorax
- ❑ C cataracts
- ❑ D renal papillary necrosis
- ❑ E hyposplenism

11. In beta-thalassaemia major

- ❑ A symptoms and signs typically develop at about five years of age
- ❑ B in children, there is seldom marked enlargement of the spleen
- ❑ C the mongoloid facies is due to expansion of the facial bones due to marrow hyperplasia
- ❑ D the serum iron is often raised although the MCH is reduced
- ❑ E the anaemia is entirely due to decreased haemoglobin synthesis

Haemolysis

12. In patients with a cold antibody haemolytic anaemia

- ❑ A Raynaud's phenomenon may be a feature
- ❑ B a lymphoma is a recognised association
- ❑ C IgE antibody is often involved
- ❑ D IgG antibodies are sometimes involved
- ❑ E recent rubella infection may be relevant

13. Warm-type autoimmune haemolytic anaemia (AIHA)

- ❑ A is a recognised complication of acute lymphoblastic leukaemia
- ❑ B is rarely mediated by IgG immunoglobulins
- ❑ C occurs following infection with *Mycoplasma pneumoniae*
- ❑ D is usually associated with a positive Coombs' test
- ❑ E is recognised following administration of L-dopa

14. The following produce haemolysis in patients with G6PD (glucose 6-phosphate dehydrogenase) deficiency:

- ❑ A primaquine
- ❑ B penicillin
- ❑ C tetracycline
- ❑ D glandular fever
- ❑ E nitrofurantoin

15. Paroxysmal nocturnal haemoglobinuria

- ❑ A is a hereditary form of haemolytic anaemia
- ❑ B is exacerbated by acidosis
- ❑ C is associated with aplastic anaemia
- ❑ D results from heterologous complement attack
- ❑ E is due to a defect in the glycosyl-phosphatidylinositol anchor

16. The following are associated with microangiopathic blood changes:

- ❑ A haemolytic-uraemic syndrome
- ❑ B severe burns
- ❑ C meningococcal septicaemia
- ❑ D Down's syndrome
- ❑ E typhoid fever

Haematological malignancies

17. Chronic myeloid leukaemia

- ❑ A is associated with a raised serum vitamin B12 level
- ❑ B can evolve into both acute myeloid or acute lymphoid leukaemia
- ❑ C commonly presents with lymphadenopathy and massive splenomegaly
- ❑ D is associated with translocation between chromosomes 8 and 22
- ❑ E can be effectively treated by alpha-interferon

18. As compared with chronic myelocytic leukaemia, chronic lymphocytic leukaemia has

- ❑ A more marked lymphadenopathy
- ❑ B more frequent hypogammaglobulinaemia
- ❑ C a more frequent occurrence of a positive Coombs' test
- ❑ D more frequent development of a blast crisis
- ❑ E a worse prognosis

19. The following are recognised complications of Hodgkin's disease:

- ❑ A amyloidosis
- ❑ B dermatomyositis
- ❑ C Cryptococcus infection
- ❑ D haemolytic anaemia
- ❑ E asthma

20. Multiple myeloma

- ❑ A occasionally occurs in the absence of a serum paraprotein
- ❑ B is a cause of a leukoerythroblastic blood picture
- ❑ C presents with bone pain in a minority of cases
- ❑ D is a recognised cause of carpal tunnel syndrome
- ❑ E has a peak incidence in the 5th decade

21. Renal failure in multiple myeloma is associated with

- ❑ A amyloidosis
- ❑ B hyperuricaemia
- ❑ C intravenous pyelography
- ❑ D glomerular destruction by precipitation of kappa and lambda light chains in Bowman's space
- ❑ E hypercalcaemia

22. In benign monoclonal gammopathy (monoclonal hypergamma-globulinaemia)

- ❑ A there is a low level of serum albumin
- ❑ B there is a marked increase in immature plasma cells in the bone marrow
- ❑ C the 'M' band in the serum electrophoretic strip does not show a progressive rise over the course of time
- ❑ D there is no anaemia
- ❑ E there is no Bence-Jones protein in the urine

Coagulation

23. In the investigation of a patient with a bleeding tendency

- ❑ A a prolonged partial thromboplastin time could indicate haemophilia
- ❑ B a normal prothrombin time excludes thrombocytopenia
- ❑ C patients should be asked to refrain from taking aspirin for 14 days
- ❑ D Hess' test is negative with a coagulation factor deficiency
- ❑ E a prolonged prothrombin time is a characteristic finding in hereditary haemorrhagic telangiectasia (HHT)

24. Haemarthrosis is seen in

- ❑ A haemophilia B
- ❑ B sickle cell disease
- ❑ C Charcot joints
- ❑ D thrombocytopenia
- ❑ E pyrophosphate arthritis

25. Haemophilia A

- ❑ A may be unassociated with a family history
- ❑ B commonly presents with spontaneous purpura
- ❑ C results in prolongation of the activated partial thromboplastin time (APTT) and prothrombin time (PT)
- ❑ D characteristically becomes less severe with advancing age
- ❑ E is associated with a normal bleeding time

26. Protein C

- ❑ A plasma level falls in patients receiving warfarin
- ❑ B deficiency produces a prolongation in the activated partial thromboplastin time (APTT)
- ❑ C requires Protein S as a co-factor
- ❑ D plasma level falls in disseminated intravascular coagulation (DIC)
- ❑ E potentiates the activity of antithrombin III

27. The following are recognised complications of heparin therapy:

- ❑ A thrombosis
- ❑ B osteomalacia
- ❑ C hirsutism
- ❑ D thrombocytopenia
- ❑ E teratogenesis

28. Disseminated intravascular coagulation

- ❑ A is often characterised by neurological presentation
- ❑ B produces fragmented red cells
- ❑ C produces thrombocytopenia
- ❑ D responds to heparin therapy in the majority of cases
- ❑ E is characterised by raised fibrin degradation products

Other haematology

29. The cause of thrombocytopenia in the following conditions is correctly assigned in each case:

- ❑ A acute leukaemia: marrow aplasia
- ❑ B systemic lupus erythematosus: platelet antibodies
- ❑ C Gram-negative septicaemia: marrow aplasia
- ❑ D massive transfusion: platelet antibodies
- ❑ E splenomegaly from any cause: sequestration

30. In idiopathic thrombocytopenic purpura (ITP)

- ❑ A most cases are due to an immune-mediated destruction of platelets
- ❑ B if the spleen is palpable then the thrombocytopenia is likely to be due to another cause
- ❑ C maternal anti-platelet antibodies may cause neonatal thrombocytopenia
- ❑ D the disease usually becomes chronic when it presents in childhood
- ❑ E can be associated with HIV infection

31. Pancytopenia may be caused by

- ❑ A folic acid deficiency
- ❑ B paroxysmal nocturnal haemoglobinuria (PNH)
- ❑ C miliary tuberculosis
- ❑ D acute myeloblastic leukaemia
- ❑ E haemosiderosis

32. Splenectomy

- ❑ A results in increased incidence of pneumococcal septicaemia
- ❑ B is a valuable diagnostic procedure in non-Hodgkin's lymphoma
- ❑ C produces blood film appearance of acanthocytes and Howell-Jolly bodies
- ❑ D produces blood film changes which are also seen in coeliac disease
- ❑ E leads to almost invariable remission in hereditary spherocytosis

33. Marrow trephine biopsy is more satisfactory than marrow aspiration in the diagnosis of

❑ A aplastic anaemia
❑ B sideroblastic anaemia
❑ C macrocytic anaemia
❑ D marrow involvement in Hodgkin's disease
❑ E myelosclerosis

34. When giving a blood transfusion

❑ A administration of Rhesus-positive blood to a Rhesus-positive recipient can be followed by haemolytic problems due to Rhesus-group antibiodies
❑ B a fever in the recipient developing during transfusion is an indication to stop transfusing
❑ C using stored blood, the oxygen delivering capacity of the blood is not restored until about two days later
❑ D with stored blood, one can assume that no viable white blood cells remain 24 hours after the blood donation
❑ E CMV antibody-negative blood should be used for all recipients who are themselves CMV negative

35. Erythropoietin

❑ A is only produced in the kidney
❑ B production increases in response to hypoxia
❑ C therapy is associated with hypertension
❑ D acts on the colony forming units of the erythroid series in the bone marrow
❑ E is produced in an active and inactive isoform

36. In a patient with polycythaemia the following support a diagnosis of primary proliferative polycythaemia (polycythaemia rubra vera):

❑ A increased bone marrow reticulin
❑ B thrombocytopenia
❑ C palpable spleen
❑ D decreased plasma volume
❑ E iron deficient blood film

37. The following are causes of a leuko-erythroblastic blood picture:

- ❑ A carcinomatosis
- ❑ B respiratory distress in neonates
- ❑ C septicaemia
- ❑ D myelofibrosis
- ❑ E severe untreated pernicious anaemia

IMMUNOLOGY

Cellular immunity

1. The following statements on cellular immunity are correct:

❑ A cytotoxic T cells (CTL) carry CD8 glycoprotein and respond to peptides presented by HLA class 1
❑ B CTL produce interleukin 2 (IL-2)
❑ C Di George syndrome is associated with impaired cellular immunity
❑ D lymphopenia is a feature of ataxia telangiectasia
❑ E Wiscott–Aldrich disease is an autosomal recessive condition characterised by depressed cellular immunity

2. Leucocytes of the CD4 T4 phenotype

❑ A are lymphocytes
❑ B do not recirculate
❑ C are phagocytic
❑ D are infected by the Human Immunodeficiency Virus (HIV)
❑ E perform a 'helper' role in the on-going immune response

3. The following are diseases with specific defects in phagocyte function:

❑ A myeloperoxidase deficiency
❑ B purine nucleoside phosphorylase deficiency
❑ C Job's syndrome
❑ D Chediak–Higashi syndrome
❑ E Bloom's syndrome

Hypersensitivity

4. Anaphylaxis

❑ A involves mast cells and basophils
❑ B is triggered by binding of monomeric IgE alone
❑ C is manifest by vasoconstriction
❑ D can be caused by administration of antibody
❑ E is an example of a type 1 reaction

5. Urticaria may be associated with

- ❑ A Strongyloides infection
- ❑ B opiate drugs
- ❑ C paracetamol
- ❑ D systemic lupus erythematosus
- ❑ E pityriasis rosea

6. The delayed hypersensitivity reaction (Type IV)

- ❑ A is a humoral immune response
- ❑ B is dependent on T lymphocytes
- ❑ C is characterised by a mononuclear cell infiltration
- ❑ D is caused by deposition of immune complexes in tissues
- ❑ E is mediated by IgE antibodies bound to Fc receptors on mast cells and basophil granulocytes

Immunoglobulins/autoimmunity

7. Specific precipitating antibodies are present in

- ❑ A byssinosis
- ❑ B bagassosis
- ❑ C histoplasmosis
- ❑ D fibrosing alveolitis
- ❑ E bird fancier's lung

8. Anti-histone antibodies

- ❑ A are associated with thrombosis
- ❑ B are found in the absence of antibodies to native DNA in drug induced SLE
- ❑ C are associated with congenital heart block
- ❑ D are a marker for polymyositis
- ❑ E are a marker for Sjögren's syndrome

9. Characteristic features of non-familial hypogamma-globulinaemia (common variable immunodeficiency) include:

- ❑ A splenomegaly
- ❑ B bronchiectasis
- ❑ C pernicious anaemia
- ❑ D *Giardia lamblia* infestation
- ❑ E IgA levels are usually greater than IgG and IgM

10. The following have a recognised association with IgM paraprotein:

- ❑ A kala-azar
- ❑ B cold haemagglutinin disease
- ❑ C chronic lymphatic leukaemia (CLL)
- ❑ D Waldenström's disease
- ❑ E chronic myeloid leukaemia

Cytokines

11. In cytokine production and function

- ❑ A tumour necrosis factor (TNF) alpha is mainly produced by T lymphocytes
- ❑ B interferon (IFN) gamma has a strong antiviral action by inducing biochemical adaptation in infected cells
- ❑ C interleukin 1 (IL-1) induces prostaglandin synthesis
- ❑ D transforming growth factor (TGF) beta inhibits the acute inflammatory response
- ❑ E interleukin 2 (IL-2) stimulates the growth and differentiation of B cells

12. Interleukin-1 (IL-1)

- ❑ A is a lymphocyte activating factor
- ❑ B is an endogenous pyrogen
- ❑ C inhibits fibroblast proliferation
- ❑ D stimulates the synthesis of acute phase proteins in the liver
- ❑ E is not synthesised by macrophages

Miscellaneous immunology

13. Complement deficiency

- ❑ A is described for all 11 classical pathway proteins
- ❑ B affecting C1 esterase inhibitor leads to angio-oedema
- ❑ C heterozygotes have half normal levels, and homozygotes have no active proteins
- ❑ D genes are located in the MHC region
- ❑ E affecting C2 may be associated with connective tissue disease

14. Hypocomplementaemia is a feature of

- ❑ A acute pancreatitis
- ❑ B membranous nephropathy
- ❑ C systemic lupus erythematosus
- ❑ D pregnancy
- ❑ E cryoglobulinaemia

15. Pneumococcal vaccination should be given to patients

- ❑ A who are HIV positive
- ❑ B who are heterozygous for Hb S
- ❑ C who have had a splenectomy
- ❑ D every five years where indicated
- ❑ E prior to travel to countries with high rates of penicillin-resistant pneumococci

INFECTIOUS DISEASES AND TROPICAL MEDICINE

Antimicrobials

1. The following antibiotics are effective against the corresponding organism:

❑ A teicoplanin – *Escherichia coli*
❑ B cefuroxime – *Pseudomonas aeruginosa*
❑ C ciprofloxacin – *Streptococcus pneumoniae*
❑ D benzyl penicillin – *Streptococcus pyogenes*
❑ E flucloxacillin – methicillin-resistant *Staphylococcus aureus*

2. Ciprofloxacin has good activity against

❑ A *Mycobacterium tuberculosis*
❑ B *Salmonella paratyphi*
❑ C *Streptococcus pneumoniae*
❑ D *Legionella pneumophila*
❑ E *Bacteroides fragilis*

Respiratory infections

3. The following organisms are recognised causes of pneumonia:

❑ A *Chlamydia pneumoniae*
❑ B *Mycoplasma hominis*
❑ C *Chlamydia trachomatis*
❑ D *Streptococcus pyogenes*
❑ E *Legionella pneumophila*

4. *Legionella pneumophila*

❑ A is a Gram-positive bacillus
❑ B infection is associated with lymphopenia
❑ C infection may be diagnosed by urine antigen detection
❑ D causes disease by ingestion of infected water
❑ E causes Pontiac fever

5. The following are true of tuberculosis in the UK:

- ❑ A HIV-positive individuals should not receive BCG
- ❑ B it occurs in less than 5% of contacts
- ❑ C sputum-positive patients are non-infectious after two weeks of therapy
- ❑ D drug resistance is now greater than 10%
- ❑ E large pleural effusions require steroid therapy

6. In tuberculosis

- ❑ A multiple drug resistance only occurs in the immunocompromised
- ❑ B vertebral body destruction is an early radiological sign in spinal disease
- ❑ C pyrazinamide should be given for six months
- ❑ D the response to treatment in HIV-positive patients is poor
- ❑ E steroids should be given for pericardial disease

Gastrointestinal infections

7. The following are true of *E. coli* gastroenteritis:

- ❑ A enterotoxigenic strains are a common cause of travellers' diarrhoea
- ❑ B enteropathogenic strains are associated with the haemolytic uraemic syndrome
- ❑ C enteroadherent strains are non-pathogenic
- ❑ D enterohaemorrhagic strains commonly belong to the serotype 0-157
- ❑ E enteroinvasive strains cause a dysenteric illness

8. Hepatitis B virus

- ❑ A e antigen is a cleavage product of core antigen
- ❑ B is an RNA virus
- ❑ C replication is inhibited by interferon
- ❑ D is required for hepatitis D infection
- ❑ E binds to hepatocytes via e antigen

9. The following are true of hepatitis C virus:

- ❑ A chronic carriage is associated with hepatoma
- ❑ B it is sexually transmissible
- ❑ C it is an RNA virus
- ❑ D infection is confirmed by a positive hepatitis C antigen test
- ❑ E chronic carriers may benefit from treatment with interferon

10. The following micro-organisms may cause chronic hepatitis:

- ❑ A *Leptospira icterohaemorrhagiae*
- ❑ B Delta virus
- ❑ C Hepatitis B virus
- ❑ D Hepatitis C virus
- ❑ E Hepatitis E virus

11. In leptospirosis

- ❑ A conjunctivitis is a frequent early symptom
- ❑ B the onset is characteristically abrupt
- ❑ C splenomegaly is found in the majority of patients
- ❑ D the transaminases are markedly elevated
- ❑ E the diagnosis is best made by serology

12. In the diagnosis of typhoid

- ❑ A the Widal test is useful
- ❑ B leucopenia supports the diagnosis
- ❑ C bone marrow aspiration has the highest yield for culturing *S. typhi*
- ❑ D stool cultures are always negative in the first week
- ❑ E rose spots are a reliable sign

13. The classical rash of typhoid fever (rose spots)

- ❑ A is a poor prognostic sign
- ❑ B begins on the extremities
- ❑ C is petechial
- ❑ D does not occur in paratyphoid
- ❑ E usually lasts a week or more

14. The following organisms are associated with both fever and jaundice:

❑ A *Entamoeba histolytica*
❑ B *Fasciola hepatica*
❑ C *Leptospira icterohaemorrhagiae*
❑ D *Clonorchis sinensis*
❑ E *Paragonimus westermani*

15. Amoebic liver abscess is commonly associated with

❑ A jaundice
❑ B splenomegaly
❑ C dysentery
❑ D pericarditis
❑ E raised hemidiaphragm

Neurological infections

16. The following are poor prognostic signs in a patient with *Neisseria meningitidis* infection:

❑ A absence of neck stiffness
❑ B widespread ecchymosis
❑ C CSF protein >2.5 g/l
❑ D leucopenia
❑ E a skin/rectal temperature difference of >3°C

17. The following may result in a lymphocytic meningitis:

❑ A *Mycobacterium bovis*
❑ B *Cryptococcus neoformans*
❑ C *Treponema pertenue*
❑ D *Brucella melitensis*
❑ E *Borrelia burgdorferi*

18. The following are features of encephalitis:

- ❑ A herpes simplex encephalitis is usually caused by HSV 2
- ❑ B chickenpox encephalitis typically coincides with the onset of rash
- ❑ C herpes simplex predominantly affects the temporal lobes
- ❑ D mycoplasma encephalitis only occurs in the immunocompromised
- ❑ E Japanese B encephalitis is preventable by vaccination

19. The following conditions are transmissible spongiform encephalopathies (prion diseases):

- ❑ A subacute sclerosing panencephalitis (SSPE)
- ❑ B Creutzfeldt-Jakob disease (CJD)
- ❑ C Gerstmann-Straussler-Sheinker disease (GSSD)
- ❑ D kuru
- ❑ E progressive multifocal leucoencephalopathy (PML)

20. Features of borreliosis include

- ❑ A hepatic enlargement and tenderness
- ❑ B petechial rash
- ❑ C meningism
- ❑ D myocarditis
- ❑ E Jarisch–Herxheimer reaction

21. The following are features of listeriosis:

- ❑ A progressive focal neurology
- ❑ B osteomyelitis
- ❑ C cholecystitis
- ❑ D resistance to cephalosporins
- ❑ E low mortality with septicaemia

22. Botulism

- ❑ A is most commonly due to types A, B and E
- ❑ B is caused by spore-forming anaerobic organism
- ❑ C is usually associated with fever
- ❑ D usually spares the pupillary reactions
- ❑ E is invariably fatal

Tropical infections

23. *Plasmodium vivax*

- ❑ A causes quartan malaria
- ❑ B is associated with relapsing disease
- ❑ C is often resistant to chloroquine
- ❑ D is transmitted by culicine mosquitoes
- ❑ E infection should be eradicated with primaquine

24. Characteristic features of acute falciparum malaria include

- ❑ A splenomegaly
- ❑ B rigors every 72 hours
- ❑ C eosinophilia
- ❑ D renal failure
- ❑ E recurrence of symptoms after one year in untreated survivors

25. The following may occur in severe falciparum malaria:

- ❑ A hypoglycaemia
- ❑ B hyponatraemia
- ❑ C haemoglobinuria
- ❑ D raised intracranial pressure
- ❑ E liver failure

26. Life cycles of the following helminths involve the lung:

- ❑ A *Ascaris lumbricoides*
- ❑ B *Strongyloides stercoralis*
- ❑ C *Necator americanus*
- ❑ D *Ankylostoma braziliensis*
- ❑ E *Schistosoma japonicum*

27. *Schistosoma mansoni* infection

- ❑ A is common in the Indian subcontinent
- ❑ B may present with spastic paraparesis
- ❑ C does not cause cercarial dermatitis
- ❑ D predisposes to recurrent salmonella bacteraemia
- ❑ E is treated with praziquantel

28. Periorbital oedema is a feature of

- ❑ A Chagas disease
- ❑ B trichinosis
- ❑ C gnathostomiasis
- ❑ D loa-loa infection
- ❑ E group A streptococcal infection

Other infectious diseases

29. *Pneumocystis carinii* infection

- ❑ A is the most common opportunist lung infection in AIDS
- ❑ B responds to treatment with co-trimoxazole (*Septrin*)
- ❑ C can usually be diagnosed by bronchoalveolar lavage
- ❑ D should be treated with prednisolone if moderate or severe
- ❑ E now has a first exposure mortality of less than 15%

30. The following are commonly associated:

- ❑ A *Staph. aureus* and toxic epidermal necrolysis
- ❑ B *Staph. aureus* bacteraemia and toxic shock syndrome
- ❑ C group A strep. and erysipelas in the elderly
- ❑ D streptococcal ecthyma and rheumatic fever
- ❑ E streptococcal cellulitis and rapid onset septicaemia

31. The following are true of toxic shock syndrome:

- ❑ A a maculo-papular rash is common
- ❑ B *Staphylococcus aureus* elaborating enterotoxin C may be isolated
- ❑ C hypotension occurs in all patients
- ❑ D non-menstrual cases account for one quarter of the total
- ❑ E alopecia is common

32. The following rashes may result from *Streptococcus pyogenes* infection:

- ❑ A erysipelas
- ❑ B erythema marginatum
- ❑ C erythema nodosum
- ❑ D slapped cheek syndrome
- ❑ E ecthyma gangrenosum

33. The following are true of urinary infection in adults:

- ❑ A *Proteus mirabilis* is the most common offending organism in general practice
- ❑ B renal damage by analgesics is a predisposing factor
- ❑ C bladder neck obstruction predisposes to infection
- ❑ D bacterial colonisation of bladder urine is usually due to descending infection from the kidney
- ❑ E chronic renal failure is a common feature

34. The following diseases can be diagnosed by examination of a blood film:

- ❑ A rat-bite fever
- ❑ B relapsing fever
- ❑ C Lyme disease
- ❑ D African trypanosomiasis
- ❑ E Oroya fever

35. The following infections may be contracted from dogs:

- ❑ A dysgonic-fermenter 2
- ❑ B *Pasteurella multocida*
- ❑ C *Echinococcus granulosis*
- ❑ D *Leptospira canicola*
- ❑ E *Campylobacter foetus*

36. Rabies

- ❑ A is invariably fatal
- ❑ B is caused by a bullet-shaped DNA virus
- ❑ C may be diagnosed by a corneal smear
- ❑ D can be passed from person to person
- ❑ E always causes hydrophobia

37. The following are true of Hantavirus infection:

- ❑ A it is transmitted by arthropod vectors
- ❑ B it causes haemorrhagic fever with renal syndrome
- ❑ C it has been associated with acute respiratory illness
- ❑ D treatment with ribavirin is of benefit
- ❑ E it causes nephropathia epidemica

38. Mumps virus infection

❑ A is asymptomatic in 40%
❑ B with raised amylase is diagnostic of pancreatitis
❑ C is complicated by meningitis in less than 1% of cases
❑ D is due to an RNA virus
❑ E is a recognised cause of oophoritis

39. Parvovirus B19

❑ A has tropism for red blood cells
❑ B infection usually spreads by the faeco–oral route
❑ C is associated with aplastic anaemia
❑ D increases the risk of birth defects
❑ E is associated with an erythematous rash

40. Intracellular inclusion bodies are seen in the following conditions:

❑ A Alzheimer's disease
❑ B rabies
❑ C sarcoidosis
❑ D yellow fever
❑ E cytomegalovirus infection

41. Fungal arthritis is suggested by

❑ A indolent synovitis
❑ B compromised host
❑ C recent travel in endemic area
❑ D discoloration of synovium
❑ E unpleasant smelling synovial fluid

42. *Candida albicans*

❑ A may cause endophthalmitis
❑ B infection is encouraged by renal glycosuria
❑ C responds to griseofulvin when affecting the nail bed
❑ D causing deep infection is more likely with lymphopenia
❑ E endocarditis most commonly involves the tricuspid valve

43. Actinomycosis

- ❑ A may be caused by *Actinobacillus actinomycetemcomitans*
- ❑ B can be associated with intrauterine devices
- ❑ C most commonly affects the lung
- ❑ D may be disseminated
- ❑ E is best treated with vancomycin

METABOLIC DISEASES

Disorders of purine metabolism

1. Hyperuricaemia occurs in

- ❑ A Lesch-Nyhan syndrome
- ❑ B polycythaemia rubra vera
- ❑ C primary hyperparathyroidism
- ❑ D starvation
- ❑ E thyrotoxicosis

2. Indications for hypouricaemic therapy include

- ❑ A tophi
- ❑ B bone erosion
- ❑ C urate levels at upper limit of normal
- ❑ D a single, severe attack
- ❑ E nephrosclerosis

Disorders of metals and metalloproteins

3. The following statements are true of attacks of acute intermittent porphyria (AIP):

- ❑ A Ehrlich's aldehyde reagent is of value in diagnosis
- ❑ B postural hypotension is a characteristic finding
- ❑ C pain in the limbs is a characteristic complaint
- ❑ D diazepam is a typical precipitant
- ❑ E carbohydrate infusions are of value in management

4. The following are recognised features of Wilson's disease:

- ❑ A band keratitis
- ❑ B low urinary copper
- ❑ C liver disease resembling chronic active hepatitis
- ❑ D reduced plasma caeruloplasmin
- ❑ E osteomalacia

Disorders of bone, mineral metabolism and inorganic ions

5. Delayed bone age (skeletal maturity) is found in the following conditions:

❑ A growth hormone deficiency
❑ B precocious puberty
❑ C hypothyroidism
❑ D metatarsus varus
❑ E familial short stature

6. In the treatment of postmenopausal osteoporosis

❑ A measurement of lumbar spine density rather than the density of the proximal femur by dual-energy X-ray absorptiometry is the most useful method of monitoring response to treatment
❑ B bisphosphonates affect bone resorption without affecting bone formation
❑ C bone density continues to increase for five years after the start of bisphosphonates
❑ D fluorides stimulate new bone formation
❑ E there is a good correlation between the increase in bone mineral density and reduction in risk of fracture

7. Glucocorticoid effects on bone metabolism include

❑ A increased osteoblastic activity
❑ B reduced gastrointestinal absorption of calcium
❑ C reduced 25-hydroxylation of vitamin D
❑ D reduced calcitonin levels
❑ E increased renal excretion of calcium

8. Recognised features of Paget's disease of bone include

❑ A hypercalcaemia
❑ B nerve deafness
❑ C angioid streaks in the retina
❑ D brain stem compression
❑ E osteopenia

9. Avascular necrosis of bone is a recognised complication of

❑ A systemic lupus erythematosus
❑ B renal transplantation
❑ C sickle cell disease
❑ D congestive cardiac failure
❑ E Cushing's syndrome

10. Hypocalciuric hypercalcaemia

❑ A is an X-linked recessive trait
❑ B occurs in the milk-alkali syndrome
❑ C is corrected by parathyroidectomy
❑ D is associated with pituitary tumours
❑ E is masked by thiazide diuretic use

11. In hypercalcaemia

❑ A serum alkaline phosphatase is always elevated in primary hyperparathyroidism
❑ B malignancy can be a cause in the absence of bone metastases
❑ C severe hypocalcaemia may follow removal of a single parathyroid adenoma
❑ D detectable parathyroid hormone (PTH) levels indicate hyperparathyroidism and the need for surgical treatment
❑ E peritoneal dialysis is effective in severe cases

12. Hypomagnesaemia is a feature of

❑ A diabetic ketoacidosis
❑ B chronic diarrhoea
❑ C loop diuretic toxicity
❑ D acute myocardial infarction
❑ E primary hyperparathyroidism

13. A high plasma inorganic phosphate level is a characteristic finding in

❑ A diabetic ketoacidosis
❑ B the osteodystrophy of chronic renal failure
❑ C hypoparathyroidism
❑ D nutritional rickets
❑ E Paget's disease

Acid-base disorders

14. A plasma bicarbonate level of 34 mmol/l would be an unexpected finding in a patient with

❑ A Conn's syndrome
❑ B vomiting due to pyloric stenosis
❑ C untreated diabetic ketoacidosis
❑ D chronic cor pulmonale
❑ E chronic renal failure

15. The anion gap

❑ A is reduced in maple syrup urine disease
❑ B is elevated in ureterosigmoidostomy
❑ C is elevated in hyponatraemia
❑ D is reduced in the nephrotic syndrome
❑ E is elevated in salicylate poisoning

16. Serum K^+ 2.5 mmol/l and HCO_3^- 14 mmol/l suggests

❑ A acetazolamide treatment
❑ B bulimia
❑ C Conn's syndrome
❑ D uretero-colonic fistula
❑ E methanol poisoning

Lipid disorders

17. Apoprotein A1

❑ A is directly related to risk of ischaemic heart disease
❑ B levels are increased in nephrotic syndrome
❑ C is associated with high density lipoprotein
❑ D is a component of chylomicrons
❑ E has beta mobility on an electrophoretic strip

18. Apolipoprotein E

- ❑ A is not present in normal brain
- ❑ B is associated with mobilisation of cholesterol in tissue repair and growth
- ❑ C is encoded on chromosome 19
- ❑ D polymorphic variants are associated with Alzheimer's disease
- ❑ E is metabolised to an amyloid precursor protein

19. The LDL receptor

- ❑ A is restricted to the cell surface of tissues
- ❑ B catalyses HDL at a lower rate than LDL
- ❑ C is defective in familial hypercholesterolaemia
- ❑ D mediates down regulation of HMG CoA reductase
- ❑ E is encoded on the X chromosome

20. Characteristic features of heterozygous familial hypercholesterolaemia include

- ❑ A autosomal recessive inheritance
- ❑ B normal ischaemic heart disease risk in affected females
- ❑ C raised plasma LDL concentration at birth
- ❑ D tendon xanthomas in early childhood
- ❑ E defective hepatic LDL receptors

Other metabolic disorders

21. Concerning pyridoxine (vitamin B6)

- ❑ A vitamin B6 status can be assessed by the tryptophan loading test
- ❑ B prolonged use of penicillamine can lead to vitamin B6 deficiency
- ❑ C its use is contraindicated in pregnant women
- ❑ D it should not be given to patients with Parkinson's disease being treated with L-dopa and carbidopa
- ❑ E it is extensively metabolised within the liver

22. Homocystinuria

❑ A is associated with aortic dilation
❑ B pyridoxine does not reduce homocystine levels but does improve symptoms
❑ C is an X–linked disorder
❑ D can be treated with penicillamine
❑ E causes renal stones

23. The neuroleptic malignant syndrome

❑ A can occur with benzodiazepines
❑ B is frequently complicated by rhabdomyolysis
❑ C pyrexia is uncommon
❑ D may respond to bromocriptine
❑ E can complicate antiparkinsonian therapy

24. Secondary (reactive) amyloidosis

❑ A results from an inability to mount an acute phase response
❑ B causes ulceration of the tongue
❑ C characteristically presents as a glomerulonephritis
❑ D only complicates rheumatic diseases in adults
❑ E can be reversed by controlling the underlying disease

25. Recognised features of hypothermia include

❑ A pancreatitis
❑ B left shift of the haemoglobin-oxygen dissociation curve
❑ C myotonia
❑ D impaired shivering thermogenesis
❑ E acute hepatic necrosis

MOLECULAR MEDICINE

Vascular mediators

1. Renin

- ❑ A is synthesised by cells of the distal tubule
- ❑ B cleaves the two N-terminal amino acids of angiotensin I
- ❑ C release is stimulated by a decrease in chloride delivery from the loop of Henle
- ❑ D transcription is stimulated by ACE inhibitors
- ❑ E concentration in blood is a high positive predictive value for renal artery stenosis

2. Endothelium derived relaxation factor

- ❑ A acts via specific receptors on vascular smooth muscle cells
- ❑ B is nitric oxide
- ❑ C is formed from L-citrulline
- ❑ D is stored in the endoplasmic reticulum of endothelial cells
- ❑ E increases intracellular cyclic GMP

3. Endothelin-1

- ❑ A is secreted as a prohormone
- ❑ B selectively constricts the glomerular efferent arteriole
- ❑ C serum concentration is elevated in heart failure
- ❑ D is a short acting local vasoconstrictor
- ❑ E has bronchoconstrictor activity

Mediators of inflammation and repair

4. Transforming growth factor beta

- ❑ A promotes wound healing
- ❑ B is released from platelets during degranulation
- ❑ C has one active isoform
- ❑ D has autocrine activity
- ❑ E stimulates lymphocyte proliferation

5. Tumour necrosis factor-alpha

- ❑ A is predominantly synthesised by activated T cells
- ❑ B circulates bound to soluble receptors
- ❑ C predominantly acts in a paracrine fashion
- ❑ D is released in response to endotoxin stimulation
- ❑ E promotes fibrotic reactions

6. Haemopoietic growth factors

- ❑ A act on colony forming units
- ❑ B include interleukin 3
- ❑ C are members of the immunoglobulin superfamily
- ❑ D are encoded for by genes on chromosome 3
- ❑ E do not affect mature cell function

The cell and signalling

7. G Proteins

- ❑ A phosphorylate guanosine diphosphate
- ❑ B include Ras oncoproteins
- ❑ C deactivation occurs via hydrolysis
- ❑ D are transmembrane signal-receptor molecules
- ❑ E are found in all cell types

8. Nuclear factor kB

- ❑ A binds to cytoplasmic proteins
- ❑ B activates tumour necrosis factor-alpha
- ❑ C regulates the expression of inflammatory response genes
- ❑ D is inhibited by glucocorticoids
- ❑ E enhances inducible nitric oxide synthase

9. In the cell cycle

- ❑ A cytoplasmic cleavage occurs in G2
- ❑ B DNA is replicated in S phase
- ❑ C organelles are synthesised in metaphase
- ❑ D interphase occupies the largest part of the cell cycle
- ❑ E the chromatids separate in anaphase

10. Apoptosis

- ❑ A causes necrotic cell death
- ❑ B is involved in embryological remodelling
- ❑ C releases proinflammatory mediators
- ❑ D is characterised by condensation of nuclear chromatin T
- ❑ E is associated with endonuclease activation

11. Adhesion molecules

- ❑ A are not present on eosinophils
- ❑ B form tight junctions between cells
- ❑ C include leucocyte integrins
- ❑ D are upregulated in inflammatory diseases
- ❑ E prevent monocyte transmigration

12. Steroid hormone receptors

- ❑ A interact with RNA to cause their effect
- ❑ B are located on the cell membrane
- ❑ C are similar to vitamin D receptors
- ❑ D are blocked by aminoglutethimide
- ❑ E are stabilised by heat shock proteins

13. Antisense oligonucleotides

- ❑ A consist of 13 to 20 amino acids
- ❑ B hybridise with native DNA to reduce gene expression
- ❑ C lead to expression of 'nonsense' proteins
- ❑ D block transcription factors
- ❑ E increase messenger RNA degradation

Miscellaneous

14. Concerning cardiac sarcomere

- ❑ A contraction is calcium-dependent
- ❑ B tropomyosin is a component of the thick filaments
- ❑ C relaxation is ATP-dependent
- ❑ D troponin I inhibits the interaction between actin and myosin
- ❑ E the thin filament is made of actin

15. Dystrophin

- ❑ A is abnormal in the limb girdle muscular dystrophies
- ❑ B binds to actin
- ❑ C is coded for by a gene on the X chromosome
- ❑ D is a transmembrane protein
- ❑ E is absent in Duchenne muscular dystrophy

16. The *P53* gene

- ❑ A is frequently mutated in lung cancer
- ❑ B inhibits apoptosis
- ❑ C is induced by alcohol
- ❑ D develops specific mutations in response to tobacco smoke carcinogens
- ❑ E suppresses tumour growth

17. Plasma proteins

- ❑ A migrate towards anode or cathode at different rates because of differences in electrical charges
- ❑ B are mostly in the form of cations
- ❑ C concentration falls early in starvation
- ❑ D are involved in the transportation of thyroid, adrenocortical, and gonadal hormones
- ❑ E are responsible for about 15% of the buffering capacity of the blood

18. Proto-oncogenes

- ❑ A are carcinogenic retroviruses
- ❑ B are only expressed in malignant tissues
- ❑ C control cell growth and differentiation
- ❑ D are transiently upregulated by growth factors
- ❑ E inactive oncogenes

19. Correct associations of tumours and circulating markers include

❑ A ovarian carcinoma and CA125
❑ B hepatoma and human chorionic gonadotrophin
❑ C teratoma and alpha fetoprotein
❑ D medullary thyroid carcinoma and thyroglobulin
❑ E osteosarcoma and PTH-related peptide

20. Angiotensin converting enzyme

❑ A is a glycoprotein
❑ B activates bradykinin
❑ C blood concentration may be raised in primary biliary cirrhosis
❑ D is raised in tuberculosis in less than 10% of cases
❑ E levels in active sarcoidosis are unaffected by ACE inhibitor therapy

21. The following pathological lesions are characteristic of the following conditions:

❑ A hepatic centrilobular necrosis in Budd-Chiari syndrome
❑ B myocardial Aschoff nodules in acute rheumatic fever
❑ C neurofibrillary tangles and cerebral amyloid plaques in Alzheimer's disease
❑ D centrilobular emphysema in alpha-1 anti-trypsin deficiency
❑ E transmural colonic inflammation with histiocytic granulomata in Crohn's disease

22. The following are characteristic features of malignant tumours:

❑ A abnormal mitoses
❑ B anaplasia
❑ C reactive hyperplasia in the regional lymph nodes
❑ D increased fibrous stroma
❑ E invasiveness

NEPHROLOGY

Basic nephrology and renal investigation

1. Renal blood flow

- ❑ A is about 1/5 of the total cardiac output
- ❑ B is distributed evenly to medulla and cortex
- ❑ C is increased by sympathetic nervous system overactivity
- ❑ D rises with anaemia
- ❑ E is constant over the range of blood pressure 90–200 mmHg

2. Atrial natriuretic factors (ANF)

- ❑ A provoke aldosterone secretion
- ❑ B inhibit Na/K ATPase in the distal tubular cells
- ❑ C may cause renal arteriolar vasoconstriction
- ❑ D are undetectable in end-stage renal failure
- ❑ E are released from atrial myocytes in concentrations directly proportionate to the atrial pressure

3. The ureter

- ❑ A contains circular and longitudinal smooth muscle arranged in spirals
- ❑ B is lined with columnar epithelium
- ❑ C receives its sympathetic nerve supply from L2, L3 and L4
- ❑ D develops from the mesonephric duct
- ❑ E radiologically lies on the tips of the transverse processes of the lumbar vertebrae

4. In the radiological investigation of patients with renal disease the following are true:

- ❑ A IVU is the most useful first-line investigation in both acute and chronic renal failure
- ❑ B DMSA will demonstrate cortical scarring in reflux nephropathy
- ❑ C ultrasound, DTPA and MAG3 scanning may well demonstrate urinary tract obstruction
- ❑ D IVU may be more useful than ultrasound in the investigation of haematuria
- ❑ E serial isotope scanning may be more reliable than IVU in the detection of renal artery stenosis

5. Microalbuminuria in a diabetic patient

- ❏ A is best assessed with a 24 hour urine sample
- ❏ B is reduced by ACE inhibition
- ❏ C follows the development of hypertension
- ❏ D indicates the presence of proliferative retinopathy
- ❏ E predicts ischaemic heart disease in NIDDM

6. Urobilinogen in urine is

- ❏ A not detectable in health
- ❏ B distinguished from porphobilinogen by Ehrlich's aldehyde reagent
- ❏ C diagnostic of intrahepatic obstruction
- ❏ D increased in pernicious anaemia
- ❏ E reduced by haemolysis

Acid-base balance, water and electrolyte disorders

7. A urine sodium concentration of 10 mmol/l is likely

- ❏ A following relief of bilateral ureteric obstruction
- ❏ B in severe dehydration
- ❏ C in cranial diabetes insipidus
- ❏ D in a patient with chronic pyelonephritis
- ❏ E in acute tubular necrosis due to burns

8. The following are recognised associations of some hypokalaemic states:

- ❏ A juxta-glomerular hypertrophy
- ❏ B vacuolation of glomerular epithelial cells
- ❏ C acidosis in fulminant colitis
- ❏ D hypotension
- ❏ E hypovolaemia

9. Serum osmolality might be considerably greater than the osmolarity in the following conditions:

- ❑ A renal failure
- ❑ B ethanolic intoxication
- ❑ C severe nephrotic syndrome
- ❑ D monoclonal gammopathy
- ❑ E diabetic ketoacidosis

10. With metabolic acidosis a normal anion-gap may suggest

- ❑ A renal tubular acidosis
- ❑ B treatment with acetazolamide
- ❑ C diarrhoea
- ❑ D salicylate poisoning
- ❑ E uraemia

11. In classical (distal type I) renal tubular acidosis (RTA) in adults, the following are characteristic findings:

- ❑ A polyuria
- ❑ B aminoaciduria
- ❑ C hyperchloraemia
- ❑ D uraemia
- ❑ E ureteric colic

Renal failure and renal replacement therapy

12. An increase in the ratio of plasma urea to creatinine is found in patients

- ❑ A on corticosteroid therapy
- ❑ B with severe liver disease
- ❑ C with intestinal haemorrhage
- ❑ D with uretero-colic anastomosis
- ❑ E with extensive burns

13. Concerning acute renal failure

- ❑ A serum complement levels are usually low
- ❑ B acute renal inflammatory disease (glomerular or interstitial) is the commonest cause
- ❑ C mortality is low if dialysis is instituted early
- ❑ D it may result from paracetamol poisoning
- ❑ E renal recovery is rarely expected

14. In a patient with renal impairment, the following would indicate acute, as opposed to chronic, renal failure

- ❑ A recent commencement of captopril for hypertensive treatment
- ❑ B Hb of 6 g/dl with RBC fragmentation and reticulocytosis
- ❑ C renal bipolar diameters of 13 cm
- ❑ D presence of an abdominal aortic aneurysm
- ❑ E recurrent urinary infections

15. Uraemic osteodystrophy is associated with

- ❑ A hyperparathyroidism
- ❑ B hyperphosphataemia
- ❑ C decreased 1,25 dihydroxycholecalciferol
- ❑ D increased osteoclastic activity within bone
- ❑ E increased calcium absorption from the gut

16. Anaemia in chronic renal failure

- ❑ A becomes evident when glomerular filtration rate falls below 30 ml/min
- ❑ B is reversed by dialysis
- ❑ C is least marked in patients with polycystic kidneys
- ❑ D is tolerated by most patients because of an increase in red cell 2,3 diphosphoglycerate (2,3 DPG)
- ❑ E due to iron deficiency is recognised by a low serum iron

17. Concerning the use of erythropoietin in patients with end-stage renal failure

❑ A adequate haemoglobin response is anticipated within the first month
❑ B oral iron supplementation is sufficient to maintain the response
❑ C the response to intravenous administration is better than to the subcutaneous route
❑ D secondary hyperparathyroidism may reduce the haemoglobin response
❑ E haemodialysis and continuous ambulatory peritoneal dialysis (CAPD) patients respond equally well

18. A 35-year-old male with chronic renal failure due to focal glomerulosclerosis has a blood pressure of 170/100 mmHg, a creatinine clearance of 40 ml/min and no oedema. Treatment should include

❑ A an ACE inhibitor
❑ B a low potassium diet
❑ C a low sodium diet
❑ D a low protein diet
❑ E fluid restriction and diuretics

19. Dosages of the following drugs should be reduced in patients with a GFR of less than 20 ml/min

❑ A enalapril
❑ B methylprednisolone
❑ C metronidazole
❑ D nifedipine
❑ E digoxin

20. Dialysis-related amyloidosis

❑ A results from beta 2 microglobulin deposition
❑ B does not occur in patients managed by peritoneal dialysis
❑ C can result in renal transplant failure
❑ D frequently presents as carpal tunnel syndrome
❑ E is more frequent in patients with diabetes

21. The following are important factors in determining the suitability of a patient for renal transplantation:

- ❑ A hepatitis B surface antigen positive status
- ❑ B previous membranous glomerulonephritis
- ❑ C high titres of lymphocytotoxic antibodies in the patient
- ❑ D full matching at HLA-A locus between patient and potential donor
- ❑ E evidence of peripheral vascular disease

22. The following may occur after renal transplantation:

- ❑ A necrosis of the femoral head
- ❑ B hirsutism
- ❑ C visual impairment due to macular degeneration
- ❑ D retardation of growth
- ❑ E squamous cell carcinoma of the skin

Glomerulonephritis and associated syndromes

23. The following are true of the nephrotic syndrome:

- ❑ A a better prognosis in children
- ❑ B an association with chronic liver disease
- ❑ C it is rare in tropical countries
- ❑ D remission of proteinuria may occur with cyclosporin A
- ❑ E there may be an accompanying hypercoagulable state

24. In rapidly progressive glomerulonephritis

- ❑ A anti-neutrophil cytoplasmic antibodies (ANCA) are often detected
- ❑ B there may be evidence of preceding or underlying infection
- ❑ C renal prognosis is rarely affected by therapeutic intervention
- ❑ D a linear IgM immunofluorescence pattern may be seen on renal biopsy
- ❑ E patients often have non-oliguric acute renal failure

25. The following statements about Goodpasture's syndrome are correct:

- ❑ A pulmonary haemorrhage occurs in less than half the patients
- ❑ B the serum complement level is generally normal
- ❑ C renal transplantation is contraindicated
- ❑ D plasma exchange is effective in controlling nephritis but not lung haemorrhage
- ❑ E intercurrent infection may lead to disease relapse

26. A low level of serum complement (C_3) is a characteristic finding in

- ❑ A minimal change glomerulonephritis
- ❑ B mesangio-capillary (membrano-proliferative) glomerulonephritis
- ❑ C sub-acute infective endocarditis
- ❑ D interstitial nephritis
- ❑ E microscopic polyarteritis

27. The following are true of membranous glomerulonephritis:

- ❑ A immune-complex mediated aetiology
- ❑ B 35% chance of progression to renal failure
- ❑ C strong association with Hodgkin's disease
- ❑ D the disease does not recur in renal allografts
- ❑ E it is a common renal lesion in patients with rheumatoid arthritis

Urinary tract infections, calculi and obstruction

28. Incontinence of urine

- ❑ A may respond to treatment of a urinary infection
- ❑ B is a feature of chronic retention of urine
- ❑ C may be induced by a diuretic
- ❑ D in the geriatric population, is less common in mobile patients
- ❑ E is commonly due to disease of the posterior pituitary

29. The following are recognised associations of patients with calcium containing urinary stones:

- ❑ A a positive family history
- ❑ B a persistently low urinary pH
- ❑ C hyperuricosuria
- ❑ D small bowel malabsorption
- ❑ E medullary-sponge kidney

30. Ureteric obstruction is a characteristic complication of

- ❑ A gastrojejunostomy
- ❑ B analgesic nephropathy
- ❑ C schistosomiasis
- ❑ D renal transplantation
- ❑ E aortic aneurysm

Renal involvement in systemic disorders

31. In the haemolytic-uraemic syndrome

- ❑ A the prognosis is worse in those with diarrhoea
- ❑ B case to case transmission is frequent
- ❑ C *E. coli* 0157 is the commonest cause in the UK
- ❑ D fragmentation of red cells may occur
- ❑ E haemodialysis and peritoneal dialysis are equally effective

32. The following are features of unilateral renal artery stenosis

- ❑ A hypokalaemic alkalosis
- ❑ B renal glycosuria
- ❑ C normochromic, normocytic anaemia
- ❑ D treatment with captopril results in a rise in blood urea
- ❑ E increased concentration of radiographic contrast on the contralateral side

33. Recognised features of renal amyloid deposition

- ❑ A are monoclonal gammopathy
- ❑ B are histology showing intra-glomerular and tubular staining with Sudan black
- ❑ C are heavy proteinuria
- ❑ D occurs as a long-term complication of haemodialysis
- ❑ E are serum amyloid P component (SAP) scan allows assessment of the extent of systemic deposition

Other nephrology

34. The following are typical associations of polycystic disease of the kidneys in adults:

- ❑ A subarachnoid haemorrhage
- ❑ B nephrolithiasis
- ❑ C polycythaemia
- ❑ D liver failure
- ❑ E nephrotic syndrome

35. Autosomal dominant polycystic kidney disease

- ❑ A has a gene frequency of 1 in 10,000
- ❑ B is associated with polycythaemia
- ❑ C usually causes end-stage renal disease by the age of 40
- ❑ D is due to an abnormality in polycystin
- ❑ E liver involvement is more frequent in females

36. Alport's syndrome

- ❑ A is an X-linked dominant condition
- ❑ B is due to a mutation of the type III collagen gene
- ❑ C is associated with retinitis pigmentosa
- ❑ D post-transplant antiglomerular basement membrane nephritis develops in 50% of patients
- ❑ E is associated with cardiac conduction abnormalities

37. The following are true statements:

- ❑ A angiotensin converting-enzyme inhibitors should never be prescribed in cases of renovascular hypertension
- ❑ B renal failure is the commonest cause of death in non-insulin dependent diabetes
- ❑ C in IgA nephropathy (Berger's disease) haematuria typically follows 2–3 weeks after an upper respiratory tract infection
- ❑ D a transplanted renal allograft will function provided donor warm ischaemic time is kept below two hours
- ❑ E in chronic reflux nephropathy there is usually a history of previous recurrent urinary infection

NEUROLOGY

Cerebral circulation and vascular disorders

1. Thrombosis of the posterior inferior cerebellar artery causes

- ❑ A infarction of the medial medulla oblongata
- ❑ B contralateral partial ptosis
- ❑ C ipsilateral loss of pain and temperature sensation in the limbs
- ❑ D diplopia
- ❑ E contralateral hemiplegia

2. Characteristic features of occlusion of the left middle cerebral artery in a right-handed individual include

- ❑ A hemiplegia that affects the leg more than the arm
- ❑ B paralysis of conjugate gaze towards the left
- ❑ C anosognosia
- ❑ D acalculia
- ❑ E alexia

3. The following are associated with increased likelihood of stroke:

- ❑ A mitral annular calcification
- ❑ B atrial fibrillation in non-rheumatic heart disease
- ❑ C atrial fibrillation in rheumatic heart disease
- ❑ D coarctation of the aorta
- ❑ E patent foramen ovale

4. Infarction in the territory of the anterior cerebral artery

- ❑ A causes more severe hand than shoulder weakness on the affected side
- ❑ B produces predominant weakness of the lower limb
- ❑ C is most frequently seen after subarachnoid haemorrhage due to berry aneurysm rupture
- ❑ D causes transcortical motor aphasia when affecting the dominant hemisphere
- ❑ E usually occurs as a result of cerebral embolism

5. In lacunar syndromes

❑ A diagnosis is based on clinical signs
❑ B about half are pure motor strokes
❑ C ataxic hemiparesis may occur
❑ D visual field defects occur in about 30%
❑ E visuospatial disturbance should not be present in order to make the diagnosis

6. In aneurysmal subarachnoid haemorrhage

❑ A multiple aneurysms are detected in about 20% of patients
❑ B vertebrobasilar circulation aneurysms are detected in about 30% of patients
❑ C dementia is a late complication
❑ D stroke may be precipitated by angiography
❑ E ST segment elevation may be present on electrocardiography

Other disorders of the brain

7. The following features typically occur in complex partial seizures of temporal lobe onset:

❑ A aura of fear accompanied by an epigastric sensation
❑ B primitive visual aura
❑ C jamais vu phenomenon
❑ D automatisms
❑ E versive seizures

8. Causes of periodic (repetitive) complexes on the EEG include

❑ A Pick's disease
❑ B hepatic coma
❑ C Creutzfeldt-Jakob disease
❑ D subacute sclerosing panencephalitis (SSPE)
❑ E progressive multifocal leukoencephalopathy (PML)

9. A 16-year-old girl presents with jerks of the arms on waking and three generalised tonic-clonic seizures. The treatment of choice is

- ❑ A carbamazepine
- ❑ B phenytoin
- ❑ C sodium valproate
- ❑ D clonazepam
- ❑ E any of the above

10. The following restrictions with respect to driving apply to patients at risk of having seizures

- ❑ A patients are obliged to contact the DVLC if they believe themselves to be at risk of seizures
- ❑ B a patient's doctor is obliged to inform the DVLC of a patient at risk of seizures
- ❑ C a patient may continue to drive following a single nocturnal seizure
- ❑ D a recent diagnosis of cerebral glioma prohibits driving
- ❑ E a recent diagnosis of bronchogenic carcinoma prohibits driving

11. In patients affected with HIV-1 related dementia

- ❑ A dementia may be the presenting feature
- ❑ B language disturbance and visuoconstructive difficulties are early features of the dementia
- ❑ C intracerebral Kaposi's sarcoma is rarely the cause of dementia
- ❑ D *Cryptococcus* is the most common opportunistic cause of dementia
- ❑ E the majority of demented patients have a raised CSF protein

12. In Alzheimer's disease

- ❑ A social misconduct and personality change are typical features
- ❑ B the plantar response is typically extensor
- ❑ C myoclonus is common in the late stages
- ❑ D neurofibrillary tangles are diagnostic
- ❑ E temporo-parietal hypometabolism on positron emission tomography is a typical finding

13. The following statements are true of Creutzfeldt-Jakob disease:

- ❑ A it is slowly progressive over many years
- ❑ B myoclonus is an early clinical feature
- ❑ C EEG is usually normal
- ❑ D it is associated with a spongiform histological change in the brain
- ❑ E approximately 10% of cases are familial

14. The following diseases are associated with subcortical dementia:

- ❑ A Binswanger's disease
- ❑ B Alzheimer's disease
- ❑ C Huntington's disease (chorea)
- ❑ D Pick's disease
- ❑ E progressive supranuclear palsy (Steele-Richardson-Olszewski syndrome)

15. The following are typical features of Pick's disease:

- ❑ A behavioural disturbance
- ❑ B prominent grasp reflexes
- ❑ C extrapyramidal rigidity
- ❑ D abnormal EEG
- ❑ E familial in approximately 80% of cases

16. Benign intracranial hypertension is typically associated with

- ❑ A enlarged blind spots
- ❑ B reduced visual acuity
- ❑ C a presentation in the puerperium
- ❑ D is characterised by normal or enlarged lateral ventricles on CT or MR scan
- ❑ E sixth nerve palsy

17. The following statements are true of Normal Pressure Hydrocephalus (NPH):

- ❑ A it causes a cortical dementia
- ❑ B spasticity in the lower limbs is greater than that in the upper limbs
- ❑ C urinary incontinence is a late clinical manifestation
- ❑ D structural imaging (CT and MRI) reveals 'slit-like' lateral ventricles
- ❑ E clinical improvement may follow a CSF shunting procedure

18. The following are true of transient global amnesia (TGA):

- ❑ A it usually occurs in individuals over the age of 40
- ❑ B personal identity is typically preserved
- ❑ C there is no associated reduction of consciousness
- ❑ D it has a low recurrence rate
- ❑ E it is typically associated with precipitating factors

19. The following favour a lesion of the cerebral cortex rather than of the brain stem:

- ❑ A dysarthria
- ❑ B diplopia
- ❑ C dysphasia
- ❑ D hemianopia
- ❑ E extensor plantar response

20. The following are correctly matched:

- ❑ A pineal tumours and hypopituitarism
- ❑ B expressive dysphasia and frontal lobe lesions
- ❑ C poor two point discrimination and a parietal lobe lesion
- ❑ D upper quadrantic homonymous hemianopia and a parietal lobe lesion
- ❑ E apraxia and a dominant parietal lobe lesion

21. The following are true with regard to speech:

- ❑ A complete aphonia may be due to a dominant parietal lobe lesion
- ❑ B spastic dysarthria is commonly due to middle cerebral artery occlusion
- ❑ C extrapyramidal disease may cause hyperkinetic speech
- ❑ D poliomyelitis will cause a pseudobulbar dysarthria
- ❑ E cerebellar 'ataxic' speech is usually due to a vermis lesion

Cranial nerve anatomy and lesions

22. Unilateral ptosis is a recognised finding in

- ❑ A syringobulbia
- ❑ B cluster headache
- ❑ C Bell's palsy
- ❑ D cavernous sinus thrombosis
- ❑ E thoracic outlet syndrome

23. A lesion of the III cranial nerve causes

- ❑ A an afferent pupillary defect
- ❑ B a divergent strabismus
- ❑ C inability to adduct the affected eye
- ❑ D contralateral hemiplegia
- ❑ E miosis

24. In Horner's syndrome

- ❑ A the pupil on the affected side will dilate with hydroxyamphetamine drops if the lesion is distal to the cervical ganglion
- ❑ B lateral medullary infarction is a recognised cause
- ❑ C the affected pupil dilates more widely than the normal one with phenylephrine drops if the lesion is preganglionic
- ❑ D the affected pupil fails to dilate with cocaine drops
- ❑ E injury to the upper trunks of the brachial plexus is a recognised cause

25. In a young person with an internuclear ophthalmoplegia

- ❑ A oligoclonal bands in the CSF confirm the diagnosis of multiple sclerosis
- ❑ B unilateral delay in the visual evoked potentials is strong evidence of the diagnosis of multiple sclerosis
- ❑ C the presence of extrinsic brain stem compression is indicated
- ❑ D high doses of intravenous steroids will speed recovery if demyelination is the cause
- ❑ E the lesion is in the median longitudinal fasciculus in the brain stem

26. Bilateral facial weakness is a feature of

- ❑ A myasthenia gravis
- ❑ B myotonic dystrophy
- ❑ C sarcoidosis
- ❑ D Guillain-Barré syndrome
- ❑ E a unilateral pontine lesion

27. Recognised associations of an VIII nerve schwannoma include

- ❑ A a similar lesion on the contralateral side
- ❑ B Lisch nodules (iris haematomatas)
- ❑ C meningiomas
- ❑ D phaeochromocytomas
- ❑ E ash-leaf spots

28. A unilateral pontine lesion may produce

- ❑ A ipsilateral hemiplegia
- ❑ B diplopia
- ❑ C pseudobulbar palsy
- ❑ D ipsilateral III cranial nerve palsy
- ❑ E ipsilateral upper motor neurone lesion of VII cranial nerve

29. The following are typical of a unilateral lesion affecting the medial aspect of the medulla oblongata:

❑ A ipsilateral XII cranial nerve palsy
❑ B contralateral hemiplegia
❑ C ipsilateral loss of touch and joint position sense
❑ D ipsilateral Horner's syndrome
❑ E ipsilateral ataxia

30. Pseudobulbar palsy

❑ A is caused by bilateral lesions of the corticospinal tracts
❑ B may cause nasal speech
❑ C causes an absent gag reflex
❑ D may be caused by multiple sclerosis
❑ E may cause fibrillation of the tongue

Spinal cord and peripheral nerve anatomy and lesions

31. A lesion of the right half of the seventh cervical segment of the spinal cord may

❑ A impair position sense in the right leg
❑ B cause a positive Hoffman's sign on the right
❑ C abolish the right abdominal reflexes
❑ D impair temperature sensation below the level of the lesion on the right
❑ E cause clonus at the right ankle

32. Absent ankle jerks are associated with extensor plantar responses in

❑ A tabes dorsalis
❑ B vitamin B12 deficiency
❑ C motor neurone disease
❑ D lesions of the conus medullaris
❑ E ataxia telangiectasia

33. Following surgery for abdominal aortic aneurysm, a 63-year-old man developed weakness of the legs. Likely signs on examination two weeks later include

- ❑ A the presence of a urinary catheter
- ❑ B impaired temperature sensation in the legs
- ❑ C fasciculation of the quadriceps
- ❑ D weakness of hip extension greater than hip flexion
- ❑ E impaired position sense at the great toe

34. The following are typical of syringomyelia:

- ❑ A Horner's syndrome
- ❑ B pseudobulbar palsy
- ❑ C loss of pain and temperature sensation
- ❑ D loss of proprioception
- ❑ E loss of reflexes in the upper limbs

35. In Guillain-Barré syndrome

- ❑ A sensory symptoms in the digits are a frequent early feature
- ❑ B the CSF cell count is frequently elevated in the first few days of the illness
- ❑ C the peak flow rate is the clearest guide to the need for artificial ventilation
- ❑ D limb ataxia frequently occurs in severely affected patients
- ❑ E there may be an underlying lymphoma

36. With regard to the normal autonomic nervous system

- ❑ A 2.5% methacholine causes pupillary constriction
- ❑ B the parasympathetic outflow to the ciliary muscle is via the superior colliculus
- ❑ C beat to beat variations of the heart rate may be used to assess vagal integrity
- ❑ D parasympathetic innervation of the bladder and lower bowel is via the dorsal nucleus of the vagus
- ❑ E postganglionic sympathetic activity is mediated by noradrenaline

37. The median nerve

- ❑ A supplies the muscles of the hypothenar eminence
- ❑ B supplies adductor pollicis
- ❑ C typically supplies the 1st and 2nd lumbricals
- ❑ D lies deep to the extensor retinaculum at the wrist
- ❑ E supplies the 1st and 2nd palmar interossei

38. The anterior interosseous nerve

- ❑ A is a branch of the ulnar nerve
- ❑ B supplies flexor pollicis longus
- ❑ C supplies abductor pollicis brevis
- ❑ D supplies extensor pollicis longus
- ❑ E supplies the first and second lumbricals

39. Carpal tunnel syndrome is

- ❑ A often bilateral in amyloidosis
- ❑ B a cause of wasting of abductor pollicis brevis
- ❑ C diagnosed by finding delayed ulnar nerve conduction
- ❑ D a possible cause of pain in the forearm
- ❑ E associated with diabetes

40. In distinguishing between a C7 nerve root lesion and a radial nerve palsy

- ❑ A weakness of triceps is more suggestive of a C7 nerve root lesion
- ❑ B weakness of brachioradialis indicates a radial nerve palsy
- ❑ C weakness of wrist flexion suggests a C7 nerve root lesion
- ❑ D sensory loss affecting the medial aspect of forearm and medial two fingers suggests a C7 nerve root lesion
- ❑ E an absent brachioradialis reflex does not help to distinguish between a C7 nerve root lesion and a radial nerve palsy

41. The following are correctly matched:

- ❑ A biceps brachialis and the musculocutaneous nerve
- ❑ B internal rotation of the shoulder and teres minor
- ❑ C brachioradialis and the median nerve
- ❑ D elbow supination and a lateral movement of the thumb
- ❑ E pinching of thumb and index finger and the anterior interosseous nerve

42. Diabetic amyotrophy

- ❑ A causes predominantly distal weakness and wasting
- ❑ B is associated with raised CSF protein levels
- ❑ C has a poor prognosis for recovery
- ❑ D causes loss of the ankle jerks
- ❑ E causes impotence

43. The sciatic nerve

- ❑ A divides into the tibial and common peroneal nerves at a variable level in the lower limbs
- ❑ B is derived from the L4, 5 and S1, 2 and 3 spinal nerves
- ❑ C supplies adductor brevis, longus and magnus
- ❑ D supplies quadriceps femoris
- ❑ E supplies gluteus maximum

44. A lesion of the common peroneal nerve may

- ❑ A be produced by a fracture of the neck of the fibula
- ❑ B cause weakness of foot plantar flexion
- ❑ C abolish foot inversion
- ❑ D cause loss of sensation affecting skin over the medial aspect of lower leg
- ❑ E cause loss of ankle reflex

45. The following are true:

- ❑ A C fibre activation usually causes a sharp pain
- ❑ B trigeminal neuralgia is best treated surgically
- ❑ C causalgia usually occurs after complete nerve transection
- ❑ D itch is C fibre mediated, unlike touch
- ❑ E sympathetic block with guanethidine is used in the treatment of some chronic pains

Dyskinesias and disorders of muscle

46. In a 70-year-old man with tremor of the upper limbs, essential tremor rather than Parkinson's disease is more likely to be the cause if:

- ❑ A the tremor is worst at rest
- ❑ B the tremor is relieved with alcohol
- ❑ C the tremor is exacerbated by anxiety
- ❑ D the tremor is predominantly postural
- ❑ E there is rigidity

47. Extrapyramidal rigidity may be caused by

- ❑ A butyrophenone tranquillisers
- ❑ B B12 deficiency
- ❑ C abuse of synthetic pethidine derivatives
- ❑ D carbon monoxide poisoning
- ❑ E the neuroleptic malignant syndrome

48. Myotonia

- ❑ A is typically exacerbated by exercise
- ❑ B occurs in hyperkalaemic periodic paralysis
- ❑ C and muscle hypertrophy may be associated
- ❑ D may be associated with cataracts
- ❑ E produces characteristic EMG findings

49. Chorea is a recognised manifestation of

- ❑ A pregnancy
- ❑ B L-dopa medication
- ❑ C choreoacanthosis
- ❑ D hypoparathyroidism
- ❑ E polycythaemia rubra vera

50. Huntington's chorea

- ❑ A is inherited as an autosomal recessive characteristic
- ❑ B may present with extrapyramidal rigidity in younger victims
- ❑ C always becomes clinically apparent by the third decade of life
- ❑ D is associated with loss of volume of the caudate nucleus on CT scans
- ❑ E usually responds to L-dopa therapy

51. The following are typical features of Parkinson's disease:

- ❑ A pseudobulbar palsy
- ❑ B hypophonia
- ❑ C supranuclear gaze palsy
- ❑ D intention tremor
- ❑ E rigidity

52. A Parkinsonian syndrome may be produced by

- ❑ A magnesium poisoning
- ❑ B N-methyl-4-phenyl-1,2,3,6-tetrahydropyridine
- ❑ C carbon dioxide poisoning
- ❑ D Wilson's disease
- ❑ E Huntington's disease

53. Muscle fasciculations

- ❑ A occur with reinervation of partially denervated muscles
- ❑ B in the calf muscles are often benign
- ❑ C may be seen during an edrophonium test for myasthenia gravis
- ❑ D are diagnostic of motor neurone disease (MND)
- ❑ E occur in spinal muscular atrophy

54. In muscular dystrophies

- ❑ A the Becker dystrophy is X-linked
- ❑ B Duchenne dystrophy may be seen in Turner's syndrome
- ❑ C cardiac involvement is usually subclinical in Becker dystrophy
- ❑ D pseudohypertrophy occurs in 80% of Duchenne muscular dystrophy (DMD)
- ❑ E EMG is useful in detecting female carriers

55. In myasthenia gravis

- ❑ A most patients will become symptom-free following thymectomy
- ❑ B anti-acetylcholine receptor antibodies are detected in about 50% of patients
- ❑ C anti-smooth muscle antibody is associated with an increased risk of thymoma
- ❑ D there is damage to the nicotinic acetylcholine receptors
- ❑ E increased weakness may follow the introduction of treatment with corticosteroids

56. Myoclonus is a typical clinical feature of

- ❑ A Pick's disease
- ❑ B subacute sclerosing panencephalitis
- ❑ C primary generalised epilepsy
- ❑ D post anoxic brain damage
- ❑ E Creutzfeldt-Jakob disease

Miscellaneous neurology

57. CSF pleocytosis with normal CSF glucose is often seen in

- ❑ A TB meningitis
- ❑ B chronic meningeal fungal infection
- ❑ C multiple sclerosis
- ❑ D Guillain-Barré syndrome
- ❑ E torticollis

58. In the chronic fatigue syndrome

- ❑ A previous psychiatric illness is a recognised risk factor
- ❑ B a mild rise in creatine phosphokinase is commonly detected
- ❑ C persistent viral antigen is detected in a minority of patients
- ❑ D decreased physical activity is a risk factor for the continuation of fatigue
- ❑ E the majority of affected patients fulfil psychiatric criteria for depression

59. There is a known association between chronic alcoholism and

- ❑ A painful myopathy
- ❑ B auditory hallucinosis
- ❑ C cerebellar degeneration
- ❑ D hypoglycaemia
- ❑ E downbeat nystagmus

60. The following treatments may reduce the severity of relapse in multiple sclerosis (MS):

- ❑ A pulsed high dose methylprednisolone
- ❑ B adrenocortical trophic hormone (ACTH)
- ❑ C hyperbaric oxygen
- ❑ D azathioprine
- ❑ E linoleic acid supplementation

61. In multiple sclerosis, plaques of demyelination characteristically occur in

- ❑ A cerebral cortex
- ❑ B subcortical white matter
- ❑ C optic nerves
- ❑ D anterior horn cells
- ❑ E cervical cord

62. In motor neurone disease

- ❑ A sphincters are involved late in the disease
- ❑ B there may be associated dementia
- ❑ C root pain is common
- ❑ D the extraocular muscles are spared
- ❑ E familial cases are described

63. The following are true:

❑ A meningiomas enhance with contrast on CT scans
❑ B T1 weighted MR scans are useful in diagnosing multiple sclerosis
❑ C a T1 nerve root lesion is often diagnosed by plain X-ray examination
❑ D PET scanning can pick up blood flow changes over a few milliseconds
❑ E functional MRI is now the investigation of choice for carotid stenosis

OPHTHALMOLOGY

1. A patient presents with a painful red eye. The following findings are more suggestive of anterior uveitis than acute conjunctivitis:

- ❑ A blurring of vision
- ❑ B profuse discharge
- ❑ C small pupil
- ❑ D photophobia
- ❑ E clear media

2. Primary open-angle (simple) glaucoma

- ❑ A characteristically gives rise to signs before symptoms
- ❑ B is a familial disorder
- ❑ C may present as an acute painful red eye
- ❑ D gives characteristic visual field defects
- ❑ E is usually treated initially by surgery

3. Anterior uveitis is the most characteristic ocular manifestation of

- ❑ A rheumatoid arthritis
- ❑ B sarcoidosis
- ❑ C systemic lupus erythematosus
- ❑ D Behçet's disease
- ❑ E ankylosing spondylitis

4. Abnormalities of the optic lens are recognised in

- ❑ A homocystinuria
- ❑ B hypoparathyroidism
- ❑ C dystrophia myotonica
- ❑ D hepato-lenticular degeneration (Wilson's disease)
- ❑ E congenital rubella

5. Unilateral exophthalmos is a feature of

- ❑ A Wegener's granulomatosis
- ❑ B orbital tumour
- ❑ C cigarette smoking
- ❑ D contralateral Horner's disease
- ❑ E Graves' disease

6. The following statements about the orbit are correct, the

- ❑ A trochlear (4th cranial) nerve supplies the inferior oblique muscle
- ❑ B levator palpebrae superioris has a nerve supply from two different sources
- ❑ C superior ophthalmic vein drains into the cavernous sinus
- ❑ D ophthalmic artery is an end artery
- ❑ E inferior rectus is supplied by the oculomotor (3rd cranial) nerve

7. Diabetic maculopathy

- ❑ A is more common in NIDDM than IDDM
- ❑ B impairs peripheral vision
- ❑ C is treated by panretinal photocoagulation
- ❑ D is characterised by drusen at the macula
- ❑ E causes painful visual loss

8. The following would characteristically result in visual field defects:

- ❑ A craniopharyngioma
- ❑ B retrobulbar neuritis
- ❑ C tertiary syphilis
- ❑ D Gaucher's disease
- ❑ E Weber's syndrome

9. A macular sparing hemianopia

- ❑ A indicates a lesion in the optic radiation
- ❑ B indicates a vascular lesion in the parietal lobe
- ❑ C does not prevent a patient from reading
- ❑ D will exclude a patient from holding a driving licence
- ❑ E suggests a lesion in the posterior cerebral artery territory

PSYCHIATRY

Schizophrenia

1. In schizophrenia

- ❑ A the age of onset is on average five years earlier in females
- ❑ B outcome is better in developed compared with non-developed countries
- ❑ C the risk of developing the disorder is higher amongst lower social class families
- ❑ D the 'expressed emotion' of close family members is predictive of relapse
- ❑ E functional deterioration usually continues insidiously over the whole illness course

2. The following are recognised features of schizophrenia:

- ❑ A disorientation in time
- ❑ B incongruity of affect
- ❑ C suspiciousness
- ❑ D perseveration
- ❑ E hearing one's own thoughts spoken aloud

3. The following are Schneiderian first rank symptoms of schizophrenia:

- ❑ A thought insertion
- ❑ B visual hallucinations
- ❑ C suicidal ideas
- ❑ D passivity phenomena
- ❑ E thought broadcast

4. Predictors of poor outcome in schizophrenia include

- ❑ A early onset
- ❑ B asocial premorbid personality
- ❑ C family history of affective disorder
- ❑ D clear consciousness
- ❑ E negative symptoms

5. Delusions

❑ A only occur in schizophrenia
❑ B are not modified by contrary experience
❑ C are obsessions
❑ D are perceived as emanating from the external world
❑ E are false ideas

Mood disorders

6. The following are true of affective disorders:

❑ A the male:female ratio in unipolar depression is 1:1
❑ B 70% of those with major depression receive treatment
❑ C bipolar disorder is more frequent amongst social class V
❑ D the prevalence of depression is reduced in non-Judeo-Christian cultures
❑ E lifetime prevalence of bipolar disorder is approximately 1%

7. Recognised features of depression in the elderly include

❑ A delusions of poverty
❑ B pseudodementia
❑ C a strong association with bereavement
❑ D agitated movements
❑ E retarded movements

8. The following features suggest a normal bereavement reaction rather than depressive illness:

❑ A complaints of physical symptoms
❑ B emotional numbness
❑ C suicidal thoughts
❑ D searching behaviour
❑ E feelings of worthlessness

9. The following features are more likely to occur in depressive pseudodementia than in dementia:

- ❑ A recent onset of symptoms
- ❑ B extensive complaining by the patient about memory loss
- ❑ C worsening of cognitive symptoms in the evening
- ❑ D 'don't know' answers
- ❑ E past history of depression

10. The following are characteristic features of hypomania

- ❑ A flight of ideas
- ❑ B thought insertion
- ❑ C sexual promiscuity
- ❑ D delusions of bodily illness
- ❑ E sleep disturbance

11. Puerperal psychosis

- ❑ A usually begins within two weeks after childbirth
- ❑ B is commonly accompanied by clouding of consciousness
- ❑ C has a favourable prognosis
- ❑ D characteristically includes auditory hallucinations
- ❑ E characteristically includes obsessional ruminations

Neurotic, stress-related and somatoform disorders

12. The following are true of anxiety states:

- ❑ A chest pain may be a presenting symptom
- ❑ B may present with persistent memory impairment
- ❑ C difficulty in exhaling is common
- ❑ D low mood and early morning wakening are invariably present
- ❑ E sweating is common

13. Agoraphobia

- ❑ A usually starts before puberty
- ❑ B occurs more often in women than men
- ❑ C can be effectively treated by systematic desensitisation
- ❑ D becomes worse during periods of depression
- ❑ E can usually be traced back to traumatic events in childhood

14. In obsessive-compulsive disorder

❑ A obsessional thought is recognised by the patient as being their own
❑ B women are more commonly affected than men
❑ C obsessional thoughts are usually pleasant in nature
❑ D depression is usual
❑ E two-thirds of cases have improved at the end of one year

15. The following are true about somatization disorder:

❑ A onset occurs usually after 30 years of age
❑ B the condition is more common in men than in women
❑ C the course tends to be fluctuating but chronic
❑ D anxiety and depression occur frequently
❑ E menstrual dysfunction in women is common

16. Post-Traumatic Stress Disorder (PTSD) following a disaster

❑ A affects primarily those with premorbid 'brittle' personalities
❑ B must by definition commence within six months of the traumatic event
❑ C is associated with alcohol and drug dependence
❑ D may provoke true hallucinations in clear consciousness
❑ E is characterised by regression to a child-like state

17. Hysterical amnesia

❑ A typically is a patchy loss of memory
❑ B typically resolves within 48 hours
❑ C is a conscious reaction
❑ D has a recognised association with head injury
❑ E is usually provoked by stress

18. The following are true of 'hysteria':

❑ A the physical symptom is produced deliberately
❑ B it may be associated with a depressive illness
❑ C it is associated with 'la belle indifference'
❑ D it characteristically occurs for the first time in middle age
❑ E the physical symptoms and signs closely resemble those of organic disease

19. The following statements regarding compensation neurosis are correct:

- ❑ A it has a recognised association with major rather than minor accidents
- ❑ B it occurs particularly after head injuries sustained at work
- ❑ C settlement of a compensation claim is followed by improvement in patients with severe symptoms.
- ❑ D malingering accounts for at least 30% of cases
- ❑ E irritability is a recognised feature

Eating disorders

20. Anorexia nervosa

- ❑ A occurs exclusively in females
- ❑ B tends to be accompanied by episodes of over-eating
- ❑ C is characterised by apathy and lassitude
- ❑ D may lead to hypokalaemia
- ❑ E is a cause of primary amenorrhoea

21. Common features of bulimia nervosa include

- ❑ A low body weight
- ❑ B recurrent episodes of binge eating
- ❑ C distorted body image
- ❑ D self-induced vomiting
- ❑ E laxative abuse

Deliberate self-harm

22. The following are true of suicide:

- ❑ A two-thirds of those who die by suicide have told someone of their intention
- ❑ B asking about suicidal intent will increase the risk of suicide
- ❑ C patients with chronic physical illness are at increased risk
- ❑ D it is associated with alcohol abuse
- ❑ E it is most common in young women

23. Factors which increase the risk of suicide include

- ❑ A advancing age
- ❑ B social class I
- ❑ C the presence of hopelessness
- ❑ D antisocial personality disorder
- ❑ E talking about suicidal ideas

Organic psychiatry

24. Clinical features of delirium often include

- ❑ A decreased motor activity
- ❑ B diurnal variation in symptoms
- ❑ C perseveration
- ❑ D a catastrophic reaction
- ❑ E hallucinations

25. An acute confusional state is

- ❑ A often responsive to tricyclic antidepressant drug therapy
- ❑ B a characteristic feature of myxoedema
- ❑ C characterised by loss of memory for recent events
- ❑ D typically reversible
- ❑ E more common with pre-existing brain disease

26. Typical features of dementia include

- ❑ A selective impairment of recall
- ❑ B perseveration of themes
- ❑ C generalised cortical atrophy
- ❑ D disorientation in place
- ❑ E depression

27. Confirmed risk factors for Alzheimer's disease include

- ❑ A head injury
- ❑ B smoking
- ❑ C aluminium
- ❑ D nose picking
- ❑ E Down's syndrome

Alcohol-related disorders

28. The following statements about alcohol dependence are true:

❑ A withdrawal symptoms typically occur in the morning
❑ B the commonest withdrawal symptoms are perceptual disturbances
❑ C most alcohol-dependent patients develop liver cirrhosis
❑ D intensive counselling has a significant effect on outcome
❑ E chlormethiazole deters impulsive drinking via the acetaldehyde reaction

29. Typical features of alcohol withdrawal include

❑ A dehydration
❑ B visual hallucinations
❑ C passivity feelings
❑ D tremor
❑ E confabulation

30. Korsakoff's syndrome is

❑ A a recognised complication of alcoholism
❑ B due to vitamin B12 deficiency
❑ C characterised by generalised deterioration of intellect
❑ D characterised by recent memory defect
❑ E associated with nystagmus

Miscellaneous psychiatry

31. The following drugs of abuse not infrequently induce paranoid psychoses:

❑ A lysergic acid diethylamide (LSD)
❑ B temazepam
❑ C heroin
❑ D volatile solvents
❑ E amphetamine

32. Morbid jealousy (delusions of infidelity)

- ❑ A is associated with hypersexuality
- ❑ B is a significant cause of wife murder
- ❑ C is a recognised symptom of alcoholism
- ❑ D has a good prognosis when treated early
- ❑ E was attributed to unconscious homosexual urges by Freud

33. In sleep disturbance the following statements are valid:

- ❑ A 55% of insomnias are secondary
- ❑ B alcohol increases total sleep time
- ❑ C benzodiazepines may cause akathisia
- ❑ D narcolepsy usually presents in the first to second decade
- ❑ E patients with hypersomnia have an irresistible urge to sleep

34. The following factors increase the risk of psychiatric sequelae to head injury:

- ❑ A prolonged retrograde amnesia
- ❑ B a family history of mental disorder
- ❑ C the complete absence of post-traumatic amnesia
- ❑ D younger age
- ❑ E where the circumstances of the injury prohibit compensation

35. Twin studies have demonstrated the heritability of

- ❑ A schizophrenia
- ❑ B male homosexuality
- ❑ C juvenile delinquency
- ❑ D life events
- ❑ E unipolar depression

36. Features of psychogenic pain include

- ❑ A muscular tension
- ❑ B good response to analgesics
- ❑ C benefit from antidepressants
- ❑ D inconsistency with anatomical patterns of innervation
- ❑ E a prolonged course of unusual severity

37. Section 5(2) of the Mental Health Act (MHA) 1983

❑ A on medical wards should only be recommended by the duty psychiatrist
❑ B lasts for 72 hours
❑ C allows the appropriate psychiatric treatment to be commenced
❑ D allows surgical or medical treatments in the absence of patient consent
❑ E may be appealed against by the next of kin

RESPIRATORY MEDICINE

Respiratory physiology

1. A shift in the haemoglobin-oxygen dissociation curve to the right

- ❑ A means that for a given pO_2 there is less oxygen per gram of haemoglobin
- ❑ B occurs in anaemia
- ❑ C occurs when the pCO_2 is increased
- ❑ D could result from an increased concentration of 2,3 diphosphoglycerate in the erythrocytes
- ❑ E is favoured by a fall in temperature

2. Transfer factor

- ❑ A increases throughout childhood
- ❑ B is higher in males than females
- ❑ C is reduced by exercise
- ❑ D is a precise measure of the diffusion characteristics of the alveolar membrane
- ❑ E is transiently elevated in idiopathic pulmonary haemosiderosis (IPH)

3. The following statements are true:

- ❑ A the vagus nerve is responsible for normal bronchial tone
- ❑ B there are 18 bronchopulmonary segments
- ❑ C most of the alveoli in the adult lung are present at birth
- ❑ D the surface markings of the right middle lobe approximate to the axilla
- ❑ E the major component of surfactant is dipalmitoyl lecithin

4. Lung compliance is

- ❑ A reduced by pulmonary congestion
- ❑ B a measure of change in lung volume per unit change in airway pressure
- ❑ C decreased by emphysema
- ❑ D approximately half in a person with one lung
- ❑ E determined by use of a peak flow meter

Interstitial lung disease

5. The following are typical features of cryptogenic fibrosing alveolitis (diffuse idiopathic interstitial fibrosis):

❑ A recurrent haemoptysis
❑ B stridor
❑ C finger clubbing
❑ D 'honeycomb' lungs radiologically
❑ E circulating rheumatoid factor

6. In alpha$_1$-antitrypsin deficiency

❑ A emphysema is usually most marked in the lower lobes
❑ B the mode of inheritance is autosomal recessive
❑ C the onset of pulmonary symptoms typically occurs in childhood
❑ D atopy is a characteristic association
❑ E smoking plays a synergistic role in the development of emphysema

7. In heart-lung transplantation (HLT) for cystic fibrosis

❑ A pleurectomy is a recognised contraindication
❑ B the recipient's heart is not usually suitable for re-transplantation
❑ C azathioprine is included in maintenance immunosuppression
❑ D obliterative bronchiolitis is a major long-term complication
❑ E the ion transport defect responsible for cystic fibrosis typically develops in the transplanted lungs within 18 months

8. The following dusts are highly fibrogenic to the lungs:

❑ A silica
❑ B iron oxide
❑ C tungsten carbide
❑ D aluminium
❑ E tin

9. The following statements concerning asbestosis are true:

- ❑ A it occurs only after heavy occupational exposure
- ❑ B pleural plaques are pre-malignant
- ❑ C carcinoma of the bronchus is a recognised complication
- ❑ D it is frequently associated with positive anti-nuclear factor
- ❑ E it produces pulmonary nodules as well as marked fibrosis

10. Typical features of farmer's lung are

- ❑ A history of exposure to mouldy hay
- ❑ B reduced diffusion capacity
- ❑ C cough with profuse expectoration
- ❑ D pronounced eosinophilia
- ❑ E seasonal incidence May to July

11. Characteristic features of early diffuse interstitial fibrosis include

- ❑ A cyanosis at rest
- ❑ B reduced vital capacity
- ❑ C reduced FEV_1/FVC ratio
- ❑ D bilateral reticular shadowing on chest X-ray
- ❑ E reduced pulmonary diffusing capacity

12. In bronchoalveolar lavage

- ❑ A normally 90% of cells are macrophages
- ❑ B extrinsic allergic alveolitis typically produces a high neutrophil percentage
- ❑ C sarcoid causes an increase in T4-lymphocytes
- ❑ D alveolar proteinosis may produce a diagnostic appearance
- ❑ E smokers have a higher neutrophil percentage than normals

Lung cancer

13. Surgical resection of carcinoma of the bronchus is contraindicated in the presence of the following:

- ❑ A SVC obstruction
- ❑ B hoarseness with immobile left vocal cord
- ❑ C mediastinal nodes > 1.5 cm in diameter on CT scan
- ❑ D hypercalcaemia
- ❑ E raised mobile right hemi-diaphragm

14. The following statements apply to bronchial carcinoma:

- ❑ A screening is of little benefit
- ❑ B it is more common in urban areas
- ❑ C nickel is a recognised risk factor
- ❑ D the incidence in females is rising
- ❑ E haemoptysis suggests a poor prognosis

15. Recognised findings in a Pancoast tumour are

- ❑ A erosion of the first rib
- ❑ B ipsilateral Horner's syndrome
- ❑ C paralysis of muscles in the arm
- ❑ D pain in the arm radiating to the 4th and 5th fingers
- ❑ E gangrene of the fingers on the same side

16. The following statements about hypertrophic osteoarthropathy are correct:

- ❑ A oat cell carcinoma of the bronchus is the commonest cause
- ❑ B the arthropathy is typically symmetrical
- ❑ C the joint pain is relieved by vagotomy below the origin of the recurrent laryngeal nerve
- ❑ D gynaecomastia is a recognised association
- ❑ E pretibial myxoedema is a recognised association

Asthma

17. In asthma

- ❑ A mortality has been falling steadily over the past ten years
- ❑ B the long-acting inhaled bronchodilators are recommended for first-line therapy
- ❑ C bacterial infections are a common cause of acute attacks
- ❑ D more than 90% of patients have hyperreactive airways
- ❑ E salbutamol and terbutaline act on adrenergic nerve endings to relax airway smooth muscle

18. Recognised occupational causes of asthma include

- ❑ A isocyanates
- ❑ B platinum salts
- ❑ C soldering flux
- ❑ D asbestos
- ❑ E beryllium

Infections

19. In the acquired immunodeficiency syndrome

- ❑ A the lung is affected at some stage in the illness in over two-thirds of cases
- ❑ B pneumocystis pneumonia (PCP) is an acute onset, rapidly progressive illness
- ❑ C atypical mycobacterial infection is usually due to *M. xenopii* or *M. kansasii*
- ❑ D broncho-alveolar lavage (BAL) plus transbronchial biopsy (TBB) are diagnostic in up to 90% of cases with pneumocystis pneumonia
- ❑ E *mycobacterium tuberculosis* typically occurs at an earlier stage than pneumocystis pneumonia

20. Tuberculosis of the respiratory tract may cause

- ❑ A wheezing
- ❑ B ARDS
- ❑ C pleural effusion
- ❑ D unilateral hilar lymphadenopathy
- ❑ E massive haemoptysis

Chest X-ray

21. Cavitating lung lesions are characteristic of

- ❑ A systemic lupus erythematosus
- ❑ B squamous cell carcinoma
- ❑ C Wegner's granulomatosis
- ❑ D progressive massive fibrosis
- ❑ E 'shock lung'

22. Pulmonary nodules are found in

- ❑ A rheumatoid arthritis
- ❑ B systemic sclerosis
- ❑ C systemic lupus erythematosus
- ❑ D Wegener's granulomatosis
- ❑ E polyarteritis nodosa

23. Pleural calcification occurs in

- ❑ A silicosis
- ❑ B asbestosis
- ❑ C haemothorax
- ❑ D tuberculosis
- ❑ E haemosiderosis

24. On chest X-ray the upper zone is more commonly affected than the lower zone in

- ❑ A asbestosis
- ❑ B silicosis
- ❑ C cryptogenic fibrosing alveolitis
- ❑ D ankylosing spondylitis
- ❑ E systemic sclerosis

25. Recognised causes of pulmonary eosinophilia (chest X-ray shadowing and peripheral blood eosinophilia) include

❑ A *Ascaris lumbricoides* infestation
❑ B systemic lupus erythematosus
❑ C sarcoidosis
❑ D polyarteritis nodosa
❑ E cryptogenic fibrosing alveolitis

Miscellaneous respiratory disease

26. Recognised causes of stridor include

❑ A foreign body in the left main bronchus
❑ B *Haemophilus influenzae* infection
❑ C vascular ring
❑ D hypercalcaemia
❑ E *C. diphtheriae* infection

27. Haemoptysis is a characteristic of

❑ A byssinosis
❑ B idiopathic pulmonary haemosiderosis
❑ C aspergilloma
❑ D Goodpasture's syndrome
❑ E asbestosis

28. Cheyne-Stokes breathing is a recognised feature of

❑ A uraemia
❑ B head injury
❑ C meningitis
❑ D diabetic ketoacidosis
❑ E left ventricular failure

29. Bilateral basal crackles are a typical finding in the following:

❑ A emphysema due to alpha-1 anti-trypsin deficiency
❑ B bronchiectasis following childhood whooping cough
❑ C pulmonary sarcoidosis
❑ D fibrosing alveolitis
❑ E acute attack of asthma

30. In the obstructive sleep apnoea syndrome

❑ A complete obstruction typically occurs during non-REM sleep
❑ B there is an association with obesity and hypertension
❑ C oximetry alone is a useful screening procedure
❑ D sustained pulmonary hypertension is a rare occurrence
❑ E tracheostomy is the definitive treatment

31. The following are recognised associations:

❑ A small left pneumothorax and audible systolic 'click'
❑ B acute pancreatitis and adult respiratory distress syndrome
❑ C sarcoidosis and bronchial obstruction
❑ D Dressler's (post-myocardial infarction) syndrome and pleural effusion
❑ E nitrofurantoin and chronic pulmonary fibrosis

32. Characteristic features of pulmonary hypertension include

❑ A dominant S wave in ECG lead V_1
❑ B large 'a' wave in jugular venous pulse
❑ C exertional dyspnoea
❑ D angina
❑ E clubbing

33. The following associations are correct in pulmonary disease:

❑ A basal fibrosis and ankylosing spondylitis
❑ B pleurisy with effusion and Sjögren's syndrome
❑ C basal pneumonia and systemic sclerosis
❑ D chylothorax and yellow nails
❑ E lymphangiitis carcinomatosa and carcinoma of the pancreas

34. The following are recognised treatments of choice:

❑ A lung lavage in alveolar proteinosis
❑ B oral corticosteroids in symptomatic bronchopulmonary aspergillosis
❑ C nebulised pentamidine in severe pneumocystis pneumonia (PCP)
❑ D ampicillin in psittacosis
❑ E methylprednisolone in sepsis-induced ARDS

35. Pleural effusion

- ❏ A is a common feature of *Pneumocystis carinii* pneumonia (PCP)
- ❏ B may be blood stained following pulmonary embolus
- ❏ C in asbestosis is almost always due to a mesothelioma
- ❏ D characteristically has a low glucose content in rheumatoid arthritis
- ❏ E usually responds to steroid therapy in SLE

RHEUMATOLOGY

Rheumatoid arthritis

1. D-Penicillamine therapy in rheumatoid arthritis may

❑ A induce a lupus-like syndrome
❑ B lower rheumatoid factor titres
❑ C cause Goodpasture's syndrome
❑ D produce ageusia (altered taste sensation)
❑ E cause malabsorption

2. The following may be manifestations of rheumatoid arthritis:

❑ A erythema multiforme
❑ B erythema nodosum
❑ C episcleritis
❑ D digital gangrene
❑ E amyloidosis

3. In the treatment of rheumatoid arthritis

❑ A indomethacin is the safest NSAID when used in conventional doses
❑ B the proteinuria caused by gold is irreversible
❑ C patients on D-penicillamine need regular ophthalmic examination
❑ D methotrexate can cause a life-threatening pneumonitis
❑ E trimethoprim increases the antifolate effect of methotrexate

SLE

4. Concerning anti-nuclear factors:

❑ A antibodies to ds-DNA are highly specific for SLE
❑ B they may be detected by use of a haemoflagellate
❑ C anti ss-DNA occurs in 90% of SLE patients
❑ D immunofluorescence staining is of great diagnostic value
❑ E titres reliably reflect disease activity

5. Drug-induced systemic lupus erythematosus is

- ❑ A equally common in men and women
- ❑ B significantly more common in fast than slow acetylators
- ❑ C not generally complicated by renal disease
- ❑ D caused by sulphonamides
- ❑ E irreversible, even after drug withdrawal

6. In a patient suspected of having a connective-tissue disorder, the following findings favour systemic lupus erythematosus:

- ❑ A joint deformities
- ❑ B cavitating lung lesion
- ❑ C peripheral neuropathy
- ❑ D anti-ribonucleoprotein (RNP) antibodies
- ❑ E severe Raynaud's phenomenon

7. Anti-phospholipid antibodies

- ❑ A prolong the bleeding time
- ❑ B are associated with recurrent spontaneous abortion
- ❑ C have a high positive predictive value for SLE
- ❑ D occur in culture negative endocarditis
- ❑ E are associated with Addison's disease

Other connective tissue disorders

8. Extractable nuclear antigens (ENA) are usually found in the following:

- ❑ A pernicious anaemia
- ❑ B Sjögren's syndrome
- ❑ C rheumatoid arthritis
- ❑ D SLE
- ❑ E mixed connective tissue disease

9. The following are features of systemic sclerosis:

- ❑ A calcinosis
- ❑ B an association with intra-abdominal malignancy
- ❑ C myopathy
- ❑ D central nervous system involvement
- ❑ E an association with primary biliary cirrhosis

10. Mixed connective tissue disease

❑ A commonly presents with Raynaud's phenomenon
❑ B is diagnosed by the presence of anti-ribonucleoprotein antibodies
❑ C typically has raised titres of anti-DNA antibodies
❑ D carries a better prognosis than systemic sclerosis
❑ E typically causes renal impairment

11. In the vasculitides

❑ A cANCA has a high sensitivity for Wegener's granulomatosis
❑ B neurological symptoms are a common feature of Churg–Straus
❑ C the pathological hallmark of Henoch-Schönlein purpura (HSP) is IgG in the skin and renal messangium
❑ D microscopic polyangiitis is more common in women
❑ E glomerulonephritis is a common feature of polyarteritis nodosa

12. Polymyalgia rheumatica

❑ A is characteristically associated with shoulder girdle muscle wasting
❑ B is characterised by a positive rheumatoid factor test
❑ C is invariably 'burnt-out' after two years
❑ D is significantly associated with underlying malignancy
❑ E typically gives rise to raised blood muscle enzyme levels

Miscellaneous rheumatology

13. The following statements about synovial fluid are true:

❑ A it is often blood-stained in acute pyrophosphate arthropathy
❑ B the greater the inflammation, the more viscous the fluid
❑ C a turbid fluid indicates the presence of infection
❑ D synovial fluid lactate levels are higher in infected than in non-infected effusions
❑ E crystals may be visualised by holding a specimen against a dark background in natural daylight

14. The following are typical features of reactive arthritis:

❑ A onset after *E. coli* enteritis
❑ B presence of viable organisms within the joint
❑ C asymmetric limb joint involvement
❑ D episcleritis
❑ E Achilles' tendonitis

15. Radiological bone erosions are a typical finding in

❑ A hyperparathyroidism
❑ B Wegener's granulomatosis
❑ C gout
❑ D systemic lupus erythematosus
❑ E psoriatic arthritis

16. Joint pain is a recognised feature of

❑ A idiopathic thrombocytopenic purpura
❑ B Christmas disease (factor IX deficiency)
❑ C acute post-streptococcal glomerulonephritis
❑ D sarcoidosis
❑ E amyloidosis

17. The following statements regarding pseudo-gout (chondrocalcinosis) are correct:

❑ A acute arthritis involves the knee more often than other joints
❑ B hydroxyapatite crystals are found in the synovial fluid
❑ C the disease may mimic osteoarthritis of the hands
❑ D there is a recognised association with primary hyperparathyroidism
❑ E colchicine provides effective prophylaxis against acute attacks

18. Sacroiliitis commonly occurs in the following diseases:

❑ A ulcerative colitis
❑ B Crohn's disease
❑ C gout
❑ D ankylosing spondylitis
❑ E Reiter's syndrome

19. Characteristic features of Behçet's disease include

❑ A thrombophlebitis
❑ B glomerulonephritis
❑ C scrotal ulceration
❑ D pyoderma gangrenosum
❑ E myocarditis

20. The following statements are true:

❑ A radiological sacroiliitis is characteristically unilateral in ankylosing spondylitis
❑ B periostitis is a frequent radiological finding in psoriatic arthropathy
❑ C juxta-articular osteoporosis does not occur with gouty erosions
❑ D erosions are characteristically periarticular in systemic lupus erythematosus (SLE)
❑ E gouty tophi are radio-opaque

21. The following are characteristically involved:

❑ A the MCP joints in psoriatic arthropathy
❑ B the hip in ankylosing spondylitis
❑ C the DIP joints in pyrophosphate arthropathy
❑ D the MTP joints in haemophilia
❑ E the hand and foot in sickle cell disease

STATISTICS

Clinical trials

1. The following are often desirable when carrying out a clinical trial of a new drug:

- ❑ A apparatus with which to make reproducible observations
- ❑ B use of a double-blind cross-over method
- ❑ C administration of the drug to patients undergoing treatment with other drugs
- ❑ D the drug should have been tested extensively in animals
- ❑ E a pilot study

2. In the clinical trial of a new treatment

- ❑ A the null hypothesis is true if there are significant differences between the response of the treatment and placebo group
- ❑ B the patients should be randomised
- ❑ C stratum matching of patients is necessary if the groups are small
- ❑ D in a type one error the null hypothesis is wrongly rejected
- ❑ E the number of subjects required decreases as the power of the trial increases

3. A new antibiotic X is compared with amoxicillin in a clinical trial. A higher proportion of those patients treated with X respond in a given time (chi-squared 4.2; $p < 0.05$). The following are true:

- ❑ A the improved response to X is clinically significant
- ❑ B treatment with X cannot be worse than treatment with amoxicillin
- ❑ C the results would be invalidated if there was a significant difference in the ages of the two treatment groups
- ❑ D the trial implies that a difference in response of 4.2 times was observed
- ❑ E the results may have occurred by chance one time in twenty

Statistical populations

4. The following are true:

- ❑ A the annual prevalence of a condition reflects the number of new cases reported annually
- ❑ B cohort studies are generally used to study a group of subjects with a particular disease and compare them with normal controls
- ❑ C in a frequency distribution, the mode is the most frequently observed value
- ❑ D if a measurement has a skewed distribution, then the mean and mode are always different
- ❑ E the standard deviation of population may be smaller than the standard error of a sample mean from that population

5. If a set of values are normally distributed the following are true:

- ❑ A the median value will be less than the mean
- ❑ B 2.5% of the values will have numerical values which are smaller than the mean value minus 1.96 standard deviations
- ❑ C the standard deviation of the values is a measure of how accurately the calculated mean approaches the true population mean
- ❑ D student's t-test may be used to compare this set of value with a second set provided they are also normally distributed
- ❑ E the values may be used to calculate chi-squared

6. The median is used in preference to the arithmetic mean when

- ❑ A the variance is large
- ❑ B the sample size is small
- ❑ C the observations are from a population with a skew distribution
- ❑ D observer error is likely to be large
- ❑ E chi-squared is to be calculated

7. The time taken to walk 10 metres was recorded in 50 patients who had suffered a stroke. The observations were found to be distributed symmetrically about the mean (47 seconds)

- ❑ A the observations, being symmetrical about the mean, must follow a Normal distribution
- ❑ B if the observations had been found to be positively skewed, their mode would have been less than the mean
- ❑ C the median time to walk 10 metres is equal to the 50th percentile
- ❑ D computing the variance of the observations would provide a measure of their spread about the mean
- ❑ E computing the standard deviation of the observations would provide a measure of the reliability of the mean

8. In a study of 54 patients with symptoms of non-ulcer dyspepsia, 27 were treated with bismuth alone and 27 were treated with metronidazole plus amoxicillin. The presence or absence of *H. pylori* infection and a global symptom score (range 0–24) was obtained for each patient both before and after the treatment period.

- ❑ A if the pre-treatment symptom scores have Normal distribution, the two groups are best compared by use of a non-parametric test
- ❑ B the post-treatment symptom scores for the two treatment groups can be compared by use of either Student's unpaired t-test or the Mann-Whitney U-test as these two techniques are equivalent
- ❑ C Student's paired t-test can be used to enhance the change in symptom score within either treatment group only if the median scores are known
- ❑ D the proportions of patients in the two groups with *H. pylori* infection can be compared by use of a chi-squared test
- ❑ E a chi-squared test is valid only if all of the expected frequencies are greater than 5

Miscellaneous

9. The average height of two groups of subjects are compared and are stated to be significantly different ($p < 0.05$). The following are true:

- ❑ A Student's paired test may have been used to calculate p
- ❑ B this result may have arisen by chance alone less than one time in twenty
- ❑ C if the t-test is used the number of degrees of freedom is the total number of observations in both groups minus two
- ❑ D even if the difference is large it has not reached conventional levels of statistical significance
- ❑ E to apply tests of significance validly the groups need to have been chosen randomly

10. In an assay for serum sodium

- ❑ A the coefficient of variation of the measurement allows the sensitivity of the assay to be determined
- ❑ B the accuracy of the assay is the degree to which repeated observations conform to each other
- ❑ C the specificity of the assay is a measure of the degree to which other substances may interfere with the serum sodium result
- ❑ D the precision of the assay is a measure of how close the assay result is to the true value
- ❑ E the sensitivity of the assay is the closeness to which the lower limits of the assay approach zero

11. For the correlation coefficient r, the following are correct:

- ❑ A the value of r lies between –1 and +1
- ❑ B if $r = 0.1$ this excludes a significant correlation between the variables
- ❑ C if r is negative, one value increases while the other decreases
- ❑ D r would be useful in comparing the relationship between blood pressure and cardiovascular mortality in a population
- ❑ E it can be used to predict one variable from the value of the other

12. Concerning clinical trials

- ❑ A phase II studies are usually conducted in healthy volunteers
- ❑ B placebo drugs are physiologically inert
- ❑ C the commonest criticism of negative trials is a type II error
- ❑ D cross-over studies require fewer patients than group comparisons
- ❑ E visual analogue scales are unreliable

CARDIOLOGY: ANSWERS AND EXPLANATIONS

1. In the heart **Answer: C**

The pulmonary valve is normally tricuspid like the aortic valve. It is the left bundle of His which is described as dividing into anterior and posterior hemibundles or fascicles. The heart is remarkable in that a high proportion of oxygen is extracted from the coronary blood, and so the blood returning from the coronary sinus into the right atrium between the inferior caval opening and the right atrioventricular valve is highly de-oxygenated. Therefore increased oxygen delivery is produced by increased coronary flow rather than increased oxygen extraction. The sino-atrial node lies high in the wall of the right atrium near its junction with the superior vena cava.

2. Arterial pulse **Answers: B C**

Pulsus paradoxus, a greater than the normal 10 mmHg inspiratory decrease in systolic arterial pressure, occurs in cardiac tamponade, and, less commonly, in constrictive pericarditis. It is not diagnostic of pericardial disease, but occurs in cardiomyopathies, severe asthma, superior mediastinal obstruction and shock. A bisferiens pulse is also found in hypertrophic cardiomyopathy and pulsus alternans during or following paroxysmal tachycardia. Severe mitral stenosis gives a low pulse volume and coarctation a delayed femoral pulse, which may also be diminished in volume.

3. Normal cardiac cycle **Answers: C E**

The cardiac cycle is initiated by depolarisation of the sinus node which is situated in the right atrium near the superior vena cava. Immediately prior to sinus node depolarisation all cardiac chambers are in diastole. It is during ventricular diastole that coronary flow occurs since this is the only time when aortic pressure exceeds left ventricular wall tension. Ventricular diastole extends from the closure of the aortic valve and hence the second heart sound and the aortic dicrotic notch to the subsequent ventricular depolarisation. During diastole, a third sound may be heard when ventricular filling is rapid. Generally a third heart sound is pathological, but it may be also heard in young, fit individuals.

4. Right coronary artery **Answers: All true**

The right coronary artery is found in a groove between the right atrium and right ventricle. It gives off a branch to the A-V node and goes on to supply the inferior aspect of the left ventricle via the posterior descending artery in the majority of patients. It also supplies the right ventricle.

5. Atrial natriuretic peptide (ANP) Answers: A B D

ANP is a 28 amino acid peptide secreted in response to stretching of both right and left atrial myocardium. Enlargement of the heart in congestive cardiac failure increases secretion which promotes renal sodium loss and inhibits aldosterone release.

6. Normal adult resting electrocardiogram Answers: B C D

The mean frontal plane QRS axis should lie between –30° and +90°. Left ventricular hypertrophy is present if the sum of the tallest R wave in the left precordial leads and the deepest S wave in the right precordial leads exceeds 40 mm. Left ventricular hypertrophy can also be diagnosed by the presence of a tall R wave (over 27 mm) in the left precordial leads alone. Small amplitude R waves may be due to myxoedema or a pericardial effusion. Tall P waves suggest right atrial hypertrophy and broad P waves suggest left atrial hypertrophy.

7. ST depression on ECG Answers: A B C E

Hypokalaemia (occasionally occurring with prolonged use of thiazide diuretics) causes a prominent U wave flattening, and later ST depression and T wave inversion. Acute pericarditis causes concave upward ST elevation and chronic pericarditis may reduce voltages. The strain pattern of left ventricular hypertrophy shows ST depression and digoxin toxicity shows ST depression with the reversed tick appearance. Syndrome X is characterised by anginal-type chest pain, angiographically-normal coronary arteries and ST depression on exercise.

8. T wave inversion Answers: C D E

T wave inversion occurs in V1 in 20% of normal adults and in V2 in 5% of normal adults (who also have T wave inversion in V1). T wave inversion in V3–V6 and I and II is always abnormal in adults. T wave inversion may be normal in aVL, aVf and III, but only if the mean frontal plane T wave axis does not differ greatly from the mean frontal plane QRS axis. Abnormal T wave inversion can be due to ischaemia, strain or pericarditis.

9. Heart block Answers: A B C

First degree heart block and the Wenckebach phenomenon occur in healthy individuals. Bifascicular block after an acute anterior myocardial infarction is associated with a mortality of about 50% since it means a large amount of cardiac tissue has been damaged. Complete heart block may occur with inferior myocardial infarction since the right coronary artery supplies the artery to the atrioventricular node, but the heart block usually resolves in a few days without requiring permanent pacing. (The atrioventricular node receives a dual blood supply with additional perfusion from the septal perforating branch of the left anterior descending artery.) Isoprenaline should not be used as first-line therapy to treat episodes of complete heart block. It may precipitate ventricular arrhythmias and permanent pacing is preferable. Intravenous isoprenaline may be of temporary use in a haemodynamically comprised patient with complete heart block whilst pacing is being arranged/attempted.

10. Complete atrioventricular (heart) block **Answers: C E**

A variable first heart sound occurs and is a sign of the asynchrony of atrial and ventricular contraction. This also gives rise to irregular giant 'a' ('cannon') waves. In acquired complete heart block the majority of cases have a pacemaker in the Purkinje system which responds poorly to exercise, vagal or sympathetic effects. In congenital heart block, the block and subsidiary pacemakers are higher and the ventricular response, particularly in the young, may be near normal. The arterial pulse has a wide pulse pressure with a large stroke volume and thus tends to feel collapsing. The volume of the blood pressure will vary with the atrial contribution.

11. Patients with heart block **Answers: C E**

In pacing nomenclature the first letter refers to the chamber(s) paced, (A = atrium, V = ventricle, D = both), the second to the chamber(s) sensed (A, V, D), the third is the response of the pacemaker to a sensed impulse (I = inhibit, T = trigger, D = both inhibit and trigger) and the fourth to programmable functions, e.g. rate response (R). Dual chamber (D. . .) pacing is inappropriate for permanent atrial fibrillation as the atrium cannot be paced. Rate response (. . . R) is needed to prevent bradycardia in patients with complete heart block where there is sinus node disease or in atrial fibrillation with frequent pauses. In sinus node disease there is no need for ventricular pacing if AV conduction is intact. For physiological pacing an attempt should be made to ensure sequential activation of both chambers where possible and to maintain an adequate rate response to exercise. VVI pacing for atrial fibrillation with a persistent bradycardia and DDD pacing for complete heart block and sinus node disease are not appropriate since these modes do not allow for a rate response with exercise (i.e. should be VVIR and DDDR respectively).

12. Cardiac syncope **Answers: A B D E**

The principal differential diagnosis is from epilepsy, which is usually characterised by a preceding aura and prolonged unconsciousness and recovery. Owing to cerebral hypoxia, tonic/clonic seizures may occur with cardiac syncope. Tachyarrhythmias (ventricular and supraventricular) may profoundly reduce cardiac output due to the sheer rapidity or by further compromising myocardial perfusion. Ventricular tachycardia may be an 'escape' rhythm precipitated by a primary bradyarrhythmia.

13. Right bundle branch block **Answers: A B E**

Right bundle branch block (RBBB) results in delayed right ventricular activation which is manifest on the ECG by a broad QRS (> 0.12 sec) an R wave in V1 and a deep S wave in V6. Incomplete or complete RBBB occurs in 95% of patients with an ASD. Left axis deviation with RBBB is associated with a primum defect. The indications for temporary pacing prior to anaesthesia are complete heart block, bifascicular block with type II second degree heart block and transient complete heart block.

14. Causes of atrial fibrillation **Answers: A B C D**

Recent infarction and cardiac surgery both predispose to atrial fibrillation which is usually transient. Sinus tachycardia is typical in anxiety, while in hyperthyroidism, sinus tachycardia or atrial fibrillation may occur. Long standing hypertension is the setting in which atrial fibrillation most often occurs in the UK.

15. Atrial flutter **Answers: A B C E**

The atrial flutter rate ranges from 250 to 350/min, usually 300/min. In the untreated state there is usually 2:1 A-V block giving a ventricular rate of 150/min. The block may occasionally be variable, giving enough ventricular irregularity to simulate atrial fibrillation. The degree of A-V block can be increased by vagal stimulation (carotid sinus pressure) slowing the ventricular rate suddenly, and making the flutter waves more obvious in the ECG. Adenosine, which results in temporary block of A-V conduction, can again help with diagnostic difficulties by temporarily slowing the ventricular rate. It does not result in cardioversion to sinus rhythm.

16. Wolff-Parkinson-White syndrome Answers: A B D

Wolff-Parkinson-White syndrome is due to an anomalous pathway (the bundle of Kent). Retrograde conduction via this pathway causes an AV re-entrant tachycardia. Atrial fibrillation is present in up to one-third of cases and the rapid ventricular response due to antegrade conduction down the anomalous pathway may give rise to ventricular fibrillation and sudden death. Digoxin and verapamil may enhance conduction down the anomalous pathway and increase the risk of sudden death. Treatment with flecainide or amiodarone is effective as is radiofrequency ablation of the anomalous pathway. The condition is associated with Ebstein's anomaly, mitral valve prolapse and hypertrophic obstructive cardiomyopathy.

17. Electromechanical dissociation Answers: D E

Electromechanical dissociation causes cardiac arrest. The ECG shows complexes but there is no mechanical activity or pulse. It has a worse prognosis than either ventricular fibrillation or asystole. It may be due to cardiac rupture. Other causes are cardiac depressant drugs, tension pneumothorax and cardiac tamponade. It is treated with drugs, particularly adrenaline, but also isoprenaline and calcium. Adrenaline may be injected down the trachea and will be absorbed into the pulmonary veins and so reach the heart if effective external cardiac massage is being performed.

18. Cardiac murmur Answers: B E

Innocent murmurs tend to be ejection systolic. Diastolic or pansystolic murmurs are pathological. An exceptional innocent murmur is a venous hum, which is continuous and often occurs in children. It may disappear on neck vein compression or on lying down. An innocent pulmonary flow murmur is common in children. A thrill or associated added sound makes any murmur unlikely to be innocent.

19. A third heart sound Answers: A C D E

A third heart sound reflects rapid ventricular filling in early diastole and may be a consequence of ventricular decompensation or A-V valve regurgitation. Significant mitral stenosis prevents rapid left ventricular filling but beware, a right-sided third heart sound may co-exist with mitral stenosis. In constrictive pericarditis the restrictive effect of the adherent pericardium halts diastolic filling abruptly, producing a third heart sound (pericardial knock).

20. Isolated calcific aortic stenosis Answers: B D

The majority of cases are secondary to bicuspid valves or to non-rheumatic calcification of a tricuspid aortic valve seen in the very old. The presence of mitral valve disease or significant aortic regurgitation would suggest a rheumatic origin. A relatively quiet murmur may be present with severe disease, particularly if the patient is in heart failure or has emphysema; severe disease is suggested by an aortic systolic thrill. Elderly patients may present with cardiac failure rather than classically with dyspnoea, angina or syncope. Significant aortic stenosis prolongs left ventricular ejection time but this is often difficult to appreciate. A click is unusual in clinically significant calcific disease.

21. Aortic regurgitation Answers: D

The Austin-Flint murmur may be distinguished from that caused by mitral stenosis because of the absence of a mitral opening snap. Significant compensated aortic regurgitation is usually associated with an aortic ejection murmur due to the increased stroke volume required to maintain cardiac output. As regurgitation worsens there is a tendency to a shortening of the early diastolic murmur, and a reduction of diastolic blood pressure. Antibiotic prophylaxis is indicated.

22. A rumbling apical diastolic murmur Answers: B C E

A fourth heart sound is usual in hypertension. A murmur mimicking mitral stenosis may occur when there is a greatly increased flow across a normal mitral valve in mitral regurgitation, VSD, patent ductus and occasionally in thyrotoxicosis and other hyperdynamic circulatory conditions. Similar murmurs occur in aortic regurgitation (Austin-Flint), acute rheumatic fever (Cary Coombs) and with atrial myxomas. The murmur of tricuspid stenosis and tricuspid flow murmurs may occasionally be heard at the apex. Complete heart block usually presents with an ejection systolic murmur due to a large stroke volume.

23. Mitral stenosis in sinus rhythm Answers: A D

The intensity of the first heart sound and the opening snap reflects the mobility of the mitral valve leaflets and not the severity of the stenosis. In more severe mitral stenosis the LV pressure falls below that of the LA earlier in diastole, leading to an early opening snap and long diastolic murmur. The murmur of pulmonary regurgitation (Graham-Steel) occurs with severe pulmonary hypertension. A third heart sound indicates rapid filling of the left ventricle and this excludes severe mitral stenosis (unless it is a right ventricular sound, when there would be obvious signs of tricuspid regurgitation).

24. Mitral valve prolapse syndrome **Answers: B C**

The characteristic murmur is ejection or late systolic. The murmur is often preceded by an ejection mid-systolic click. Liability to infective endocarditis relates to the amount of mitral reflux. The prognosis is generally good, although severe mitral regurgitation can occur requiring mitral valve replacements or repair. The condition was believed to be more common in females, but the sex incidence is now thought to be equal.

25. Mitral regurgitation **Answers: B C D**

The first heart sound is characteristically soft; when loud it excludes severe mitral regurgitation. The third heart sound and diastolic murmur (in the absence of any stenosis) reflect rapid diastolic filling of the left ventricle. Left atrial distension in systole may produce a left sternal heave. The second heart sound is usually normal; with severe regurgitation early aortic valve closure causes wide (but not reversed) splitting of the second heart sound. A mid systolic click suggests mitral leaflet prolapse as the cause of the regurgitation. Acute mitral regurgitation, which may produce an apical thrill, may be due to papillary muscle infarction and rupture.

26. Pulmonary stenosis **Answers: C**

Coarctation of the aorta is the commonest cardiovascular abnormality in Turner's syndrome. Pulmonary stenosis is common in Noonan's syndrome, which is superficially similar. The chest X-ray is usually normal but may be oligaemic if the stenosis is severe, if there is right ventricular failure or right-to-left shunt. Carcinoid secretions of serotonin cause fibrous plaques, giving pulmonary stenosis and tricuspid regurgitation. An ejection click points to valvular stenosis, as in aortic stenosis. With increasing severity the pulmonary component of the second sound becomes more delayed and softer, and the systolic murmur extends later into systole.

27. Ostium secundum atrial septal defect **Answers: B D**

This is the commonest type of ASD and may well present in adult life. Unless pulmonary hypertension is present pregnancy is well tolerated. A tricuspid mid-diastolic murmur indicates a large left-to-right shunt. This murmur, and the classical pulmonary area systolic murmur, lessen and disappear as pulmonary hypertension develops, and the shunt is reduced. Haemodynamic deterioration is often heralded by the onset of atrial fibrillation, flutter or tachycardia. Left axis deviation is the ECG hallmark of ostium primum ASD which involves the A-V valves.

28. Ventricular septal defects Answers: A B

Ventricular septal defects usually involve the membranous septum. A Gerbode defect occurs when the defect passes between the left ventricle and the right atrium and it occurs because the mitral valve is normally attached to the interventricular septum higher than the tricuspid valve. Pulmonary hypertension and the Eisenmenger syndrome can occur at an early age if the defect is large. Right bundle branch block is more characteristic of atrial septal defects and the electrocardiogram seen in patients with ventricular septal defects may vary from normal to gross ventricular hypertrophy.

29. Infective endocarditis Answer: E

The most frequently observed evidence of renal involvement in endocarditis is asymptomatic proteinuria and haematuria, caused by an immune-complex mediated focal proliferative glomerulonephritis which may also be associated with renal failure and nephrotic syndrome. *S. faecalis* is a common cause of subacute endocarditis, whilst *S. aureus* and *Strep. pneumoniae* are commonly responsible for the acute form of the disease. Petechiae occur in the skin, retina and under the nails, and are probably due to immunological changes. Such changes account for low serum complement levels and positive rheumatoid factor tests, but ANF is not found. Thrombocytopenia is rare. Treatment started within two weeks after onset of symptoms gives a 90% survival. If treatment is delayed longer than eight weeks survival drops to 74%.

30. Surgery in infective endocarditis Answers: B C D E

Indications for surgery following endocarditis include: congestive cardiac failure due to valve dysfunction, refractory sepsis despite adequate antibiotic therapy, fungal aetiology, recent onset heart block, aortic root abscess, recurrent emboli and valve obstruction. Development of new AV block on ECG is 85% specific for the development of an aortic root abscess. 70% of vegetations do not resolve despite adequate antibiotic therapy.

31. Heart disease **Answers: C D E**

Both false-positive and false-negative exercise tests occur but a normal test makes it unlikely that a major cardiac event will occur in the next year. Exercise testing is potentially hazardous in significant aortic valvular stenosis. This is also true for severe LV outflow tract obstruction due to hypertrophic cardiomyopathy. Exercise testing is useful in assessment of ventricular ectopic activity and in revealing ventricular tachycardia and atrial tachyarrhythmias. Any resting ST segment change, bundle branch block pattern or left ventricular hypertrophy makes interpretation of an exercise test difficult. A fall in blood pressure on exercise, (except if exercising soon after a myocardial infarction), suggests a poor prognosis.

32. Risk of atheromatous coronary disease **Answers: C D E**

Although there is severe hypertriglyceridaemia, WHO type 1 disease is not associated with increased ischaemic heart disease risk. HDL cholesterol (reverse cholesterol transport) values above 1.1 mmol/l appear to be protective. In angiographic studies, LDL cholesterol values below 3.4 mmol/l seem to be associated with atheroma regression and values above 4.1 mmol/l with progression. Familial hypercholesterolaemia is an autosomal dominant condition with affected heterozygotes expressing defective hepatic LDL receptors (hence reduced LDL clearance from plasma). Proteinuria and microalbuminuria are markers for later development of atheromatous disease in type 2 diabetes.

33. Angina pectoris **Answers: A E**

Angina with normal coronary arteries is found in cardiomyopathies, severe aortic stenosis and pulmonary hypertension, as well as in otherwise normal hearts when coronary artery spasm or coronary blood flow abnormalities are implicated. The resting ECG is normal in 50% or more of patients between attacks. Many patients get angina on getting up in the morning and become symptom-free later in the day. ST segment elevation during an attack is the major feature of Prinzmetal's 'variant' angina. The mechanism of angina decubitus is unknown but this symptom usually indicates severe coronary disease.

34. Intravenous streptokinase **Answer: E**

In the ISIS-2 study, intravenous streptokinase given alone within 12 hours reduced mortality by 25% at 35 days and this benefit increased to 42% when aspirin was added. Alteplase given as an accelerated regime with heparin is more effective than streptokinase alone in patients with anterior infarcts (GUSTO). Streptokinase prolongs the APTT. Efficacy is reduced by neutralising antibodies which may be a result of recent streptococcal infection or recent administration of streptokinase. Hypertension is a contraindication as it increases the risk of haemorrhagic complications, particularly stroke.

35. Myocardial infarction **Answers: A D E**

LV aneurysm formation and ventricular septal defects are more common in anterior myocardial infarction. Impaired LV function is associated with an approximate 8% mortality at 1 year and is a more important prognostic indicator than a positive exercise test. Although a high frequency of ectopic beats is associated with an increased mortality, treatment with flecainide (as in the CAST study) increases mortality compared with placebo. HGV drivers have to complete three stages of the Bruce protocol without symptoms or ECG changes off medication in order to qualify for their licence.

36. Coronary revascularisation and cardiac surgery **Answer: A**

Coronary angioplasty is associated with restenosis in 30–40% of cases and usually occurs in the first three months. Coronary artery bypass grafting (CABG) has been shown to improve survival in patients with triple vessel disease and impaired LV function and in those with triple vessel disease with proximal left anterior descending artery involvement. Internal mammary artery grafts are preferable to saphenous vein grafts as they have greater long-term patency rate. CABG is associated with an overall mortality of 1–2%. All patients should be considered for valve replacement in aortic stenosis regardless of the degree of LV impairment.

37. Congestive (dilated) cardiomyopathy **Answers: A B D**

Congestive cardiomyopathy is characterised by a dilated heart with functional mitral and tricuspid regurgitation, and congestive heart failure. Emboli are common even in the absence of arrhythmias which also frequently complicate the picture. There are many causes of congestive cardiomyopathy including alcoholism, but the majority of cases in the UK are idiopathic, occurring in the middle-aged and elderly. Septal hypertrophy and familial sudden death are features of hypertrophic cardiomyopathy (HOCM).

38. Dilated cardiomyopathy — Answers: A C E

Dilated cardiomyopathy is characterised by dilatation and impaired left and right ventricular function. Evidence of a myocarditis is found in less than 20% of cases. Anticoagulation is indicated despite sinus rhythm if there is significant left ventricular dilatation. Cardiac failure develops in around 15% of patients with haemochromatosis and tends to occur late; the earliest and commonest presentation is with diabetes mellitus (80%). A familial incidence of idiopathic cardiomyopathy is found in 20% of cases although the mode of inheritance is not well defined.

39. Left ventricular failure — Answers: B C

In left ventricular failure, interstitial pulmonary oedema interferes with gas transfer. Alveolar PCO_2 is increased only when the fluid has entered terminal airways. As the left ventricle fails, left ventricular end-diastolic pressure and pulmonary venous pressure rise. X-ray changes may antedate auscultatory findings by 24 hours, depending on the rapidity of onset.

40. Refractory heart failure — Answers: A C D E

Hyponatraemia is often due to diuretic therapy but occurs especially with advanced disease. Of the vasodilators used for heart failure, enalapril (an ACE inhibitor) acts primarily on arteries, nitrates on veins and nitroprusside and prazosin on both sides of the circulation. Some antacids, such as magnesium trisilicate mixture, contain substantial amounts of sodium chloride. Splenomegaly occurs with long-standing liver congestion usually associated with tricuspid regurgitation. Heart failure is a catabolic process with tissue breakdown contributing to uraemia and to cardiac cachexia.

41. Hypertrophic cardiomyopathy — Answers: A E

The development of atrial fibrillation or identification of ventricular tachycardia indicates a poor prognosis. The clinical findings are usually of left ventricular hypertrophy, a long ejection systolic murmur at the left sternal edge due to outflow obstruction, and often some mitral regurgitation. However, significant myopathy may be present without outflow gradient when no murmur may be apparent. If in sinus rhythm a loud fourth heart sound is present. A third heart sound is common but a diastolic murmur is uncommon and would indicate mixed aortic valve disease. Outflow obstruction is liable to increase with GTN as this reduces ventricular volume and also lowers arterial pressure. The echo shows combinations of asymmetric septal hypertrophy (ASH), systolic anterior motion of the mitral apparatus (SAM), a high ejection fraction with early closure of the aortic valve, and an outflow gradient which can be measured by Doppler.

42. Coarctation of the thoracic aorta **Answers: C D**
Males outnumber females by more than 2:1. It is common in Turner's syndrome, which should be suspected in all females with coarctation. The commonest site for a coarctation is just distal to the left subclavian artery. If the lumen is very narrow, flow through it may occur throughout the cardiac cycle. The commonest cause of a diastolic murmur is, however, aortic regurgitation due to a bicuspid valve. Other associated malformations are PDA, VDS and mitral abnormalities. Left ventricular failure, cerebral haemorrhage, aortic dissection and infective endocarditis are all serious hazards of untreated coarctation.

43. Dissecting aneurysms of the aorta **Answers: C D E**
The factors that predispose to dissection are cystic medial necrosis, which occurs in Marfan's syndrome, and increased haemodynamic stress on the aorta as in hypertension, pregnancy and coarctation of the aorta.

44. Abdominal aortic aneurysms **Answers: B C D**
The majority of abdominal aortic aneurysms are atherosclerotic and arise below the renal arteries. Expansion may compress contiguous structures and cause ureteric obstruction. The majority of patients are asymptomatic at the time of diagnosis. Pain from the aneurysm usually means impending or actual rupture, which is more likely to occur in larger aneurysms; 50% of aneurysms with diameters greater than 6 cm rupture within one year.

45. Pulmonary embolism **Answers: A C D**
Pulmonary emboli usually originate from thrombi in the lower limbs and pelvis. When recurrent, they may produce pulmonary hypertension and right heart failure. However, more characteristically there are single episodes of dyspnoea, chest pain and haemoptysis, at which time arterial gases show a reduced PO_2 and reduced PCO_2. The jugular venous pressure is often raised and right atrial pressure may exceed left atrial pressure. Pulmonary emboli can be demonstrated by lung scanning or angiography, but neither technique is entirely free from risk of sudden deterioration and death of the patient.

46. Acute rheumatic fever **Answer: C**

Significant murmurs indicating carditis are those of mitral and aortic regurgitation and an apical mid-diastolic rumbling murmur (Carey Coombs) which is often associated with mitral regurgitation. Mitral and aortic stenosis only develop after months or years. Rheumatic nodes are painless. The most frequent conduction defect is prolongation of the P-R interval. The classical cutaneous manifestation of rheumatic fever is erythema marginatum found mainly on the trunk and proximal parts of the limbs.

47. Acute pericarditis **Answers: A B D**

Acute pericarditis is a recognised feature of all the connective tissue diseases and can complicate any septicaemia. It is a serious complication of amoebic abscesses of the left lobe of the liver. Although pericardial fluid accumulates in congestive cardiac failure, the amount is rarely significant and is not inflammatory.

48. Dressler's syndrome **Answers: C D**

Dressler's syndrome usually occurs in the first weeks after myocardial infarction. The incidence is up to 5%. It is characterised by pain, fever, a raised ESR and ST and T wave changes on the ECG. It responds well to non-steroidal anti-inflammatory drugs. Constrictive pericarditis is an extremely rare complication.

49. Constrictive pericarditis **Answers: A B E**

Atrial fibrillation is present in about one-third of cases. Cardiomegaly is often absent but when present is usually only moderate. The chest X-ray occasionally suggests considerable cardiomegaly due to gross thickening of the pericardium. Acute pulmonary oedema and pulsus alternans would suggest myocardial disease. The third heart sound of constrictive pericarditis (pericardial knock) represents rapid, but suddenly abbreviated, ventricular filling.

50. Left atrial myxoma **Answers: All true**

A pedunculated left atrial myxoma may fall into the mitral orifice and obstruct blood flow into the left ventricle; thus syncope and acute pulmonary oedema may occur. Less often the findings resemble those produced by combined mitral stenosis and regurgitation or even pure mitral regurgitation. Embolic manifestations are common resulting in stroke, peripheral gangrene, etc. There is often a raised sedimentation rate and high serum globulin.

CLINICAL PHARMACOLOGY: ANSWERS AND EXPLANATIONS

1. Drug absorption **Answers: C E**

The small intestine is the principal site of absorption for most drugs. Most drugs are absorbed by passive transport. In contrast to active absorption, passive absorption shows no structural specificity, is usually down a concentration gradient and cannot be saturated. For those drugs that have high pre-systemic elimination (i.e. undergo breakdown in the gut wall) loss of surface area from diseases such as coeliac disease will increase bioavailability. In general, however, such diseases are associated with reduced bioavailability. A delay in gastric emptying decreases the rate of absorption but not the amount absorbed.

2. High first-pass effect **Answers: C D E**

A drug with a high first-pass effect will undergo extensive metabolism within the gut wall and liver, and will therefore have low bioavailability. If the patient has severe liver impairment for whatever reason, then the first-pass effect (and thus the extraction ratio), will be diminished. First-pass metabolism is seen with the following drugs: propranolol, GTN, pethidine, pentazocine, imipramine, nortriptyline, amitriptyline, cyclosporin, chlorpromazine, chlormethiazole, oxprenolol, metoprolol and labetalol. For pro-drugs such as isosorbide dinitrate, terfenadine and enalapril, a high first-pass effect is required to convert them to their active metabolites.

3. Bioavailability **Answers: B C E**

Bioavailability after oral administration depends on drug absorption from the gut and first-pass metabolism in the bowel wall and liver. First-pass metabolism is reduced in hepatic cirrhosis, resulting in increased bioavailability. Drugs with high first-pass metabolism therefore have increased bioavailability in the presence of cirrhosis. Examples are lipid soluble beta-blockers (e.g. propranolol), most opioids, metoclopramide, most tricyclic antidepressants, lignocaine, and natural oestrogens.

4. Enterohepatic recirculation **Answers: A C**

Enterohepatic recirculation is the process whereby some drugs are excreted in the bile and then reabsorbed from the gastrointestinal tract back into the circulation. If drugs are excreted as conjugates, the conjugate must be broken down by bacterial enzymes to release the parent drug.

5. Blood-brain barrier **Answers: C E**

The blood-brain barrier is more easily soluble to lipid- than to water-soluble drugs. Highly polar drugs have lower concentrations of unionised molecules at pH 7.4 and penetrate slowly. The penetration of acid and basic drugs also depends on the lipid solubility of the unionised molecules. Adrenaline (acid) penetrates poorly but amphetamine (base) much more easily as it has fewer polar groups.

6. Polymorphic metabolism **Answers: B C D**

Many drug metabolising enzymes are polymorphically expressed: that is, the gene coding for them contains nucleotide changes such that the less frequent variant occurs at a frequency of at least 1% in the population. Polymorphisms can be important in determining the toxic or therapeutic actions of a drug. Metoprolol is metabolised by debrisoquine hydroxylase (CYP2D6) which is absent in 5–10% of the Caucasian population. Patients with the defective enzyme can develop bradycardia. Hydralazine is metabolised by N-acetyl transferase: slow acetylators can develop systemic lupus erythematosus (SLE). 6-Mercaptopurine is metabolised by thiopurine methyltransferase; variation in this enzyme may determine response to the drugs in children with acute lymphoblastic leukaemia.

7. Slow acetylators **Answers: C D E**

Hydralazine lowers blood pressure and slow acetylators have a more marked response. Isoniazid hepatitis may be related to a metabolite since it is more common in fast acetylators. The remaining adverse effects are dose dependent and are more commonly seen in slow acetylators.

8. Enzyme induction **Answers: A C D E**

Enzyme induction may occur with several drugs and hydrocarbons. There is an increase in the activity of the enzymes which metabolise drugs and natural compounds. Osteomalacia may occur because of increased breakdown of vitamin D metabolites. Low dose oestrogen pills may be metabolised too quickly such that the lower plasma concentrations fail to inhibit ovulation. Smoking increases the activity of liver enzymes other than those induced by most drugs. Bilirubin conjugation is increased by enzyme induction with a resulting fall in plasma concentration.

9. Competitive enzyme inhibitors **Answers: A B C E**

Metyrapone inhibits the enzyme 11 β hydroxylase, the final step in cortisol synthesis. Finasteride is a competitive inhibitor of 5 α reductase, which converts testosterone to the active dihydrotestosterone. This agent is effective in benign and malignant prostatic disease. Enalaprilat is the active form of enalapril, which inhabits the angiotensin converting enzyme. Pyridostigmine is a competitive inhibitor of the enzyme cholinesterase and is used in the management of myasthenia gravis. Pralidoxime is used to reactivate cholinesterase following organophosphorus poisoning (sheep dip, insecticide).

10. Sympathomimetic amine actions **Answer: A**

Sympathomimetic actions at the α-receptor include vasoconstriction, production of viscous saliva, constriction of systemic veins, contraction of alimentary and bladder sphincters, decrease in gut motility, contraction of pregnant uterus, decreased exocrine secretion by pancreatic acini, decreased endocrine secretion by β cells of the pancreas, and contraction of the radial muscle of the iris. Decreased bronchial secretions and stimulation of gluconeogenesis is mediated via the β_2-receptor, while contraction of the ciliary muscle of the iris is mediated by the parasympathetic system.

11. α-receptor antagonists **Answers: A B E**

Phenoxybenzamine is an irreversible α-receptor antagonist used for the treatment of phaeochromocytoma. Doxazosin, used for hypertension, blocks the α_1-receptor. Chlorpromazine has a large number of actions, and has effects on the muscarinic, histamine, and α-receptors. Blockade of the α-receptor by chlorpromazine can lead to peripheral vasodilatation, postural hypotension (particularly in the elderly) and hypothermia. Both phenytoin and lignocaine act on sodium channels.

12. β-adrenoceptor antagonists **Answers: A E**

β-blockers have many different properties, which can be used to differentiate their actions and side-effect profile. These include lipophilicity, cardioselectivity and intrinsic sympathomimetic activity (ISA). β-blockers with ISA are less likely to cause bradycardia. β-blockers such as atenolol are cardio-selective but not cardio-specific; this means that they can still affect β_2-receptors especially when used in high dosage. β-blockers have class II antiarrhythmic properties and apart from sotalol (which also has class III properties) are unlikely to affect the Q-T interval. Celiprolol is a 'vasodilating' β-blocker and usually decreases total peripheral resistance. Esmolol is a short-acting β-blocker which can be given intravenously to treat supraventricular arrhythmias.

13. Drug combinations **Answers: A B C D**
Pharmacodynamic interactions between drugs having similar or opposite effects are common and often predictable. Metoclopramide and chlorpromazine, both dopamine antagonists, increase the risk of extrapyramidal adverse effects. Levodopa and nifedipine summate their hypotensive effects.

14. Warfarin metabolism **Answers: A C**
Warfarin is a narrow therapeutic index drug. It undergoes extensive metabolism with the P450 isoform CYP2C9 being the major enzyme responsible for metabolism. Inhibitors of CYP2C9 such as zafirlukast, omeprazole, cimetidine, amiodarone, disulfiram and metronidazole can cause an increase in International Normalised Ratio, and predispose to bleeding. Bezafibrate enhances the anticoagulant effect of warfarin, although the mechanism of this is unclear.

15. Aspirin **Answers: A C**
Aspirin in large doses is hypoprothrombinaemic. In smaller doses, it increases the bleeding tendency by its antiplatelet and gastric irritant effects. Also, in large doses, aspirin is uricosuric, but in therapeutic doses of 1–2 g/day or less, it reduces urate excretion. Again, in large doses aspirin is hypoglycaemic.

16. Increase in plasma digoxin levels **Answers: A B C**
Amiodarone and nifedipine displace digoxin from plasma-binding protein, and quinidine and nifedipine reduce renal clearance of digoxin. Cholestyramine binds digoxin, and rifampicin induces hepatic metabolism.

17. Risk of pregnancy **Answers: C D E**
Carbamazepine, phenytoin and rifampicin are potent inducers of hepatic mixed function oxidase. The clearance of the steroids is increased, the plasma concentrations fall and break-through bleeding may occur. Neither diazepam nor isoniazid induces steroid metabolism.

18. Cigarette smoking **Answers: A D E**
Cigarette smoking induces the P450 isoform CYP1A2, and can therefore increase the metabolism of those compounds metabolised by this enzyme. Smoking accelerates the metabolism of paracetamol, amitriptyline, dextropropoxyphene, chlorpromazine, theophylline, imipramine and caffeine.

19. Chronic alcohol intake **Answers: A E**

Alcohol taken acutely inhibits various enzymes including the P450 enzymes. In contrast, chronic alcohol intake induces the P450 isoform CYP2E1. Alcohol is metabolised mainly by alcohol dehydrogenase and to a lesser extent by CYP2E1. Induction of CYP2E1 by alcohol will increase the proportion of alcohol undergoing metabolism via this pathway. Alcohol also increases the metabolism of paracetamol to its toxic metabolite, and provides an explanation as to why chronic alcoholics are more susceptible to paracetamol hepatotoxicity. The metabolism of phenytoin, tolbutamide and warfarin is also increased in chronic alcoholics.

20. Breast milk **Answers: A B C E**

Toxicity to the infant can occur if the drug enters the breast milk in pharmacologically significant quantities. The British National Formulary is a valuable source of information on drugs to avoid in breast-feeding mothers. Cyclosporin, phenindione (but not warfarin), tetracycline and mefloquine are excreted in amounts significant enough to cause toxicity in the infant. Digoxin is safe in breast-feeding mothers.

21. Drugs and renal diseases **Answers: A D**

The tetracyclines (except doxycycline) can aggravate uraemia dangerously and should be avoided in patients with anything other than minimal renal impairment. Penicillamine, like gold, produces an immune-complex membranous glomerulonephritis, usually presenting with proteinuria. Although procainamide is often responsible for a lupus syndrome, glomerulonephritis is usual in drug-induced SLE.

22. Renal failure **Answers: B E**

Tetracyclines, apart from doxycycline, should be avoided in renal failure as they are antianabolic, causing salt and water loss, raise the blood urea and can lead to permanent loss of nephrons. Nitrofurantoin is prone to give toxic levels and peripheral neuropathy in renal failure. It is also likely to be ineffective for urinary infections. Although aluminium hydroxide is used for phosphate lowering, there are concerns about aluminium retention with prolonged usage.

23. Chronic liver disease **Answers: B D E**

The ability of the diseased liver to detoxify drugs is maintained to a considerable degree. Known hepatotoxins like some anti-TB drugs and phenothiazines should not be used. Drugs that are CNS depressants are likely to have increased efficacy and prolonged duration of action; antidepressants should also be avoided.

24. Acute intermittent porphyria **Answers: A B C E**

Other drugs that should be avoided include sulphonamides, sulphonylureas, barbiturates and griseofulvin. These agents may precipitate acute porphyria by hepatic microsomal enzyme induction of ALA-synthetase, so stimulating the first step in the porphyrin synthetic pathway.

25. Amiodarone **Answers: B E**

Amiodarone has a long half-life (13–102 days). It is a class III anti-arrhythmic which also has some anti-anginal properties. It blocks potassium channels and also has some effects on inactivated sodium and calcium channels. It contains iodine which can affect thyroid function: it can cause both hyperthyroidism and hypothyroidism, the latter being more common than the former. Other adverse effects include hepatotoxicity, skin rashes, pulmonary fibrosis, peripheral neuropathy and corneal microdeposits. It interacts with digoxin by inhibiting its renal and non-renal excretion. It also interacts with warfarin by inhibiting its metabolism.

26. Adenosine **Answers: B D**

Adenosine stimulates adenosine A1 receptors within the heart. It is particularly effective in terminating junctional tachycardias. Arrhythmias arising within the atria are rarely affected by adenosine, although there may be transient AV block, which may aid in making a diagnosis. Adenosine has no effect on ventricular arrhythmias. This property can be used in the diagnosis of true ventricular tachycardia and differentiate it from supraventricular tachycardia with aberrant conduction. Adenosine should be administered while the patient is being monitored and therefore can usually only be used in a hospital setting. It can induce bronchospasm and facial flushing.

27. Negative inotropic action **Answers: A C D**

All calcium channel blockers have some negative inotropic action but this is minimal for some of the dihydropyridine derivatives. Verapamil has most negative inotropic and AV blocking action and diltiazem has intermediate effects. Lisinopril has beneficial effects on cardiac function without intrinsic negative inotropic action. Propafenone, an anti-arrhythmic agent has significant negative inotropic effect and weak beta adrenoceptor blocking action. Bisoprolol is a highly selective beta-1 adrenoceptor antagonist. Thyroxine increases myocardial contractility and oxygen consumption in hypothyroid patients.

28. Calcium channel blockers **Answers: B D**

Calcium channel blockers are mainly used for the treatment of angina and hypertension. There is little correlation between serum levels and the clinical effect in patients. Dihydropyridines may worsen angina via a 'steal' phenomenon, and the short-acting agents may increase mortality in patients with cardiovascular disease. In general, calcium antagonists have not been shown to reduce mortality following myocardial infarction. Like other antihypertensives, calcium antagonists reduce left ventricular mass in hypertensive patients. Verapamil blocks the AV node and will block an increase in heart rate with exercise.

29. Calcium channel blocking drugs **Answers: B C D**

There is much greater variability in this group of drugs than with e.g. beta blockers. Verapamil has the most potent anti-arrhythmic and negatively inotropic activity; dihydropipones like nifedipine are the most potent vasodilators with little direct effect on the heart. Diltiazem has the midway position between them.

30. Enalapril **Answers: A B D**

The most common side-effect is cough which may be dose-dependent. The cough is dry and may require the drugs to be stopped. Acute renal failure is a serious problem but is usually reversible if it is recognised early and the drug stopped. It is thus essential to monitor renal failure.

31. Patients with heart failure **Answers: A D**

ACE inhibitors such as enalapril have been shown to improve prognosis in patients with heart failure. Studies to date have not consistently shown that frusemide and digoxin have a beneficial effect on mortality in patients with heart failure. Verapamil is negatively inotropic and is likely to worsen heart failure. Carvedilol is a mixed α_1 and non-cardioselective β-blocker, with some calcium channel blocking properties. It has the same effects as labetalol in that it causes bradycardia and leads to peripheral vasodilatation. It is licensed for use in hypertension and angina. A recent study has found that carvedilol improved survival in patients with heart failure, followed up for an average of 6.5 months.

32. Nicorandil **Answers: A E**

Nicorandil is a nitrate derivative (and therefore has actions similar to nitrates) which also activates potassium channels in vascular smooth muscle, increasing efflux of potassium ions and inhibiting calcium entry. This results in vasodilatation of venous and arterial vessels including the coronary arteries. Nicorandil is indicated for the prevention and long-term treatment of angina pectoris. Most efficacy studies have been monotherapy studies, and its role as add-on therapy in patients with angina uncontrolled by more conventional treatments is unknown. The effects on the circulation resemble those of an organic nitrate and a calcium channel blocker: thus, nicorandil will reduce vascular resistance, LV filling pressure, and blood pressure. In patients with heart failure, nicorandil has been shown to increase cardiac output by 17–55%. Tolerance does not occur probably because of the effects of the drug on potassium channels.

33. Moxonidine in hypertension **Answers: C D**

Moxonidine is a centrally-acting antihypertensive; it acts as an agonist at the imidazoline (I1) receptor. Unlike the $\alpha 2$ receptor agonists such as clonidine, it does not induce sedation and drowsiness. Tolerance to the antihypertensive effects of moxonidine does not occur, and there is no rebound hypertension on stopping the drug. It is as efficacious as the other first-line agents, and may have an additive effect with thiazide diuretics. It has the advantage of having a beneficial effect on insulin sensitivity and glucose metabolism, and causes regression of LV hypertrophy, and functional improvement in congestive cardiac failure.

34. Minoxidil **Answers: A D E**

Minoxidil is a prodrug, the active metabolite of which dilates arterioles selectively rather than veins. Inactivation is by further liver metabolism. A compensatory increase in heart rate prompts combination therapy. Oedema is common and most patients require a diuretic. Hypertrichosis is troublesome in women: it resolves about three months after drug withdrawal. The tachycardia can induce angina but the ECG changes are seldom accompanied by symptoms.

35. Alteplase **Answer: B**

Alteplase is a serine protease which has a low affinity for free plasminogen but rapidly activates plasminogen bound to fibrin in a thrombus. Streptokinase and urokinase in contrast act on both free and fibrin-bound plasminogen. It has higher fibrin specificity and lower antigenicity when compared with streptokinase. Its half-life is shorter (about 5 min) than that of streptokinase (30 min). Trials to date have suggested that there may be a higher incidence of cerebral haemorrhage compared with streptokinase, although it may show higher efficacy in certain patient groups (i.e. young patients with anterior myocardial infarction). It is approved for treatment in acute ischaemic stroke; this has not been shown to reduce mortality but may reduce long-term disability.

36. Platelet function **Answers: A C D**

Aspirin, ticlopidine and abciximab all affect platelet function, and thus are being used in patients with ischaemic heart disease. Aspirin, by inhibiting cyclo-oxygenase, prevents the formation of thromboxane, a potent aggregator of platelets. Abciximab is a monoclonal antibody which is a potent inhibitor of the platelet glycoprotein IIb/IIIa receptor. This receptor binds fibrinogen, which promotes the aggregation of platelets. Hirudin is a potent direct inhibitor of thrombin.

37. Serum LDL cholesterol **Answers: A B D**

By inhibiting the synthesis of cholesterol in the liver from acetate, HMG CoA reductase inhibitors (statins) reduce hepatic secretion of LDL cholesterol. Cholestyramine binds bile acids in the gut, preventing their reabsorption and encouraging the synthesis of new bile acids from hepatic cholesterol. All fibrates reduce LDL cholesterol by a variety of mechanisms and also reduce plasma triglyceride. Marine oils lower triglyceride concentrations and may exacerbate hypercholesterolaemia. Propranolol produces a small rise in LDL cholesterol and a small fall in HDL cholesterol.

38. Simvastatin **Answers: A D**

Simvastatin is a HMG-CoA reductase inhibitor, which is highly effective in reducing cholesterol levels, and triglycerides to a lesser extent. It is less effective at raising HDL levels than fibrates. Its major adverse effects are muscle pain, increase in creatine phosphokinase levels and occasionally rhabdomyolysis. Several cases of rhabdomyolysis have been reported on co-prescription of simvastatin with the novel T-type calcium channel blocker mibefradil (which has now been withdrawn). It should not be used in patients with acute porphyria. Cholestyramine indirectly increases the faecal loss of cholesterol.

39. Glibenclamide **Answer: B**

Glibenclamide has a relatively long biological half life although it is shorter than chlorpropamide. Unfortunately, it also has biologically active metabolites with a long half life which are excreted by the kidney. This therefore precludes the use of glibenclamide in patients with renal impairment. It should be used with caution in the elderly. Gliclazide is metabolised by the liver to inactive metabolites and is therefore the sulphonylurea of choice in patients with renal impairment. Despite strong protein binding, all sulphonylureas cross the placenta, producing fetal hyperinsulinaemia and predisposing to macrosomia and neonatal hypoglycaemia. All sulphonylureas act by stimulating insulin secretion which inhibits gluconeogenesis.

40. Anti-thyroid drugs **Answers: A D**

The mainstay of treatment for thyrotoxicosis is the thionamides (carbimazole and propylthiouracil). Both inhibit the iodination of tyrosine and coupling of iodotyrosines. In addition, propylthiouracil inhibits the peripheral conversion of T4 to T3. It usually takes 4–8 weeks for these drugs to have an effect. In that time, β-blockers are useful: they block the adrenergic effects of excess thyroid hormone such as sweating and tremor, but have no effect on basal metabolic rate. In euthyroid subjects, an excess of iodide from any source can cause a goitre. Radioactive iodine emits mainly β radiation (90%) which penetrates only 0.5 mm of tissue. It does emit some of the more penetrating γ rays which can be detected with a Geiger counter.

41. Radioiodine therapy **Answer: A**

A woman should avoid breast-feeding for at least eight weeks following radioiodine therapy to ensure that the level of radioactivity in breast milk is down to background values. Pregnancy should be avoided for at least four months after radioiodine therapy. Radioiodine is not suitable for patients with thyroiditis or those with iodine-induced hyperthyroidism, because iodine uptake by the thyroid is low in these disorders. Radioiodine may exacerbate Graves' ophthalmopathy, although this is controversial. About 50–75% of patients have normal thyroid function and shrinkage of thyroid goitre within 6–8 weeks of being given radioiodine. Radioiodine can be used in the treatment of thyroid cancer; metastases cannot be treated simultaneously since they will not take up iodine in the presence of functioning thyroid tissue.

42. Status epilepticus **Answers: A C**

Seizures are stopped by first-line therapy in 80% of patients if treatment is begun within 30 minutes of the onset of seizures, while the response rate drops down to less than 40% when treatment is begun two hours after the onset of seizures. Both lorazepam and diazepam are equally effective in controlling seizures; although diazepam has a quicker onset of action, lorazepam has a longer duration of anti-seizure effect (12–24 hours) than diazepam (15–30 minutes). Out of hospital, diazepam should be administered rectally; it is 80% effective in controlling prolonged seizures in children, usually within 15 minutes. Intravenous phenytoin can cause thrombophlebitis, hypotension (28–50%) and cardiac arrhythmias (bradycardia and ectopic beats, 2%).

43. Phenytoin **Answers: B E**

Adverse effects with a frequency of > 1 in 100 can be defined as common. Phenytoin commonly causes various dose-dependent toxicities such as ataxia, nystagmus and dizziness. Like other anticonvulsants, phenytoin is also associated with cognitive deficits such as memory impairment. Skin rashes may occur in up to 16% of patients on beginning therapy; starting at a low dose and increasing the dose slowly may reduce the frequency of rashes. Aplastic anaemia and IgA deficiency are rare adverse effects of phenytoin.

44. Migraine **Answers: A B E**

Migraine can be prevented by β-blockers (propranolol, metoprolol, atenolol, nadolol and timolol), pizotifen, methysergide, flunarizine and sodium valproate. The triptans are used in the treatment of an acute attack. Sumatriptan has no effect on the aura of migraine and it should be taken as soon as the headache starts. Triptans exhibit highly selective and potent agonist activity at the 1B, 1D, 1F and 1A 5HT receptors. Stimulation of the 5-HT1D receptor inhibits CGRP release and thus dural vasodilatation. Sumatriptan can cause ‘chest symptoms’ in 40% of patients, and in some patients with pre-existing coronary artery disease, sumatriptan has been associated with myocardial ischaemia. It is therefore contraindicated in patients with coronary artery disease. Ergot derivatives have also been used for acute attacks but are associated with peripheral and coronary vasoconstriction.

45. Donepezil **Answer: C**

Donepezil is a new treatment for Alzheimer's disease. It inhibits acetylcholinesterase, the enzyme responsible for acetylcholine breakdown, and therefore, enhances the action of acetylcholine. Donepezil improves rating scales of cognitive function and the global rating scores in some patients with mild-to-moderate disease; however, this effect is not predictable. There is no evidence that donepezil improves either quality of life (of both patient and carer) or day-to-day functioning. Adverse effects are those associated with enhanced cholinergic activity including diarrhoea, muscle cramps, nausea, vomiting and insomnia. There have also been reports of hallucinations, agitation and aggressive behaviour, which improved when the drug was stopped or the dose reduced.

46. Guillain-Barré syndrome **Answers: A B C**

Guillain-Barré syndrome (GBS) has an incidence of 1–2 per 100,000. About 8% of patients will die and 10% are severely disabled one year later. The aetiological factors are unclear but an autoimmune pathogenesis is thought likely. Antibodies to ganglioside GM1 are present in 25% of patients; these can therefore not be used for either diagnosis or monitoring therapy. If a patient requires ventilatory support, depolarising agents such as suxamethonium should be avoided as they can open up potassium channels and induce hyperkalaemia, especially in denervated muscle. Plasma exchange and intravenous immunoglobulin are equally effective in hastening recovery in patients, although the latter is more practical and associated with fewer adverse effects. Corticosteroids have not been shown to be of benefit in randomised controlled trials.

47. Benzodiazepine anxiolytics **Answers: C E**

Negligible evidence supports the numerous claims of differences in the pharmacodynamics of the dozen or so available benzodiazepines. They do however differ in their duration of action. Triazolam, temazepam and oxazepam are short-acting (plasma concentration half time less than 10 hours). The remainder persist in the body for a long time (e.g. diazepam and its active metabolites) with a half time of up to three days in the elderly. Metabolism is mainly by oxidation then to glucuronide conjugates. The increase in body sway predisposes to falls, especially in the elderly.

48. Tricyclic antidepressants **Answers: A B C**

The tricyclic antidepressants have a number of important side-effects. There are five main groups. Autonomic effects: dry mouth, blurred vision, urinary retention, constipation, postural hypotension, tachycardia and increased sweating. Tricyclics are contraindicated in glaucoma. Psychiatric effects include sedation, acute confusional states. Cardiovascular effects include ECG changes such as prolonged PR and QT intervals, depressed ST segment and flattened T waves. Ventricular tachycardias may develop, usually where there is heart disease. Neurological effects include fine tremor, inco-ordination, headaches, epileptic fits, peripheral neuropathy. Others are allergic rashes, cholestatic jaundice and agranulocytosis. Tricyclic anti-depressants may be used in patients with ischaemic heart disease, with caution. They are safe in patients anticoagulated with warfarin.

49. Phenothiazines **Answers: A B D E**

Other clinically important side-effects of phenothiazine therapy include orthostatic hypotension and the extra-pyramidal syndromes.

50. Lithium carbonate **Answers: A C E**

Almost all patients taking lithium carbonate report polydipsia and polyuria, due to interference with ADH action in the kidney. A high serum lithium concentration causes gastrointestinal disturbances, weakness and fine tremor of the hands, but not an intention tremor. There is a risk of hypothyroidism in patients taking lithium, due to effects on intrathyroid iodine metabolism.

51. Cytotoxic chemotherapeutic agents **Answers: All true**

Cytotoxic chemotherapeutic agents act on the proliferative and not the resting phase of the cell cycle. As such, they can affect both proliferating malignant and normal cells including those in the bone marrow and gut mucosa. A dose usually kills a given percentage rather than a given number of tumour cells. Chemotherapeutic agents are often given intermittently in high doses, and are often combined, the rationale being that drugs acting by different mechanisms should enhance response and reduce toxicity. The drugs kill tumour cells by inducing programmed cell death, of which apoptosis is the most common form.

52. Chemotherapeutic agents — Answers: A B

Methotrexate is an antimetabolite which inhibits the conversion of folic acid to dihydrofolic acid and of this to tetrahydrofolic acid (essential to DNA synthesis). Alkylating agents denature preformed DNA: they include mustine, chlorambucil, melphalan and cyclophosphamide. Vinblastine and vincristine are vinca alkaloids which disrupt microtubular proteins and interfere with metaphase in dividing cells. Cytosine arabinoside is a pyrimidine analogue and azathioprine is a purine analogue: both inhibit DNA synthesis. Anti-cancer drugs have greatest activity and toxicity in rapidly dividing tissues where there is less time for DNA repair or synthesis between cell divisions.

53. Methotrexate — Answers: B D

Methotrexate is a dihydrofolate reductase inhibitor that is used in both malignant and non-malignant diseases (e.g. rheumatoid arthritis, psoriasis and graft-versus-host-disease). It is used in children for diseases such as juvenile chronic arthritis. The drug has also been used in asthma: one study has shown that methotrexate reduced prednisolone dose in 50% of patients, compared with the placebo arm where there was a reduction in steroids in 14% of patients. Like most cytotoxics, there is no relationship between plasma concentrations and therapeutic effect. Methotrexate causes mucositis which develops 3–7 days after its administration. NSAIDs such as naproxen can precipitate methotrexate toxicity: this is secondary to displacement of methotrexate from protein binding sites and inhibition of its excretion via the proximal convoluted tubule.

54. Lignocaine — Answers: B C

Lignocaine is a local anaesthetic and an antiarrhythmic (class IIb). As a local anaesthetic, it prevents conduction but not generation of nerve impulses, and is used topically or subcutaneously. As an antiarrhythmic, it is used intravenously for the treatment of ventricular arrhythmias, particularly those following myocardial infarction. It can cause CNS toxicity (tremor and convulsions) and arrhythmias. It can occasionally lead to methaemoglobinaemia (particularly in infants), but its potential to do this is much less than that observed with ester local anaesthetics such as prilocaine.

55. Halothane **Answers: B C D**

Halothane is a halogenated hydrocarbon; it is a potent anaesthetic but weak analgesic. It causes atropine-sensitive bradycardia, increases the tendency to arrhythmias (especially in patients with hypercapnia), increases the myocardial sensitivity to catecholamines, and produces hypotension (which may require treatment with a vasoconstrictor such as phenylephrine). It is also associated with a severe and often fatal form of hepatitis which occurs more frequently in patients who have had multiple exposures to halothane.

56. Inhaled corticosteroids **Answers: B C D E**

Systemic corticosteroids are associated with a large number of serious adverse effects. The use of inhaled steroids in patients with asthma has the advantage of local delivery of the steroid to the lung with minimal systemic side-effects. Inhaled steroids do have local adverse effects which include oral candida and hoarseness. More recently, they have been shown to have systemic effects including adrenal suppression with high-dose therapy. The use of inhaled steroids has also been associated with the development of posterior subcapsular and nuclear cataracts, open angle glaucoma, osteoporosis, skin thinning and bruising, and growth retardation.

57. Terfenadine **Answers: A B**

Terfenadine is a non-sedating oral antihistamine. It is a pro-drug and its levels cannot normally be detected in the plasma since it is converted by cytochrome P450 enzymes (P450 3A4 in particular) to fexofenadine, which has antihistamine actions. On administration of the P450 inhibitors such as ketoconazole, erythromycin, and grapefruit juice, the metabolism of terfenadine will be inhibited leading to an increase in plasma levels. This can affect potassium channels within the myocardium leading to QT interval prolongation and torsades des pointes (polymorphic ventricular tachycardia) in some individuals. The interaction led to a number of sudden deaths worldwide. Terfenadine is now only available on prescription in the UK.

58. Morphine **Answer: E**

Morphine is detoxicated mainly by conjugation with glucuronic acid in the liver and should be used with caution in cirrhosis. Pin-point pupils (severe miosis) are an important sign of intoxication or addiction with opiates. Intestinal smooth muscle tone is increased and propulsive waves diminished, explaining the constipating effects of these drugs. The therapeutic effect of morphine in acute left ventricular failure is probably largely due to its venodilating action.

59. Drug associations **Answers: A B D**

Drugs which may produce pulmonary fibrosis include amiodarone, busulphan, melphalan, cyclophosphamide and bleomycin. Pulmonary oedema may occur as an adverse reaction to hydrochlorothiazide, phenylbutazone, β_2 agonists and bleomycins. Barbiturates may produce profound respiratory depression. Phenytoin is one of a number of drugs which have been associated with a lupus-like syndrome; others include hydralazine, procainamide and isoniazid. Prostaglandin F2 alpha is a potent bronchoconstrictor and prostaglandin E2 is a bronchodilator although this has yet to be exploited therapeutically.

60. Antiviral therapies **Answers: B D E**

Amantadine is active against influenza A and administered prophylactically is as effective as vaccination. The role of AZT in asymptomatic HIV infection is still controversial but no trial has shown proven benefit for patients with a CD4 count of over 500.

61. Generalised pruritus **Answers: A B C**

Treatment of the underlying cause is important in patients with generalised pruritus. However, symptomatic relief may be provided by antihistamines such as hydroxyzine, which probably act via their sedative or anxiolytic effect. Chlorpromazine or trimeprazine may also provide relief. The itching of obstructive jaundice may be relieved by cholestyramine if the obstruction is partial. Codeine may cause pruritus.

62. Aminoglycosides **Answers: B C E**

Once daily aminoglycosides are recommended for simple infections such as urinary tract infections, but not for complicated infections such as endocarditis. Due to the high cardiac output in patients with Paget's disease, the half-life of aminoglycosides is reduced and thus once-daily dosing is inappropriate. They are used parenterally and are active against Gram-positive and Gram-negative organisms. Streptococci are intrinsically resistant unless the aminoglycoside is combined with a penicillin. Aminoglycosides are concentrated within the renal cortex, and levels can reach 10–50 times that found in plasma, which may cause renal damage.

63. Ciprofloxacin **Answers: C D E**

Ciprofloxacin inhibits the enzyme DNA gyrase, and in this way prevents DNA synthesis. It is particularly active against Gram-negative bacteria, including *Salmonella, Shigella, Campylobacter, Neisseria,* and *Pseudomonas.* Ciprofloxacin only has moderate activity against Gram-positive bacteria such as *Streptococcus pneumoniae* and is therefore not the drug of first choice for pneumococcal pneumonia. It is active against *Chlamydia* and some mycobacteria. Most anaerobic organisms are not susceptible. It interferes with GABA action within the CNS and may therefore lead to seizures; it should therefore be used with caution in epileptics. It can also lead to tenosynovitis (the drug should be withdrawn), and inhibits the metabolism of theophylline, which can precipitate theophylline toxicity (convulsions and arrhythmias).

64. Rifampicin **Answers: A B D**

Rifampicin is a potent enzyme inducer and can produce clinically significant interactions with cyclosporin, warfarin, oral contraceptives and methadone, to name a few. It is effective against intra- (such as mycobacteria) and extra-cellular organisms. Apart from TB, uses include leprosy, Legionnaires' disease and chemoprophylaxis of meningococcal meningitis. Intermittent dosing can lead to a flu-like illness, haemolysis and renal failure. Red discoloration of urine, tears and sputum is seen in patients on the drug. Orange discoloration is also seen in patients who wear soft contact lenses.

65. Tetracycline **Answer: E**

Tetracycline is a bacteriostatic drug whose mode of action involves binding to ribosomes and inhibition of protein synthesis. Its absorption is reduced by food and it is not extensively metabolised. It can therefore accumulate in patients with renal impairment, and apart from doxycycline, none of the tetracyclines should be used in renal failure. The following organisms are rarely susceptible to tetracycline: *Enterococcus faecalis, Pseudomonas aeruginosa, Streptococcus* Group B, *Proteus* species and *Serratia* species. The efficacy of oral contraceptives is reduced by tetracycline resulting in unwanted pregnancy. The anticoagulant effect of warfarin is enhanced. The oral absorption of tetracycline is reduced by calcium, bismuth, iron, magnesium or zinc salts, antacids or milk, or with quinapril or sucralfate.

66. Co-trimoxazole in HIV-positive patients Answers: A C E

Prophylaxis against *Pneumocystis carinii* pneumonia (PCP) is recommended in HIV-positive patients with CD4 cell counts of less than 200/ml, and also in patients with immunosuppression due to other causes. Co-trimoxazole (but not trimethoprim by itself) has been shown to be more effective for both prophylaxis and treatment than the other drugs which are available including pentamidine, dapsone-trimethoprim and clindamycin-primaquine. Sulphamethoxazole and trimethoprim inhibit sequential steps in the folic acid synthesis pathway (dihydropteroate synthetase and dihydrofolate reductase are the enzymes that are inhibited). Rash is the most common side-effect occurring in 50% of patients during treatment of acute PCP and 30% when used for prophylaxis.

67. Antibiotics and their adverse effects Answers: B C E

Fusidic acid is associated with liver dysfunction rather than nephrotoxicity. Vancomycin can cause flushing of the upper half of the body (termed 'red man' syndrome). This occurs during rapid infusion and may be due to histamine release. Cefotaxime and other cephalosporins have been reported to cause haemolysis, although this is uncommon. Metronidazole is associated with a sensory neuropathy on long-term use. Minocycline on prolonged therapy has been associated with autoimmune hepatitis which may be accompanied by arthralgia and positive antinuclear antibodies.

68. Ketoconazole Answers: A E

Ketoconazole is useful in treating systemic mycoses, but is also available for topical use. It blocks the demethylation of lanosterol to ergosterol by inhibiting C-14 a-demethylase in fungal cells. It is a broad spectrum agent, and can be either fungistatic or fungicidal depending on dose. It antagonises the effects of amphotericin. It causes hepatic toxicity rather than renal toxicity. In high doses, it inhibits the steroid synthesis enzymes in humans and can lead to endocrine adverse effects. It also inhibits the P450 enzymes and can thus lead to interactions with drugs such as terfenadine, astemizole, cyclosporin and phenytoin.

69. Hyperprolactinaemia **Answers: A B E**

Hyperprolactinaemia is associated with (a) dopamine receptor antagonists (including risperidone), (b) drugs impairing CNS dopamine function via a separate pathway (e.g. methyldopa), (c) drugs enhancing serotoninergic transmission (e.g. fenfluramine), (d) serotonin re-uptake inhibitors (e.g. fluvoxamine), (e) H_1-receptor agonists, and (f) H_2-receptor antagonists (e.g. cimetidine). Sodium valproate is a GABA-mimetic drug while ergotamine is a direct-acting dopamine receptor agonist: both actions inhibit prolactin release. Indirect-acting dopamine receptor agonists, drugs impairing serotoninergic action, histamine H_2-receptor agonists and cholinergic receptor agonists also inhibit prolactin release.

70. Glucose tolerance **Answers: A B D**

Thiazide diuretics are associated with a risk of developing diabetes. The effect is dose related being more likely with bendrofluazide in a dose of 5–10 mg daily. The low dose of 2.5 mg daily has little effect on glucose tolerance and the very low dose of 1.25 mg has no effect. Corticosteroids such as prednisolone increase blood glucose, especially if high doses are used for a prolonged period. Oestrogens are associated with impaired glucose tolerance but development of diabetes is very unlikely.

71. QT interval prolongation **Answers: B C D E**

QT interval prolongation is usually drug-induced but is also seen in patients with hypokalaemia, extreme bradycardia, or may be congenital. QT interval prolongation may sometimes lead to torsades des pointes, which can degenerate into ventricular fibrillation, causing sudden death. Drugs causing QT interval prolongation include antidepressants (particularly older generation tricyclic antidepressants), antipsychotics (including typical antipsychotics such as thioridazine, and atypical antipsychotics such as sertindole), antiarrhythmics (particularly class Ia and III drugs), antihistamines (terfenadine and astemizole), and other drugs including halofantrine, erythromycin, ciprofloxacin and cisapride.

72. Thrombocytopenia **Answers: B C D E**

Quinine, quinidine and heparin are the drugs most likely to produce thrombocytopenia. They induce production of platelet damaging antibodies. NSAIDs, gold and thiazides are a lesser risk, the mechanism being unclear. Chloramphenicol depresses platelet production.

73. Haemolysis **Answers: A B C E**

Drugs causing haemolytic anaemia in G6PD deficiency:

Antimalarials:	primaquine, chloroquine
Sulphonamides:	sulphanilamide, sulphamethoxazole, sulphapyridine
Sulphones:	dapsone
Nitrofurans:	nitrofurantoin
Miscellaneous:	ciprofloxacin, methylene blue, nalidixic acid, niridazole, naphthalene.

74. Acute renal failure **Answers: A B C D**

ACE inhibitors cause renal failure in patients with bilateral renal artery stenosis by causing vasodilatation of the efferent glomerular arteriole leading to a drop in the glomerular filtration rate. Penicillins can lead to interstitial nephritis, while sulphonamides can cause both interstitial nephritis and crystalluria. With mesalazine, the mechanism is unclear, but interstitial nephritis and papillary necrosis may be involved.

75. Parkinson-like extrapyramidal effects **Answers: A C E**

Parkinson-like effects are brought about by dopaminergic deficit in the nigrostriatal tracts. Drugs which antagonise the action of dopamine at receptors in this area and thus produce the effects, are the neuroleptics, haloperidol, prochlorperazine and trifluoperazine. Imipramine is a central muscarinic antagonist of acetylcholine and phenytoin is likewise without action at dopamine receptors.

76. Retinopathy **Answers: B C D E**

Retinopathy can be caused by chloroquine, tamoxifen, thioridazine, tacrolimus, desferrioxamine and vigabatrin. Most clinical experience has been gained with chloroquine and hydroxychloroquine when used in rheumatoid arthritis. The retinopathy is dose-dependent and is only seen when the drugs are used long-term. Patients should be warned to stop taking the drug and seek medical advice if they notice any disturbance in vision.

77. Diarrhoea **Answers: A D E**

Of the antacids, magnesium-based compounds will cause diarrhoea while aluminium-based compounds cause constipation. Verapamil affects calcium channels in the large bowel leading to constipation in about 8–10% of the population. Misoprostol and colchicine both cause diarrhoea.

78. Withdrawal syndrome **Answers: A D E**

Abrupt withdrawal of paroxetine and to a lesser extent of other selective serotonin re-uptake inhibitors has been associated with a withdrawal syndrome. Withdrawal of the serotonin noradrenaline re-uptake inhibitor venlafaxine can also lead to a withdrawal syndrome. Abrupt discontinuation of diazepam can precipitate seizures. Other symptoms of withdrawal include anxiety, agitation, irritability, confusion, tremor, headache and diarrhoea.

79. Drug-induced anaphylaxis **Answers: B D E**

Drug-induced anaphylaxis is mediated by IgE antibodies linking to Fc receptors on mast cell surface, with consequent release of vasoactive mediators. Anaphylaxis to drugs such as penicillin is more common in atopic patients. A history of prior sensitisation may not be available: for drugs such as penicillin, covert exposure may have occurred, for example through cows' milk. The severity of anaphylaxis increases with parenteral administration of the drug. Prophylactic steroids have no effect on the occurrence of such reactions.

80. Overdosage **Answers: B D**

Plasma monitoring is of prime value in the management of paracetamol and salicylate poisoning. It has a role with theophylline, barbiturates, iron and lithium. Tricyclic concentrations are difficult to measure and reflect toxicity poorly. Beta blocker and digoxin toxicity are better assessed by bioassay, i.e. pulse rate and cardiac output.

81. Aspirin overdose **Answers: C D E**

Salicylate is secreted into the stomach long after ingestion. A respiratory alkalosis is the commonest metabolic abnormality in adults, but is only transient in children who develop metabolic acidosis more readily. Although peritoneal dialysis removes salicylate effectively, it is not used unless an alkaline diuresis is not possible. Salicylates impair carbohydrate metabolism.

82. Paracetamol poisoning **Answer: D**

Paracetamol toxicity after self-poisoning is the result of increased production of an alkylating metabolite. Enzyme inducers like tobacco increase metabolite production and hence toxicity whilst enzyme inhibitors like cimetidine have the reverse effect. The earliest sign of liver damage, and the most useful prognostic indicator, is the prothrombin time; values less than 100 seconds after 3–4 days are rarely associated with death. If recovery occurs it is complete.

83. Paracetamol overdosage **Answers: A C**

Paracetamol in overdosage causes hepatotoxicity via the formation of a toxic metabolite by the cytochrome P450 enzymes, which causes depletion of glutathione in the liver. The formation of the toxic metabolite is increased in chronic alcoholics (who also have a hepatic glutathione deficiency) and in patients on enzyme-inducing anticonvulsants (phenytoin, phenobarbitone and carbamazepine). Cimetidine may potentially prevent the formation of the toxic metabolite and thus protect against hepatotoxicity. Children have higher sulphation capacity and may therefore form smaller amounts of the toxic metabolite.

84. Severe poisoning with iron **Answers: B D**

Iron overdose is more common in children than in adults. Severe poisoning is characterised by haematemesis, hypotension, coma and shock. Disintegrating tablets may make the stools grey or black in colour, and this does not necessarily indicate a gastrointestinal bleed. A white cell count of $> 15 \times 10^9$/l and blood glucose level > 8.3 mmol/l in the six hours after ingestion, together with the presence of tablets on abdominal X-ray, have been shown to correlate with serum iron concentrations > 54 mmol/l. A challenge dose of desferrioxamine, if it results in urine with a red/orange colour, indicates the presence of free circulating iron, and is an indication for further treatment with desferrioxamine.

85. Digoxin toxicity **Answers: A D**

Digoxin is a narrow therapeutic index drug. Toxicity (even when levels are within the therapeutic range) can be precipitated by hypokalaemia, hypomagnesaemia and hypercalcaemia. Changes in the plasma sodium concentration have no effect on digoxin toxicity *per se*. Digoxin toxicity may manifest with symptoms such as nausea, vomiting, xanthopsia or ECG changes such as ST depression (reversed tick pattern) or cardiac arrhythmias. Phenytoin can be used to treat digoxin-induced cardiac arrhythmias.

86. Lithium poisoning **Answers: C E**

Severe poisoning, when lithium is taken in overdose, is characterised by diarrhoea, coma, seizures, muscle tremor, cerebellar ataxia and nephrogenic diabetes insipidus. There may also be apparent hyperkalaemia.

87. Atropine poisoning **Answers: A E**

Atropine poisoning produces parasympathetic blockade and toxic psychosis characterised by mania, hallucinations and delirium. There is dry mouth, dilated pupils, a dry, flushed skin, fever, tachycardia, urinary retention and abdominal distension. Atropine-like drugs used for Parkinsonism and gastrointestinal disorders can give the same picture.

88. Theophylline overdosage **Answers: C E**

The two major problems of serious overdosage are intractable vomiting and hypokalaemia; intravenous potassium supplementation may be required. Convulsions tend to occur after moderate/severe overdosage and should be treated with repeated doses of diazepam. The most effective method of theophylline excretion is the use of repeated doses of activated charcoal after gastric lavage. Haemoperfusion should be reserved for patients unable to tolerate charcoal and for the seriously ill patient having severe acidosis, coma or circulatory instability in addition to a very high theophylline level.

DERMATOLOGY: ANSWERS AND EXPLANATIONS

1. Alopecia areata **Answers: B D E**

Hair loss, which is commonly asymptomatic in alopecia areata, may occur at any site. Most of the follicles retain the ability to form new hairs. Alopecia areata may be associated with frank or subclinical autoimmune thyroid disease and with Down's syndrome. Nail pitting or roughness is commonly found in alopecia areata.

2. Changes to the nail **Answers: A B C E**

Dilated capillaries around the distal nail fold are a feature of dermatomyositis. The nails in psoriasis show pitting and onycholysis. The nails may be deformed and lost in dystrophic forms of epidermolysis bullosa, although it is uncommon to see changes in the simple form of the disease. Beau's lines are transverse grooves across the nail plate and result from altered growth during a period of severe illness.

3. Exfoliative dermatitis **Answers: A D E**

Exfoliative dermatitis (erythroderma) will contribute to congestive cardiac failure by virtue of the increased blood flow in the skin, a factor also tending to hypo- not hyperthermia. Pruritus is common and not indicative of an underlying lymphoma. Psoriasis is responsible for about 25% of cases of exfoliative dermatitis. Lymphadenopathy is often marked with exfoliative dermatitis, constituting so-called dermatopathic lymphadenopathy.

4. Bullae **Answers: A B D E**

Orf is a pox virus which causes a stomatitis in lambs and is transmitted to the hands of humans involved in their feeding. Eczema of the palms and soles usually develops large bullae hence the term 'pompholyx' (Greek for 'bubble'). Erythema nodosum does not develop bullae, but severe erythema multiforme may do. The bullae in pemphigoid are subepidermal and are more often intact than those in pemphigus which occur within the epidermis.

5. Dermatitis herpetiformis **Answers: A B D E**

The diagnosis of dermatitis herpetiformis is confirmed by the presence of IgA antibodies deposited in a granular pattern at the dermo-epidermal junction of uninvolved skin. A rapid response to dapsone is characteristic. Although most patients have a gluten-sensitive enteropathy, malabsorption is rare. There is an increased incidence of malignancy, particularly gastrointestinal lymphoma.

6. Strawberry naevi **Answers: B E**

Strawberry naevi may be single or multiple. The lesions usually enlarge during the first year and usually resolve spontaneously over the next few years. Surgical treatment is not recommended unless the lesion involves vital structures e.g. the larynx. There is no predisposition to malignant change. Large or rapidly expanding naevi can lead to platelet consumption and depletion of circulating clotting factors (Kasabach-Merritt syndrome).

7. Erythema nodosum **Answers: A B C**

Erythema nodosum may be due to underlying systemic disease e.g. Crohn's disease, ulcerative colitis, Behçet's disease and sarcoidosis. It can be caused by various drugs, notably sulphonamides and oral contraceptives, and by preceding infection, especially streptococcal.

8. Purpuric skin lesions **Answers: B C**

Perifollicular haemorrhages are a feature of vitamin C deficiency. Hypovitaminosis A presents with dry skin, follicular hyperkeratosis and xerophthalmia. T cell lymphoma may present with purpuric skin lesions. Both long-term topical and systemic corticosteroid therapy may cause easy bruising and skin fragility.

9. Immunocompromised patients **Answers: A B C D E**

Transplant patients have an increased incidence of viral warts and squamous cell carcinoma as a result of long-term immunosuppressive therapy. Kaposi's sarcoma is a characteristic finding in sexually transmitted HIV disease, although it is unusual in patients who acquired the condition through blood transfusion or intravenous drug abuse, suggesting it may be due to a different infectious agent. Classical Kaposi's sarcoma occurs in Africans, European Jews and in people from the Po valley area of Italy. Seborrhoeic dermatitis is a feature of AIDS and may be due to overgrowth of pityrosporum yeast. Scabies infestation is more florid in the immunocompromised.

10. Drugs **Answers: A B C D E**

Virtually all drugs can cause cutaneous reactions. It is important to recognise that some drug-induced rashes may mimic specific types of skin disease. Lichen planus-like reactions may occur with gold, antimalarials, phenothiazones and captopril. Skin pigmentation may be induced by antimalarials, phenothiazines and minocycline. Oral contraceptives may produce chloasma. Exfoliative dermatitis may result from gold therapy. Aspirin may cause urticaria in patients with salicylate hypersensitivity, and can exacerbate idiopathic urticaria as a result of its pharmacological action. Thiazides, sulphonamides, tetracyclines and phenothiazines may cause a photosensitive rash.

ENDOCRINOLOGY: ANSWERS AND EXPLANATIONS

1. Actions of glucagon **Answers: A C E**

Glucagon is secreted by the pancreas in response to hypoglycaemia. It elevates blood glucose by increasing hepatic glucose production through gluconeogenesis and glycogenolysis, both actions being mediated by cyclic AMP. Paradoxically, glucagon stimulates insulin secretion. Its positive inotropic action has been exploited occasionally in the treatment of severe beta blocker poisoning.

2. Diabetes mellitus **Answer: E**

Whereas pruritus and in particular genital pruritus is a common feature of diabetes mellitus, it is not diagnostic. Similarly, diabetes insipidus, hypercalcaemia and hypokalaemia may all present with polyuria. Glycosuria is most commonly due to diabetes but renal glycosuria (low threshold) must be considered. The fasting venous plasma glucose must exceed 7.8 mmol/l to confirm the diagnosis and the value 2 hours after a 75 g glucose tolerance test must be > 11.0 mmol/l. Note that the diagnostic values differ according to whether glucose is measured in capillary whole blood, venous whole blood or venous plasma – the latter is used most commonly in the UK.

3. Insulin dependent diabetes (IDDM) **Answers: A B**

Islet cell antibodies are present in over 90% of patients with IDDM (type 1 diabetes) at presentation. 20 years after diagnosis, only 10% of patients retain islet cell antibodies and these patients are more likely to have other organ-specific autoimmune disease (type 1b diabetes). Several HLA types have been found with increased frequency in patients with IDDM, including DR3, DR4 B8 and B15. Twin studies indicate a much lower concordance in type 1 compared to type 2 (NIDDM) diabetes. Although there have been 'outbreaks' of diabetes associated with viral infection, this remains uncommon. In contrast to NIDDM complications of any form are rare at presentation in IDDM.

4. Diabetic glomerulosclerosis **Answer: C**

Mild proteinuria is the first clinical feature of diabetic glomerulosclerosis and is frequently associated with retinopathy and neuropathy. Hypertension often develops later and may exacerbate the condition, but amyloid is not a complication. Nodular sclerosis, although the most specific form of diabetic nephropathy, accounts for less than 20% of renal involvement.

5. Insulin resistance **Answers: B D**

Insulin resistance is a feature of NIDDM, obesity and hypertension. There is associated hyperinsulinaemia, hypertriglyceridaemia and reduced HDL cholesterol. The defect is thought to be post-receptor and can be improved by physical training. Acanthosis nigricans is a cutaneous marker of insulin resistance, occurring in patients with obesity, polycystic ovary syndrome and acromegaly (it is also associated with internal malignancy).

6. Hypoglycaemia **Answers: A B C E**

Hypoglycaemia is one of the characteristic biochemical findings in acute adrenal insufficiency (adrenal crisis); others include acidosis, hyperkalaemia, hyponatraemia and hypercalcaemia. Retroperitoneal tumours are always included in the differential diagnosis of spontaneous hypoglycaemia, as is an insulinoma, which may be a part of MEN type I (pancreas, pituitary, parathyroid). Alcohol impairs hepatic glucose production and may precipitate hypoglycaemia, particularly in otherwise well-controlled insulin-treated diabetics. Glycogen storage diseases that involve the liver (as in von Gierke's disease) may cause hypoglycaemia.

7. Total serum thyroxine levels **Answers: B C E**

Both pregnancy and oral oestrogen administration lead to increased secretion of thyroxine binding globulin, with a consequent rise in total serum thyroxine concentration. Phenytoin and salicylate displace thyroxine from its plasma binding sites but negative feedback ensures that free thyroxine levels remain normal. Phenytoin may additionally lower thyroxine levels by inducing hepatic metabolism. In panhypopituitarism, the thyroid is usually affected last but by definition, there must be TSH deficiency (normal sequence of pituitary hormone loss GH, LH, FSH, ACTH, TSH).

8. Thyroid hormones **Answer: D**

Over 90% of thyroxine is bound to circulating proteins, predominantly thyroxine-binding globulin which is produced by the liver. Thyroglobulin is a protein in the colloid of the thyroid follicles and does not normally appear in the blood. Its measurement may be useful in thyroid carcinoma where it is used as a tumour marker. Triiodothyronine is produced largely in the periphery as a consequence of mondeiodination of thyroxine which has a half life of about 36 hours. TSH is a potent stimulus to thyroid growth in the normal individual and is responsible for the goitre of iodine deficiency and dyshormonogenesis (negative feedback).

9. Hypothyroidism **Answers: A B C E**

Menorrhagia and normochromic anaemia are not uncommon complications of hypothyroidism. Remember that menorrhagia may lead to a microcytic picture and associated vitamin B12 deficiency may cause a macrocytic blood film. Fluid retention may occur, giving protein-rich pericardial, pleural and peritoneal effusions as well as dependent oedema in the absence of heart failure. An abnormality of lymphatic drainage from interstitial tissues has been implicated. Clinically significant ascites and cerebellar ataxia are rare. Clubbing (thyroid acropachy) and pretibial myxoedema are rare manifestations of autoimmune thyrotoxicosis (Graves' disease) and usually occur in association with severe exophthalmic eye disease.

10. Autoimmune thyroid eye disease **Answer: B**

The characteristic finding in thyroid eye disease is inflammatory swelling of the extraocular muscles. This impairs eye movements and subsequent fibrotic tethering may make ophthalmoplegia permanent. Inferior rectus is most commonly affected, leading to impairment of upward gaze in the abducted eye. The disease is both more severe and more common in males and cigarette smokers. Radioactive iodine has been associated with deterioration of the condition. Steroids are generally reserved for rapidly progressive disease where there is reduction in visual acuity due to optic nerve compression at the apex of the orbit.

11. Intact parathyroid hormone **Answer: C**

In sarcoidosis with hypercalcaemia, PTH levels are suppressed by the hypercalcaemia, which is in turn due to excess vitamin D activity as a consequence of increased 25 hydroxylation of cholecalciferol in granulomatous tissue. In primary hyperparathyroidism, the PTH level is usually high but may be in the normal range but inappropriately so in the presence of hypercalcaemia (which should suppress it). PTH stimulates renal 1-alpha hydroxylase and in the human consists of 84 amino acids. Many peptide hormones are now measured by two-site immunoradiometric or non-isotopic methods rather than the older and less sensitive displacement radioimmunoassay.

12. Primary hyperparathyroidism Answers: B C E

The hypercalcaemia of hyperparathyroidism is often associated with raised parathyroid hormone (PTH) levels. A PTH level within the normal range however, is abnormal in the presence of hypercalcaemia, as the raised calcium should inhibit PTH. This occurs in the other causes of hypercalcaemia such as sarcoidosis. Hypercalciuria is not as great as would be predicted from other causes of hypercalcaemia, as there is increased renal tubular absorption of calcium. Fetal parathyroid activity may be suppressed by maternal hypercalcaemia, resulting in tetany in the neonate. A third of patients have hypertension, in part due to renal damage, but in some, recovering when hypercalcaemia is corrected. Over 80% of patients have a solitary adenoma, 15% have diffuse hyperplasia, and a small minority a carcinoma of one gland.

13. Primary hypoparathyroidism Answers: A B

Characteristic features of hypoparathyroidism include calcification of the basal ganglia (and possible Parkinsonism), carpopedal spasm, cataract and papilloedema. Biochemistry typically shows elevated serum phosphate with low calcium and alkaline phosphatase. Delayed tendon relaxation is a feature of hypothyroidism: muscular excitability and hyperreflexia are seen in hypocalcaemic states.

14. Pituitary fossa Answers: A B C D

A number of important structures lie close to the pituitary fossa and can be encroached upon by an expanding pituitary tumour. Immediately lateral to the fossa (which does not have bony lateral walls) lies the cavernous sinus, through which runs the VI cranial nerve. The III, IV and upper two divisions of the V cranial nerves lie in the lateral wall of the sinus. The internal carotid artery lies in the sinus lateral to the dorsum sella, its siphon fitting under the 'shoulder' of the dorsum. The fossa is an indentation in the roof of the sphenoidal sinus, which may be invaded by downward growth of a pituitary tumour.

15. Pituitary gland **Answer: D**

Although chromophobe cells were previously thought to be non-secretory, direct immunostaining for pituitary hormones has indicated that many produce hormones, particularly prolactin. Radiological evidence of pituitary fossa expansion is present in over 90% of patients and extension of the tumour to involve optic chiasm and nerves, the III, IV and VI cranial nerves and hypothalamus may occur. Destruction of normal pituitary tissue by the expanding tumour typically leads to a sequence of anterior pituitary deficits: growth hormone, gonadotrophins, corticotrophin then thyrotrophin. Diabetes insipidus due to supraoptico-hypophyseal tract involvement is rare. There is an association with parathyroid hyperplasia or adenoma (MEN type 1).

16. Prolactin **Answers: A B C E**

The release of prolactin from the anterior pituitary is largely controlled by prolactin-inhibitory factor (PIF), probably dopamine, produced in the hypothalamus. When production or release of PIF is deficient, as in hypothalamic or pituitary stalk lesions hyperprolactinaemia occurs. Prolactin-secreting pituitary microadenomas are also a common cause of hyperprolactinaemia. TRH (thyrotrophin-releasing hormone) releases prolactin and may play a part in the occasional hyperprolactinaemia found in primary myxoedema. The clinical features of hyperprolactinaemia, in addition to amenorrhoea in women, include galactorrhoea, reduced libido and hypogonadism.

17. Vasopressin (ADH) **Answers: A D**

ADH is a nonapeptide believed to be synthesised in the supraoptic and paraventricular nuclei of the hypothalamus and transported along nerve axons to the posterior hypothalamus. It increases the permeability to water of the renal collecting ducts (both cortical and medullary). The osmolar gradients mean that water leaves the tubule thus concentrating the urine. ADH release stimulated by a fall in blood volume (real or 'apparent') may override osmotic changes inhibiting release, hence the paradox of the hyponatraemia observed in severe volume depletion.

18. Diabetes insipidus **Answers: A C D E**

Polyuria throughout the day and night is characteristic in the untreated patient. DDAVP, a synthetic analogue of vasopressin, has an antidiuretic effect for 10 to 12 hours when administered as a nasal spray, and is the treatment of choice. Chlorpropamide potentiates ADH action on the renal tubule, but because of its primary hypoglycaemic action, is best avoided in children. The effect of thiazides is to enhance proximal tubular reabsorption as a result of causing mild salt depletion.

19. Acromegaly **Answers: A B D**

Clinical features of acromegaly include bitemporal hemianopia due to chiasmal compression, frontal sinus hypertrophy and nerve entrapment due to soft tissue overgrowth. Biochemically, there is elevated growth hormone secretion which fails to suppress in a glucose tolerance test and elevation of insulin-like growth factor 1 (IGF-1), which is secreted by the liver in response to growth hormone. Untreated acromegaly shortens life expectancy, largely as a consequence of cardiovascular disease but there is also an increased incidence of malignancy.

20. Acromegaly **Answer: E**

Active acromegaly doubles mortality at all ages (due to associated hypertension, diabetes and atheroma) and should therefore be treated in all but the elderly or very frail. GH levels fall relatively slowly after external beam radiotherapy and are normalised in only 40% of cases at two years after treatment; interim medical treatment may be necessary. Large extrasellar tumours, especially those compressing the optic chiasma, should be treated surgically; the transfrontal route must be used to allow adequate access. Bromocriptine normalises GH in only about 30% of cases. Long-acting somatostatin analogues can suppress GH levels and cause resolution of acromegaly, and may be effective in some cases which are unresponsive to bromocriptine.

21. Aldosterone secretion **Answers: A C D**

Aldosterone secretion is largely controlled via the renin-angiotensin system, and is inversely related to plasma volume. Plasma potassium concentrations also influence aldosterone release. Aldosterone secretion is greater when the subject is on a low sodium diet. It is the adrenal medulla, not the cortex, which is controlled by the sympathetic nervous system.

22. 21 hydroxylase deficiency **Answers: A B**

21 hydroxylase deficiency leads to a block in conversion from 17 hydroxy-progesterone to 11 deoxycortisol (glucocorticoid pathway) and from progesterone to 11 deoxycorticosterone (mineralocorticoid pathway). Elevated plasma levels of the steroids proximal to the block (progesterone and 17 OH-progesterone) and their urinary metabolites (pregnanetriol) are characteristic. Accumulated 17 OH-progesterone is diverted to andro-stenedione with subsequent conversion to testosterone, which causes clitoromegaly in the female fetus and early enlargement of the genitalia in boys. In salt-losers, there is impaired mineralocorticoid action and thus reflex increase in renin secretion.

23. Cushing's disease **Answers: A B**

Depression and delusional symptoms occur in Cushing's syndrome, whatever the aetiology. Hypertension is a consequence of ACTH stimulation of cortisol secretion which has some mineralocorticoid action. Hirsutism (androgen dependent hair) but not hypertrichosis (generalised hairiness) may complicate excess androgen secretion from pituitary-dependent disease or adrenal tumour. Glucocorticoid excess in children typically slows growth. Polycythaemia is a rare accompaniment but anaemia is not a recognised manifestation.

24. Cushing's syndrome **Answers: A C**

If hypercortisolism (Cushing's syndrome) is suspected, first-line investigations include 24 hour urine free cortisol collection and morning and midnight serum cortisols to confirm loss of diurnal variation. Additionally overnight or low dose dexamethasone suppression tests may be performed. Patients with depression or alcoholism may demonstrate abnormal results with all these tests and are best evaluated after abstinence from alcohol and all neuroleptic drugs. Once hypercortisolism is confirmed, the site of overactivity – adrenal, pituitary or ectopic production of CRF or ACTH – must be determined. A suppressed ACTH level is characteristic of an adrenal source. If ACTH is detectable in the serum, suppression of steroid levels with high dose dexamethasone, an increase in ACTH after CRH stimulation and higher ACTH levels on inferior petrosal sinus sampling than in the peripheral blood suggest a pituitary tumour rather than ectopic ACTH production. MRI scanning of the pituitary is an unreliable test alone as ACTH secreting pituitary tumours are often too small to detect (< 3 mm) and up to 25% of normal people have small inactive pituitary microadenomas of no relevance.

25. Phaeochromocytoma **Answers: B D**

Extra-adrenal tumours lack the methylating enzyme needed to convert noradrenaline to adrenaline and will rarely, if ever, secrete adrenaline. The basis of medical treatment is an alpha blocker such as phentolamine or phenoxybenzamine. Beta-blockade by itself could increase the hypertension due to unopposed alpha-activity. The tumour may occur as part of the multiple endocrine adenomata syndrome (MEN-II) in association with hyperparathyroidism and medullary carcinoma of the thyroid. Hypercalcaemia is occasionally found in the absence of hyperparathyroidism or bone secondaries.

26. Hormone receptors **Answers: B D E**

Recently a syndrome of growth hormone deficiency in adults has been described comprising lack of energy, low mood, decreased muscle and increased fat mass and possibly reduced myocardial function, osteoporosis and hypercholesterolaemia. Who should receive expensive growth hormone replacement therapy remains controversial. Magnesium is lost in both urine (increased in diabetes, alcohol excess, hypercalcaemia, renal failure diuretic, amphotericin aminoglycoside, cisplatin and cyclosporin treatment) and faeces (increased with diarrhoea). Steroids, vitamin D and thyroxine all act via intracellular (cytoplasmic) receptors which after hormone binding migrate to the nucleus and bind directly to DNA. All other hormones act via cell surface receptors.

27. Endocrinopathies **Answers: C D**

Hyperparathyroidism is associated with gout, pseudo-gout and osteoporosis; hypoparathyroidism can produce a picture similar to ankylosing spondylitis. Forestier's disease and cheiroarthropathy (pseudo-scleroderma) are features of diabetes mellitis.

28. Breast development **Answer: B**

Arrhenoblastoma of the ovary is a very rare tumour, almost confined to adults, and causes androgen (not oestrogen) secretion. Breast development is frequently the first manifestation of constitutional precocious puberty in a girl, with no recognisable organic changes. (It follows, therefore, that laparotomy to examine the ovaries is rarely necessary.) The XXY chromosome constitution (Klinefelter's syndrome) results in a phenotypic male and gynaecomastia occurs at or after the usual time of puberty. Maternal oestrogens frequently cause breast enlargement in newborn babies, both male and female, but this disappears within 2–3 weeks of birth.

29. Gynaecomastia **Answers: B E**

Physiological (pubertal) gynaecomostia is a consequence of oestrogenisation of the male breast. Gynaecomastia also occurs with a number of drugs including cimetidine and spironolactone. Diabetes mellitus is not a recognised cause but gynaecomastia may be seen in men with thyrotoxicosis, due to the elevation of plasma sex hormone binding globulin caused by the excess thyroid hormones. Oestrogen treatment and orchidectomy for prostatic carcinoma may cause gynaecomastia, but the disease itself does not.

30. Testicular malfunction **Answers: B D E**

Infertility is due to failure of the Sertoli cells to produce sperm or to a 'mechanical' disorder, the testosterone-producing Leydig cells often remaining intact. However, an adequate concentration of androgen is necessary for spermatogenesis. Impotence is rarely of endocrine origin or due to testicular disease. The testicular lesion in Klinefelter's syndrome is of the tubules and the interstitial (Leydig) cells may respond to gonadotrophins to produce testosterone.

31. Polycystic ovary syndrome **Answer: B**

Polycystic ovaries are found in up to 20% of young women but the majority do not have the syndrome associated with oligomenorrhoea, hirsutism and infertility. Patients may be obese or non-obese. Infertility is characteristically due to anovulation. Biochemical findings typically include elevated LH to FSH ratio, elevated serum testosterone, androstenedione, oestrogen and a reduced concentration of sex hormone, binding globulin. Hyperprolactinaemia may interfere with gonadotrophin secretion and cause anovulation but does not produce the other abnormalities. Female athletes and ballet dancers develop amenorrhoea as a consequence of low weight and hypothalamic disturbance.

32. Female menopause **Answer: E**

Peak bone mass is achieved in the early twenties in women and declines from there, although the rate of bone loss accelerates when the patient becomes oestrogen deficient. Flushes and sweating are due to vasomotor instability which is a consequence of oestrogen deficiency. The fall in serum oestrogen leads to a rise in circulating gonadotrophins, predominantly FSH. Bowel disturbance is not a characteristic feature of the menopause. The incidence of myocardial infarction rises slowly in the years after menopause when the protective influence of oestrogen is lost.

33. Carcinoid tumour **Answers: B D E**

The commonest site for a primary carcinoid tumour, often discovered incidentally, is the ileum. With carcinoids of the gut, liver involvement (metastases) is necessary before the syndrome is said to occur. Right-sided valvular lesions (tricuspid and pulmonary stenosis and incompetence) are well described. However, the rarer bronchial carcinoids can result in a carcinoid syndrome in the absence of metastatic disease and they are also associated with left-sided cardiac valvular lesions. The tumour can produce a number of hormones e.g. VIP, and a high volume secretory diarrhoea may result.

GASTROENTEROLOGY: ANSWERS AND EXPLANATIONS

1. Diffuse oesophageal spasm **Answers: A B C**

Oesophageal spasm occurs in all ages and can mimic angina closely even to the extent of being relieved by GTN. The diagnosis is suggested by a corkscrew oesophagus on barium swallow and simultaneous non-peristaltic contractions on manometry.

2. Plasma gastrin level **Answers: A B C**

Gastrin production is stimulated by a rise in gastric intraluminal pH (i.e. reduced acidity) such as that produced by omeprazole. Elevated gastrin levels also occur in chronic renal failure as gastrin is excreted in the urine. The elevated levels found after massive small bowel resection are unexplained. Patients with duodenal ulcers do not show significant elevations of plasma gastrin as secretion is inhibited by duodenal acidification. Very high plasma gastrin is a feature of the Zollinger-Ellison syndrome which forms part of the syndrome Multiple Endocrine Adenoma (MEA) type I.

3. Rate of gastric emptying **Answers: A B D E**

Liquid gastric emptying depends on the nature and volume of the liquid, and the presence of tobacco or drugs (e.g. atropine, opiates). Migrating motor complexes clear the fasting gut.

4. *Helicobacter pylori* **Answers: A C E**

Helicobacter pylori are found in 10–30% of normal stomachs on endoscopy. It only colonises gastric tissue and causes an acute gastritis. It is poorly responsive to H_2 antagonists but show some response to bismuth. Eradication is difficult but currently triple therapy with bismuth, metronidazole and amoxicillin is the most effective. They are implicated in ulcer recurrence and possibly in the genesis of peptic ulcers.

5. Upper gastrointestinal tract **Answers: All false**

Ranitidine is a competitive inhibitor of histamine H_2 receptors. The prokinetic effects of cisapride are mediated through cholinergic stimulation and the actions of domperidone are related to blockade of dopamine receptors. Omeprazole inhibits gastric acid secretion and leads to a rise in intragastric pH. Sucralfate is an aluminium-based muco-protective agent with only weak acid neutralising properties.

6. Acute pancreatitis **Answers: A C**

Acute pancreatitis still has an appreciable mortality (up to 10%). The commonest associated factor is biliary tract stones if the patient has jaundice. An emergency ultrasound followed by an ERCP and sphincterotomy is indicated. Injecting dye into the pancreatic duct at ERCP may be dangerous. Most cases of acute pancreatitis do not go on to chronic pancreatitis. Persistent pain and hyperamylasaemia suggest a complication like pseudocyst or abscess. Some patients can become profoundly hypocalcaemic.

7. Chronic pancreatitis **Answers: A E**

The commonest known cause of pancreatitis in the UK is alcohol excess. Other known factors include hypercalcaemia and hyperlipidaemia. In up to 50% of cases no cause is found. Plasma amylase is a very non-specific and insensitive indicator of disease activity. The diagnosis rests on the history, plain X-ray and specific imaging, especially CT scan and ERCP. Histology is difficult to obtain and rarely diagnostic. Over 90% of the gland needs to be destroyed or resected before diabetes ensues.

8. Acute gastroenteritis **Answers: A B**

Gastro-enteritis in at risk groups (infants, elderly) produces dehydration. ORT, by utilising a glucose-coupled sodium absorption pathway, corrects the dehydration. Commercial preparations are adequate for the treatment of mild/moderate dehydration commonly seen in the UK. Food has little or no effect on the diarrhoea and should be encouraged as soon as practicable. Antibiotics are rarely required but erythromycin is needed for *Campylobacter* infection with systemic upset.

9. Coeliac disease **Answers: A C E**

A diagnosis of coeliac disease means life-long gluten exclusion. Gluten is found in wheat, rye and barley but not in oats, rice and maize. There are two peak ages of presentation: infancy with diarrhoea and growth failure, and 40–60+ years of age where malabsorption or metabolic bone disease may be the major features.

10. Bacterial overgrowth **Answers: B D E**

A common cause of malabsorption in the elderly is bacterial overgrowth in jejunal diverticula, but overgrowth can occur wherever there is decrease in acid production or altered motility. A breath hydrogen analysis after an oral carbohydrate load is cheap and non-invasive.

11. Malabsorption of fat **Answers: A B**

In both Crohn's disease and radiation enteritis affecting the terminal ileum, a failure of bile salt resorption may occur resulting in an overall decrease in the circulating bile acid pool. Eventually, inadequate production of bile acids leads to malabsorption of fat. Fat malabsorption in cystic fibrosis occurs as a result of impaired digestion. Mucosal lesions of the upper small intestine, such as coeliac disease and giardiasis, lead directly to malabsorption of fat without evidence of bile acid deficiency.

12. Crohn's disease **Answers: A B D**

Elemental diet alone has been shown to be as effective at inducing remission of Crohn's disease as steroid therapy. More recently 5-ASA compounds delivered in the appropriate form to the small intestine can also induce remission of active disease and maintain improvement.

13. Ulcerative colitis **Answers: A C D**

Colitis starts in the rectum and may or may not progress proximally. Distal proctitis responds better to local than to systemic drugs. The newer 5-ASA analogues are thought to be as effective as sulphasalazine at reduced toxicity. Total colectomy with ileo-anal anastomosis is very successful in colitis but may allow severe recurrence of symptoms if used in patients with Crohn's disease.

14. *Clostridium difficile* **Answers: C D**

Clostridium difficile is present in approximately 5% of the adult population and the onset and severity of colitis is unrelated to the length of antibiotic treatment. The histological changes are diagnostic. Metronidazole is recognised as the drug of first choice but should be given orally whenever possible.

15. Colonic gas **Answers: B D E**

The major factors in the production of intestinal gas are the volume of air swallowed, bacterial colonisation and ingestion of non-absorbable carbohydrates.

16. Colonic polyps **Answers: A B C E**

The development of most colon cancers from adenomatous polyps is now well established. The larger the polyp the more likely it is to be malignant but even small polyps can grow into large ones! Colonoscopy, because of the ability for polypectomy, is the investigation of choice. Diet, in particular heavy ingestion of red meat and low fibre, is thought to be an important predisposing factor.

17. Intestinal pseudo-obstruction **Answers: A C D**

Other well recognised causes of intestinal pseudo-obstruction (i.e. no mechanical lesion but clinical and radiological features of obstruction) include progressive systemic sclerosis, diabetes mellitus, hypothyroidism and chronic phenothiazine therapy. Rarely, it is the presenting manifestation of occult neoplasm, either small cell lung cancer or phaeochromocytoma.

18. Irritable bowel syndrome **Answer: A**

A significant minority of patients relate their symptoms, usually of painless diarrhoea, to an episode of infective diarrhoea often contracted abroad. The whole gut may be involved and gastric symptoms may coexist with colonic ones. A barium enema on colonoscopy is not essential in most patients especially when all the typical features are present in the young person. The diagnosis is common in the elderly but more extensive investigations are required to rule out alternative diagnoses. Despite the similarities between the irritable bowel syndrome and diverticular disease evidence is lacking that the former precedes the latter in individuals.

19. Drug-induced acute hepatitis **Answers: B D E**

Tetracycline produces steatosis. Vitamin A excess results in hepatic fibrosis. The commonest drugs causing an acute hepatitis are isoniazid, rifampicin, methyldopa, ketoconazole, verapamil and atenolol. Indomethacin and carbamazepine are quite rare causes.

20. Hepatitis C **Answers: A C E**

Hepatitis C is an RNA flavivirus. It is less likely to produce jaundice than hepatitis B but a greater percentage of those infected will have chronic active hepatitis that will progress to cirrhosis, perhaps taking 20 years or more. Hepatocellular carcinoma is well recognised. Hepatitis D only complicates infection with hepatitis B.

21. Infectious hepatitis **Answers: B C**

Hepatitis C (previously A-non B) is now the commonest blood borne hepatitis in the UK. Hepatitis D (Delta agent) co-exists with hepatitis B and is rare in the UK. Hepatitis E is food/water borne, producing an illness similar to hepatitis A. It is hoped the widespread vaccination against hepatitis B will greatly reduce the incidence of primary hepatoma.

22. Liver failure **Answers: C D E**

Liver failure is acute or acute on chronic. Acute liver failure after drugs or viruses is characterised by hypoglycaemia and a generalised bleeding diathesis. Acute on chronic failure demonstrates glucose intolerance and gastrointestinal bleeding related to portal hypertension. Any gut-specific antibiotic is effective; lactulose is useful as it produces a catharsis and an acid caecal pH. The latter reduces the formation of ammonia-dependent bacteria. Opiates are contraindicated and can cause prolonged encephalopathy.

23. Hepatic encephalopathy **Answers: A B C D**

Encephalopathy following therapeutic paracentesis is usually reversible and is uncommon. Its development is unrelated to the type of plasma expander used. Intravenous saline predisposes cirrhotic patients to fluid retention and ascites, and to encephalopathy from the resulting hyponatraemia and hypokalaemia.

24. Cholestatic jaundice **Answers: A C D E**

Erythromycin estolate causes cholestatic jaundice but other formulations of erythromycin do not. The other calcium antagonists may also rarely produce cholestasis. A number of phenothiazines and tricyclic antidepressants have been reported to produce cholestatic jaundice.

25. Haemochromatosis **Answers: B C D**

Haemochromatosis is associated with the A3 and B14 HLA antigens. There is an increase in iron absorption from the gut leading to iron deposition in many organs including the pituitary gland. Serum ferritin is often grossly raised, but as it is an acute phase protein very high concentrations can be seen in many acute conditions. Treatment can reduce complications especially if instituted in the pre-cirrhotic stage.

26. Hepatocellular carcinoma **Answers: B C**

Hepatocellular carcinoma is more common in men and associated with cirrhosis of any cause, the most common worldwide being hepatitis B. It may also occur in an otherwise histologically normal liver. Hepatomegaly is common and spontaneous rupture of the characteristically vascular tumour may lead to an acute presentation, and is a relative contraindication to liver biopsy. Hepatocellular carcinoma is one of a number of tumours that causes secondary polycythaemia. It is diagnosed by the appropriate clinical associations together with a positive ultrasound or CT scan, with high serum titre of alpha fetoprotein.

27. Artificial nutrition **Answers: D E**

A low serum albumin indicates a septic or toxic patient; severe malnutrition, e.g. starvation, does not depress the serum albumin. Enteral nutrition is preferred to parenteral nutrition as it is safer, easier, cheaper and at least as effective. The main complication of TPN is catheter sepsis.

28. Acute gastrointestinal bleeding **Answers: A C E**

An acute upper gastrointestinal bleed leads to a raised urea (increased amino acid absorption and urea generation) and a normochromic normocytic anaemia, but the blood urea will also be raised due to the volume contraction and pre-renal changes accompanying a large bleed from any site. Angiography is rarely helpful if endoscopy is negative; the patient needs to be bleeding at a rate of 0.5 ml/minute in order to be detected on an angiogram.

29. Gallstones **Answers: B D E**

Bile salt depletion may lead to gallstone formation either as a result of Crohn's disease of the terminal ileum, or following ileal resection for this condition. The unconjugated hyperbilirubinaemia of Gilbert's syndrome does not lead to gallstone formation as it is a manifestation of a failure of transport of bilirubin.

30. Carcinoid syndrome **Answer: A**

The carcinoid syndrome, due to tumour overproduction of serotonin (5-HT) may be treated with specific 5-HT antagonists or octreotide (somatostatin analogue). Right-sided heart lesions are characteristic (tricuspid and pulmonary valve thickening) and more likely with bronchial lesions. Flushing, wheeze and diarrhoea are the usual complaints, pallor and sweating being better associated with phaeochromocytoma. There may be long term survival (> 10 years). Diagnosis is best made by 24 hour urine collections for 5HIAA, a metabolite of 5-HT.

31. Ascites **Answers: B E**

Patients with the syndrome of inappropriate ADH secretion are euvolaemic and do not develop ascites. Ascites and oedema are recognised features of kwashiorkor rather than marasmus. Hepatocellular carcinoma and peritoneal mesothelioma may both produce ascites. Restrictive cardiomyopathy and constrictive pericarditis are rare causes of ascites.

GENETICS: ANSWERS AND EXPLANATIONS

1. Genetic associations **Answers: A B C D**

Klinefelter's (47,XXY) may be caused by non-disjunction (failure of the chromosomal pair to separate during meiosis) in either parent. Patients with Klinefelter's syndrome are chromatin positive (i.e. have a Barr body visible in the nuclei of their cells). Turner's syndrome is associated with the karyotype 45,XO. The karyotype 47,XYY is associated with tall stature and below average IQ (1/3) but otherwise patients lead normal lives; a small number of patients with mental retardation have anti-social behaviour. In the fragile-X syndrome there is a characteristic break on one of the Xq arms; the syndrome, which includes mental retardation and macro-orchidism, is found predominantly in males.

2. HLA molecules **Answers: A D E**

The MHC (major histocompatibility complex) on chromosome 6 encodes the polymorphic cell surface glycoproteins of the HLA (human leucocyte antigen) system. Class I molecules (HLA-A, B and C) are associated with beta-2 microglobulin and are constitutively expressed on most cells. Class II molecules (HLA-DP, DQ and DR) are constitutively expressed only on a few cell types (B lymphocytes, macrophages, monocytes and follicular dendritic cells) but can be induced by interferon in a wide variety of tissues (including endothelial cells, pancreatic beta cells and renal tubular cells) and present antigen to T cells.

3. Inheritance patterns **Answers: A D**

Nephrogenic diabetes insipidus is X-linked recessive and familial hypercholesterolaemia, autosomal dominant. Both ataxia telangiectasia and Erb's muscular dystrophy are autosomal recessive conditions.

4. Autosomal dominant inheritance **Answers: B D**

Familial Mediterranean fever, Friedreich's ataxia and haemochromatosis are autosomal recessive traits. Neurofibromatosis and dystrophia myotonica are inherited as autosomal dominants.

5. Autosomal recessively inherited conditions **Answers: B C E**

Alport's syndrome is usually inherited dominantly or as X-linked recessive, whereas nephrogenic DI is an X-linked recessive condition. Patients with cystinuria have a tendency to form semi-opaque renal calculi, due to a failure of reabsorption of filtered dibasic amino acids. Cystinosis is a more severe condition in which cystine accumulates within lysosomes, leading to major pathology in kidneys, heart, eyes and blood vessels.

6. X chromosome **Answers: B D**

Haemophilia A (factor eight deficiency) is X-linked; haemophilia B is autosomal recessive. Congenital pyloric stenosis has no simple Mendelian pattern of inheritance; rather, it is the result of a combination of environmental and gene effects so that a sibling has an increased risk of developing the illness. Nephrogenic diabetes is X-linked recessive. Ataxia telangiectasia is autosomal recessive.

7. Osteogenesis imperfecta **Answers: A B C E**

Osteogenesis imperfecta, in which there appears to be a generalised defect in the maturation of collagen, manifests in the eye (blue sclerae), ear (otosclerosis), skeleton (multiple fractures), loose jointedness and in skin. The alkaline phosphatase is normal or perhaps raised following a fracture. There is said to be a partial remission from pathological fractures during the reproductive years in women presumably owing to the effects of oestrogen. A low alkaline phosphatase is characteristic of hypophosphatasia, a rare inherited syndrome of short stature, which usually presents as rickets.

8. Huntington's disease (chorea) **Answers: C D**

The gene is localised on the distal end of the short arm of chromosome 4. The precise gene abnormality is a trinucleotide repeat (CAG). Huntington's disease is associated with a subcortical dementia and early psychiatric disturbance. L-dopa medication increases chorea in symptomatic patients and has been used as a provocative test for 'at-risk' individuals.

9. Neurofibromatosis **Answers: All true**

Neurofibromatosis (von Recklinghausen's disease) is inherited as an autosomal dominant trait. It is also associated with cutaneous fibromata and neurofibromata which may undergo sarcomatous change. Retinal phacoma also occurs in tuberous sclerosis. 'Plexiform neuroma' is the term applied to diffuse neurofibromatosis of nerve trunks.

10. Klinefelter's syndrome **Answers: A B C D**

The karyotype in Klinefelter's syndrome is characterised by one or more extra X chromosomes. The IQ and other features of disease severity are usually related to the number of X chromosomes. Patients are usually tall, long limbed, with very small testes, gynaecomastia and primary infertility due to azoospermia. FSH and LH are normally both elevated. Characteristically, they retain a good head of hair and are not prone to balding, which is androgen-dependent.

11. Cystic fibrosis **Answer: C**

Cystic fibrosis is an autosomal recessive disease affecting 1 in 2500 live births. There is a generalised epithelial defect in chloride transport due to a variety (> 300) of mutations in the CF transmembrane conductance regulator gene. The recombinant gene can be delivered to the lungs using a viral vector (or carrier) to infect the respiratory epithelium but the gene product does not incorporate into the host's genome and treatment must be repeated monthly.

12. Wilson's disease **Answers: C D E**

The characteristic ocular abnormality in Wilson's disease is the Kayser-Fleischer ring due to copper accumulation in the cornea. As the disease progresses, liver damage occurs and the pathological changes of chronic active hepatitis and cirrhosis become evident. Osteomalacia may follow phosphate wasting from the kidney, in turn due to copper-associated tubular damage. Biochemically, there is a reduced serum caeruloplasmin (copper binding protein) and an increased urinary excretion of copper.

13. Alport's syndrome **Answers: B C E**

Alport's syndrome is an hereditary glomerulonephritis (X-linked or dominant) which classically is associated with sensorineural deafness and characteristic eye lesions. It is due to mutations of the 5 chain type IV collagen of basement membrane, which is the antigen recognised in Goodpasture's syndrome. Therefore, antiglomerular basement membrane disease can occur post renal transplant but Alport's syndrome cannot recur. The disease is rarely associated with leiomyomatosis, macro-thrombocytopenia or hyperprolinaemia.

14. Turner's syndrome **Answers: C D**

In Turner's syndrome, there is loss of all or part of one of the X chromosomes and in rare cases there may be translocation of the genetic material to an autosome, hence other karyotypes are possible. Turner girls are short prepubertally due to an associated skeletal dysplasia and fail to undergo the normal pubertal growth spurt due to oestrogen deficiency. This leads to poor breast development and a small uterus. Both organs enlarge when appropriate sex steroid replacement treatment is given. Serum FSH is high as a result of negative feedback.

15. Genetic technology **Answers: A D E**

The genetic code is carried by nuclear DNA which consists of two complementary strands. Series of three nucleotides (bases: adenosine, cytosine, thymidine and guanine) on one strand code for each amino acid and also provide codes for stopping and starting transcription. In RNA, thymidine is replaced by uracil. Transcription is the process of transferring genetic code from DNA to RNA. DNA consists of exons containing genetic material and introns of apparently functionless nucleotide sequences which are not transcribed into mature messenger RNA. Southern blotting is a semi-quantitative method for measuring DNA in chromatographic gels and Northern blotting is used to measure RNA. Endonucleases are enzymes (mostly derived from micro-organisms) which digest DNA, cutting it at specific necleotide sequences, allowing detection of small mutations given appropriate complementary DNA probes. DNA polymerase is an enzyme used to replicate significant amounts of DNA from tiny samples for research and diagnosis (forensic DNA fingerprinting, prenatal genetic diagnosis from chorionic villus biopsy, etc).

16. Diagnostic genetics **Answers: C D E**

Restriction fragment length polymorphisms are inherited variations in the size of DNA fragments produced when DNA is cut with specific (restriction) enzymes. A particular fragment size can be shown to be linked to a particular genetic disorder, generally using family studies. Oligonucleotide probes recognise the normal gene or an abnormal gene but will not detect a deletion; they are most useful for detecting point mutations (e.g. sickle cell). Gaucher's disease may be detected by demonstrating abnormal enzyme function. Haemophilia A may be diagnosed using gene probes.

17. Pre-natal genetic diagnosis **Answers: A B D E**

The maternal AFP is often lower than normal in mothers carrying a fetus with Down's syndrome; a low maternal AFP in combination with maternal age is a more sensitive method of identifying pregnancies with a high risk of an affected fetus, than maternal age alone. Although chorionic villus sampling (CVS), performed between 9 and 12 weeks' gestation, carries a 1–2% risk of miscarriage, it allows first trimester diagnosis of many single gene defects using DNA analysis. Cultured cells allow many inherited metabolic defects and all chromosomal abnormalities to be detected. After 16–18 weeks cultured amniotic cells obtained by amniocentesis becomes the method of choice. Fetal blood sampling is no longer necessary to diagnose fetal haemophilia and is only used to confirm the results obtained by other methods, and for rapid chromosomal analysis.

18. Male : female dominance **Answers: A B E**

Agammaglobulinaemia and the Lesch-Nyhan syndrome are X-linked recessive, and therefore more common in males. NB Vitamin D resistant rickets is X-linked dominant. The non-organ specific autoimmune diseases such as mixed connective tissue disease, systemic lupus erythematosus, scleroderma and rheumatoid arthritis are all more common in females. The primary vasculitides, polyarteritis nodosa and Wegener's granulomatosis are commoner in males (4:1). Generally the organ-specific autoimmune diseases (e.g. Graves' disease and Addison's disease) are commoner in women; IDDM affects both sexes equally.

GENITOURINARY MEDICINE AND HIV/AIDS: ANSWERS AND EXPLANATIONS

1. HIV seroconversion illness **Answers: A C D**

Approximately 30% of patients develop an acute febrile illness in association with seroconversion. Common features are a maculopapular rash, oral ulceration and generalised lymphadenopathy. A rise in indicators of viral replication occur with the illness and antibody tests usually become positive 2–6 weeks after the onset. Increased severity of the illness is associated with a poorer prognosis.

2. HIV sero-positive patient **Answers: A C D**

Cryptosporidia and microsporidia account for 40% of infective diarrhoea; cytomegalovirus 20%, *M. avium intracellulare* 10%, and *Giardia* 5%. *Pneumocystis carinii* pneumonia is not thought to arise by reactivation of latent infection but from airborne re-infection. Early in infection the chest radiograph may appear normal. Bilateral interstitial infiltrate is common but consolidation can occur. Tuberculosis can stimulate cell-mediated immunity thereby activating HIV production in infected T cells. Most CNS infection occurs late. Early, uncommon encephalopathies and presumed autoimmune disorders are reported. Classic infections include cryptococcal meningitis, cortical (grey matter) toxoplasmosis, and demyelination by JC virus (progressive multifocal leucoencephalopathy) and generally HIV encephalopathy is a late manifestation.

3. Infection by HIV **Answers: All true**

A clinical picture resembling infectious mononucleosis, including the presence of atypical lymphocytes in the peripheral blood, can be seen at the time of primary HIV infection. ITP has been reported with increasing frequency in HIV-infected persons. Cytopenia of all peripheral blood cell lineages can be seen in HIV infection. Morphological features of myelodysplasia such as megaloblastic erythropoiesis are commonly identified in the bone marrow smears obtained from HIV-positive individuals. Circulating immunoglobulins with antiphospholipid activity such as the lupus anticoagulant have been demonstrated in patients with HIV infection, particularly in association with acute infection such as with *Pneumocystis carinii*.

4. Complications of HIV and AIDS **Answers: B C E**

Radiotherapy and resection are the best treatments for focal Kaposi lesions; systemic disease can be treated with vincristine, bleomycin and anthracycline. Large cell lymphomas in the immunocompromised transplant patient are nearly always associated with EBV. This is true of 50% of AIDS associated lymphomas except in the CNS which, like the transplant case, are nearly always positive for EBV. Peripheral nerve and muscle infection is uncommon. Cytomegalovirus (CMV) can cause a painful, ascending polyradiculopathy and mononeuritis multiplex. Cotton wool spots are seen in 50% of patients and are usually visual sparing and non-infectious, requiring no treatment. They may be associated with increased risk of CMV retinitis and confused with the latter. AIDS-related sclerosing cholangitis is caused by several agents including cryptosporidia, microsporidia and CMV.

5. Opportunistic infections **Answers: B C D**

Prophylaxis against opportunistic infections has been the main advance in the care of HIV-positive patients. Cotrimoxazole is the drug of choice for PCP prophylaxis and also gives a good prophylaxis against *Toxoplasma* encephalitis. Rifabutin delays the onset of MACBAC but has not been shown to prolong life.

6. AIDS **Answers: All true**

In AIDS primary neural damage may occur causing atrophy. Secondary infection or tumours are also common. Myopathy secondary to zidovudine is clinically indistinguishable from AIDS myopathy.

7. Intracranial space-occupying lesion **Answers: A B D E**

Toxoplasma gondii tends to cause multiple ring enhancing space-occupying lesions whereas *M. tuberculosis* causes a single enhanced SOL. Lymphoma tends to be non-enhancing and single. *Cryptococcus neoformans* most commonly causes meningitis but can cause multiple enhancing SOLs, and progressive multifocal leuco-encephalopathy, due to JC virus, shows up as non-enhancing low density lesions of the periventricular white matter. A therapeutic trial of antitoxoplasmal therapy (pyrimethamine and sulphadiazine) is indicated in patients with multiple enhancing SOLs who have positive toxoplasmal serology; response is usually quick. *Cryptococcus* can be diagnosed by looking for the antigen in serum and CSF. Failure to respond to antitoxoplasmal therapy after two weeks indicates the need for brain biopsy to elucidate the cause of the lesion.

8. Enteric pathogens **Answers: A B**

Microsporidia are being increasingly recognised as a cause of protracted small bowel diarrhoea in AIDS patients. The diagnosis has to be made by small bowel biopsy and no established treatment is available. *Isospora belli* should be especially considered in patients from the tropics and is diagnosed by observing the cyst in a stool specimen. Co-trimoxazole treatment is very effective. *H. pylori, H. nana* and *E. hartmanni* may occur in HIV infection but patients are not particularly susceptible nor is the ensuing disease severe.

9. Syphilis **Answer: B**

Mucosal ulcers occur in approximately 30% of patients with secondary syphilis. Tertiary disease develops three or more years after the primary stage and the skin, mucous membranes and bones are typically involved. Procaine penicillin is the treatment of choice for all stages. After treatment of primary and secondary disease the VDRL usually becomes negative whereas the TPHA remains positive.

10. *Neisseria gonorrhoeae* **Answers: All true**

The rash in disseminated gonococcal infection is usually sparse and often associated with tenosynovitis or septic arthritis. Acute perihepatitis (the Fitz-Hugh-Curtis syndrome) may be due to *Chlamydia trachomatis* or *Neisseria gonorrhoeae* and very rarely meningitis and endocarditis may complicate gonococcal infection. Proctitis is a particular complication in homosexuals.

11. Non-gonococcal urethritis **Answers: B C E**

Chlamydia trachomatis accounts for up to half of cases of non-specific urethritis. In the remainder, *Ureaplasma urealyticum* and *Mycoplasma genitalium* are pathogens whereas *Mycoplasma hominis* is not. Bifidobacteria are commensal faecal organisms.

12. Organisms **Answers: All false**

Calymmatobacterium granulomatosis causes granuloma inguinal, *Haemophilus ducreyi* causes chancroid and *Chlamydia trachomatis* lymphogranuloma venereum. Condylomata lata occur in secondary syphilis and condylomata acuminata are caused by papilloma virus. The pubic louse is *Phthirus pubis* whereas *Pediculosis corporis* is the body louse.

8. **Enteric pathogens** **Answers: A B**
Microsporidia are being increasingly recognised as a cause of unexplained small bowel diarrhoea in AIDS patients. The diagnosis has to be made by small bowel biopsy and [illegible] [illegible] and [illegible] [illegible] [illegible] [illegible] [illegible] [illegible] [illegible] [illegible] treatment is very effective. [illegible] in HIV [illegible] but [illegible] [illegible] [illegible] [illegible] disease.

9. **Syphilis** **Answer: E**
Neurosyphilis occurs in approximately [illegible]% of patients with untreated syphilis. [illegible] disease develops fifteen or more years after the primary [illegible] and the [illegible] of the brain [illegible] are typically involved. [illegible] [illegible] primary and secondary [illegible] the VDRL usually becomes negative whereas the TPHA remains positive.

10. **Neisseria gonorrhoeae** **Answers: All true**
The [illegible] [illegible] [illegible] [illegible] [illegible] [illegible] [illegible] associated with [illegible] [illegible] [illegible] [illegible] may be [illegible] [illegible] [illegible] [illegible] [illegible] [illegible] [illegible]

11. **[illegible]** **Answers: B C**
[illegible]

12. **[illegible]** **Answers: All false**
[illegible]

HAEMATOLOGY: ANSWERS AND EXPLANATIONS

1. Normochromic-normocytic anaemia **Answers: A C D**

Sideroblastic anaemia is associated with a hypochromic anaemia that may be either macrocytic or microcytic depending on the underlying cause. In cases of acute haemorrhage that occur prior to the development of iron deficiency the blood film may appear normochromic/normocytic if examined before the onset of a reticulocyte response (2–3 days). Long-term treatment with phenytoin can be followed by folate deficiency. Possible mechanisms include inhibition of absorption, inhibition of folate-dependent enzymes and induction of folate-utilising enzymes.

2. Macrocytosis of red cells **Answers: A C D**

The macrocytosis of coeliac disease is usually due to folate deficiency. Alcohol makes the red cells large directly, through secondary folate deficiency and with liver disease. In aplasia, younger large red cells are thrown out from the marrow. Azidothymidine may affect red cell morphology via DNA synthesis. A reticulocytosis is also a cause of macrocytosis.

3. Iron deficiency **Answers: C D E**

The serum ferritin and serum iron levels fall while that of transferrin rises due to increased hepatic synthesis. The anaemia, seen as a result of iron deficiency, is primarily due to defective haem synthesis. Glossitis and less commonly partial villous atrophy have been described in patients with iron deficiency and are believed to result from a reduction in iron-containing enzymes normally responsible for the maintenance of epithelial surfaces. Chronic intravascular haemolysis, such as occurs in PNH, can lead to excessive loss of iron in the urine.

4. Oral iron treatment **Answers: A D E**

The stool discolouration should not be confused with melaena. Oral iron produces the same increment in haemoglobin as parenteral iron (about 1 g/week) unless deficiency is due to malabsorption. Reducing the dose will usually improve side effects such as indigestion and constipation; if this does not work then change to another oral iron preparation. For patients who pay prescription charges it is cheaper to purchase oral iron at the chemist.

5. Low serum folate **Answers: A C**

All are causes of macrocytosis. Tropical sprue produces malabsorption. In pernicious anaemia, serum folate levels are normal or high. The megaloblastic anaemia of pregnancy or alcoholism is usually due to dietary deficiency. Lack of thyroxine, liver disease and chronic lung disease can produce macrocytosis with a normal B12 and folate level.

6. Vitamin B12 **Answers: A C D**

All rapidly dividing cells require B12 and folic acid, including the lining of the intestinal tract, so patients with deficiency often complain of sore mouths and mild diarrhoea and have a malabsorption type Schilling test result if this investigation is done too early in the treatment of the disease. Vitamin B12 is cheap and non-toxic, it may be given daily during the first week of treatment. In the myeloproliferative disorders the increased numbers of developing myeloid cells produce increased amounts of B12 binding protein, increasing the serum level. This may be a useful marker for myeloproliferative disorders. Parietal cell antibodies have a low diagnostic specificity for pernicious anaemia, being found in half of women over 60, but intrinsic factor antibodies are more useful. Hydroxocobalamin is derived from bacterial fermentation and may be given to vegans.

7. Falling haemoglobin **Answers: B D E**

Reticulocyte response to bleeding or iron therapy is rarely higher than 5%. Spherocytosis produces crises following infection/stress. Sideroblastosis produces ineffective erythropoiesis with a low reticulocyte count. The anaemia of lead poisoning is not due to haemolysis but impaired haem synthesis; however red cell survival is decreased and acute haemolytic anaemia occasionally occurs. Methyldopa produces a 20% incidence of positive Coombs' test but haemolytic anaemia is rare.

8. Addisonian pernicious anaemia (PA) **Answers: A C D E**

The deficiency of vitamin B12 results in a failure to transport folate from the plasma to intracellular sites. Antibodies to intrinsic factor are found in the serum of approximately half of all patients with PA; they are present in the gastric juice of 80% of patients. The pathophysiology is essentially that of an autoimmune disorder leading to gastric atrophy. Although therapy with corticosteroids improves the gastric lesion with a return of secretion of intrinsic factor the disease is best managed by life-long vitamin B12 supplements.

9. Sickle cell anaemia **Answers: A B D E**

Infection of bone infarcts occurs and tends to be with salmonella. Other problems of the adult sickler include severe anaemia, crises, pulmonary infarcts, gallstones, cerebrovascular complications and recurrent haematuria.

10. Sickle cell disease **Answers: A D E**

The sickled red cells can result in stasis of blood in the penile tissue causing priapism; this can lead to impotence unless treated effectively. Stasis in the renal medulla can cause papillary necrosis, haematuria and even nephrogenic diabetes insipidus. The cumulative effect of multiple infarcts in the spleen commonly results in hyposplenism. The 'sickle chest syndrome' can produce symptoms consistent with those of a pneumothorax although the pathology is different. Patients with sickle cell disease can develop proliferative retinopathy, especially if haemoglobin C is also present (haemoglobin SC disease).

11. Beta-thalassaemia major **Answers: C D**

In severe thalassaemia major, symptoms and signs develop in the first two years of life and marked enlargement of the spleen is very common. Mongoloid facies are typical of all the congenital haemolytic anaemias in which there is marked marrow hyperplasia. Raised serum iron occurs with iron therapy, haemochromatosis, sideroblastic anaemia and the thalassaemias. In beta-thalassaemia major, there is significant under-haemoglobinisation of red cells associated with a very low MCH. The anaemia is due to combination of ineffective erythropoiesis and haemolysis.

12. Cold antibody haemolytic anaemia **Answers: A B D E**

Raynaud's phenomenon occurs when cold antibodies cause *in vivo* agglutination at the cold peripheries. These antibodies are usually IgM or IgG in class and the IgM are often associated with lymphoma. The Donath-Landsteiner IgG cold antibody was, in the past, commonly seen with syphilis, but now viral infections such as rubella are the most frequent cause.

13. Warm-type autoimmune haemolytic anaemia (AIHA)
Answers: D E

AIHA is seen as a complication of lymphoproliferative disorders such as chronic lymphocytic leukaemia, Hodgkin's and non-Hodgkin's lymphoma. Rarely the disorder can be mediated via classes of immunoglobulin other than IgG such as IgM and IgA and in some instances the direct antiglobulin test can be negative. The AIHA seen following infection with *Mycoplasma pneumoniae* is of the cold-type. The classic example of drug-induced warm AIHA occurs following administration of methyldopa but other drugs, including L-dopa, have been associated with the disorder.

14. G6PD deficiency **Answers: A D E**

Antimalarials were the first group of drugs to be connected with the precipitation of haemolysis in G6PD deficiency. Of the antibacterial agents which can safely be given to these patients, penicillin and tetracycline are both useful whilst many sulphonamide preparations, nitrofurantoin, PAS and chloramphenicol precipitate haemolysis. Many viral infections precipitate haemolysis in G6PD deficiency and glandular fever is a good example of this.

15. Paroxysmal nocturnal haemoglobinuria **Answers: B C E**

Paroxysmal nocturnal haemoglobinuria (PNH) is an acquired genetic disorder of the glycosyl-phosphatidylinositol anchor that binds complement neutralising proteins to red cell membranes. The result is increased red cell sensitivity to autologous complement lysis. This is exacerbated by acidosis, explaining the nocturnal nature of haemolysis and is the basis for Ham's acid lysis test. PNH is associated with aplastic anaemia and a number of leukaemias.

16. Microangiopathic blood changes **Answers: A B C**

Fragmented red cells are seen in the haemolytic-uraemic syndrome and the closely related thrombotic thrombocytopenic purpura. The destruction of small superficial vessels by burns causes breaking up of the red cells as they pass through. In meningococcal sepsis the microangiopathy can be associated with DIC. Microangiopathic anaemia occurs in other conditions with DIC such as septic shock, and in malignant hypertension and polyarteritis nodosa.

17. Chronic myeloid leukaemia **Answers: A B E**

As with other myeloproliferative disorders with a raised granulocyte count, a raised transcobalamin I results in an elevation in serum vitamin B12. In up to 20% of all acute transformations seen in CML the blast cells demonstrate a lymphoid phenotype. Lymphadenopathy is uncommon in the early stages of CML but can be seen as the disease progresses. The Philadelphia chromosome involves a translocation between chromosomes 9 and 22. Alpha interferon can result in both complete haematological and cytogenetic remission in a minority of patients with CML.

18. Chronic myelocytic leukaemia **Answers: A B C**

Patients with chronic lymphocytic leukaemia also tend to be older, the splenomegaly is not as marked, and is painful much less often. Autoimmune thrombocytopenia can also complicate CLL, though less frequently than an autoimmune haemolytic anaemia.

19. Hodgkin's disease **Answers: A C D**

There is a T-cell defect in Hodgkin's disease which reflects the long-standing observation of cutaneous anergy in this condition. This probably explains the predisposition to certain infections such as TB, cryptococcosis, toxoplasmosis, pneumocystis, aspergillosis, herpes zoster and disseminated varicella. Treatment undoubtedly aggravates the predisposition. Haemolytic anaemia is much rarer in Hodgkin's disease than with lymphocytic neoplasia.

20. Multiple myeloma **Answers: A B D**

Approximately 10–15% of patients with myeloma have Bence-Jones proteinuria in the absence of a serum paraprotein. Infiltration of the bone marrow from any cause can result in a leukoerythroblastic blood picture. Up to 60% of patients with myeloma present with symptoms of bone pain. Amyloid can occur as a complication of myeloma and cause compression of the median nerve in the carpal tunnel. The incidence of myeloma rises with age, the median age at presentation is 70 years and only 2% of patients are below 40 years of age.

21. Renal failure in multiple myeloma **Answers: A B C E**

Renal failure in myeloma is characteristically associated with eosinophilic intratubular casts in the distal part of the nephron associated with a giant cell reaction. Chronic renal failure may also complicate renal amyloidosis, which occurs in about 10% of cases. Glomerular abnormalities are, however, usually minor. Acute renal failure may follow intravenous pyelography due to precipitation of light chains during dehydration. Hypercalcaemia may precipitate renal failure and if reversed may result in improvement in renal function. Uric acid crystal nephropathy can be avoided by the use of allopurinol.

22. Benign monoclonal gammopathy **Answers: C D E**

In the condition, which may occur in as many as 3% of those over age 70 years, there is an abnormal band of globulin present in the electrophoretic strip. Typically, the level of abnormal globulin (IgG in about 85% of cases) is under 30 g/l and the other serum proteins are normal. This condition is not associated with anaemia, abnormal numbers and types of plasma cells in the marrow, or the presence of Bence-Jones protein in the urine. A percentage have, however, developed multiple myeloma or lymphoma after many years of follow-up.

23. Bleeding tendency **Answers: A C D**

The partial thromboplastin time is prolonged with deficiencies of the intrinsic system factors including VIII and IX, which do not affect the prothrombin time. The prothrombin time is prolonged with deficiency of the extrinsic system factor VII as well as the common pathway factors X, V and II. Hess's test is abnormal with small vessel abnormality, thrombocytopenia and impaired platelet function. The bleeding disorder in HHT is due to the abnormal mucosal blood vessels. Aspirin causes irreversible inhibition of platelet cyclo-oxygenase and so may cause prolongation of the bleeding time.

24. Haemarthrosis **Answers: A C E**

Haemarthrosis occurs in Christmas disease (haemophilia B due to deficiency of factor IX). Locomotor symptoms are common in sickle cell disease but haemarthrosis does not occur. A low platelet count does not lead to haemarthrosis. Charcot joints may be affected by haemarthrosis as may pyrophosphate arthritis, probably as a consequence of inflammation.

25. Haemophilia A **Answers: A E**

Haemophilia A is inherited in an X-linked fashion but up to 30% of patients have no family history and presumably it results from spontaneous mutations. Classically the bleeding tendency results in spontaneous haemorrhage into joints and muscles. Bleeding into the skin is a feature but is less common. The deficiency of the coagulation factor VIIIC results in a defect in the intrinsic pathway of the clotting cascade; the extrinsic pathway is not affected. This produces a prolongation of the activated partial thromboplastin time (APTT) but not the prothrombin time (PT). The bleeding time is abnormal in disorders where there is a bleeding tendency due to thrombocytopenia, abnormal platelet function or vascular defects, it is unaffected by abnormalities of the coagulation cascade.

26. Protein C **Answers: A C D**

Protein C is a vitamin K-dependent protein and therefore plasma level falls in patients receiving warfarin. It is activated by thrombin and in association with protein S inactivates the active forms of factor VIIIC and factor V. Plasma levels fall in DIC as a consequence of increased consumption of the protein.

27. Heparin therapy **Answers: A D**

Thrombocytopenia occurs in approximately 5% of patients receiving heparin in therapeutic doses. Paradoxically arterial and venous thrombosis occurs in up to 20% of patients with heparin-induced thrombocytopenia and is associated with a 50% mortality rate. Osteoporosis and alopecia are recognised adverse effects of long-term administration with heparin. Heparin can be used with relative safety in pregnancy, coumarin anticoagulants are suspected to be teratogenic when used in the first trimester.

28. Disseminated intravascular coagulation **Answers: B C E**

Neurological presentation is rare except in thrombotic thrombocytopenic purpura. Fibrin deposition produces fragmentation and platelet consumption. Heparin frequently exacerbates the bleeding tendency with fatal results.

29. Thrombocytopenia **Answers: A B E**

In acute leukaemia there is hormonal suppression of normal cells by leukaemic cells and mechanical 'crowding out' in the bone marrow. In SLE thrombocytopenia may be an initial manifestation. Septicaemia induces consumption by immune complexes, complement activation and direct toxaemia. Massive transfusion produces thrombocytopenia by dilution.

30. Idiopathic thrombocytopenic purpura (ITP) Answers: A B C E

Although termed 'idiopathic' most cases are due to coating of the platelets with anti-platelet antibodies. Platelet surface immunoglobulin tests may be positive but these tests are technically demanding and there may be too few platelets to do them. Although the spleen may be enlarged on scan, it is rarely palpable. Children usually have an acute self-limiting form of the disease. A history of i.v. drug abuse or HIV exposure should be sought in all males presenting with ITP.

31. Pancytopenia Answers: A B C D

Important causes of pancytopenia which are potentially reversible also include vitamin B12 deficiency, SLE, hypersplenism, and drug-induced marrow aplasia.

32. Splenectomy Answers: A C D E

A is true and may be complicated by DIC, and even in Hodgkin's splenectomy is currently less popular in view of A. Splenic atrophy may occur in all inflammatory bowel disorders. E is true although spherocytes remain in peripheral blood. Howell-Jolly bodies in the presence of acanthocytosis are virtually pathognomonic of reduced splenic function.

33. Marrow trephine biopsy Answers: A D E

ADE may all result in a dry tap due to increased reticulin. Aplasia may be patchy and Reed-Sternberg cells are difficult to identify in hypercellular aspirate. Histology makes interpretation of morphology of the erythyroid series difficult.

34. Blood transfusion Answer: A

The term Rhesus positive refers to patients whose red cells bear the antigen D and does not take account of the other antigens in the Rhesus group. Thus Rhesus-positive blood which is commonly CDe/cde may induce antibody formation against C, c or e if the recipient does not possess these antigens. Fever may develop during transfusion due to non-specific pyrogens or to WBC or platelet antibodies in patients who have received previous transfusions; it is safe to continue as long as no additional signs and symptoms develop. 2,3 diphosphoglycerate is reduced in stored red cells, but is restored 4–12 hours after transfusion thus restoring oxygen delivering capacity. Dextran can cause RBC agglutination *in vitro* and so complicate the cross-match reaction. It does not cause clinical problems. Lymphocytes remain viable in stored blood for several days and can cause graft versus host disease in severely immunocompromised recipients. CMV-negative blood is only required for CMV-negative recipients who are immunocompromised, for example marrow transplantation.

35. Erythropoietin **Answers: B C D**

Erythropoietin (EPO) is a 30 kD glycoprotein produced in the single isoform by the kidney, and in fetal life, the liver. The liver continues to produce small amounts of endogenous EPO even in anephric adults. Anaemia or hypoxia stimulate EPO production and it acts on the bone marrow to increase red cell production selectively. Recombinant erythropoietin therapy in renal failure can exacerbate hypertension and is associated with increased risk of seizures.

36. Proliferative polycythaemia **Answers: A C E**

The myeloproliferative disorders (polycythaemia rubra vera, essential thrombocythaemia, myelofibrosis, chronic myeloid leukaemia) share overlapping features so that increased bone marrow reticulin may be found in any of them, though it is at its most marked in myelofibrosis. In primary proliferative polycythaemia there is often an associated thrombocytosis and neutrophilia. Decreased plasma volume is a feature of the relative (pseudo) polycythaemias. Patients with primary proliferative polycythaemia frequently have an associated iron deficiency because they may run out of iron making an expanded red cell mass, and may be bleeding from associated peptic ulcer and defective platelet function.

37. Leuko-erythroblastic blood picture **Answers: All true**

All can cause leuko-erythroblastic anaemia. This is merely a descriptive term for the presence of immature red and white cells in the peripheral blood, and does not imply aetiology.

IMMUNOLOGY: ANSWERS AND EXPLANATIONS

1. Cellular immunity **Answers: A C D**

T helper cells (Th) express CD4 and recognise HLA (major histocompatibility complex) class 2. Most CTL are CD8+ and restricted to class 1 HLA. A sub-class of Th cells produce IL-2. Di George syndrome (thymic aplasia) is associated with impaired T cell production. Immunoglobulin levels are usually adequate and there is an increased risk of autoimmune disease. Ataxia telangiectasia has several deficiencies of immunoglobulins and lymphopenia; it is autosomal recessive. Wiscott–Aldrich syndrome is X-linked, the gene defect leading to abnormalities in the regulation of sialophorin (CD43). The condition is characterised by thrombocytopenia and lymphopenia.

2. Leucocytes of the CD4 T4 phenotype **Answers: A D E**

The T4 antigen, now designated CD4 (CD=cluster of differentiation), is a marker for a subpopulation of T lymphocytes that are thought to play a 'helper' role in the immune response. Long-lived resting lymphocytes enter lymphoid tissue, such as lymph nodes, pass through the lymphoid parenchyma into efferent lymph. Thence the lymphocytes pass into the central lymphatic ducts and then back into the blood stream. This process of lymphocyte migration is called recirculation and allows each individual lymphoid organ to share the large pool of recirculating lymphocytes with the rest of the immune system, thus disseminating immunological function and memory. Most small resting T lymphocytes are considered to be recirculating cells. HIV preferentially infects T4 cells and may enter the cell by way of the T4 antigen.

3. Phagocyte function **Answers: A C D**

Purine nucleoside phosphorylase deficiency and Bloom's syndrome are associated with T cell abnormalities. Neutrophil chemotaxis and lysosome formation are defective in Job's syndrome and Chediak–Higashi syndrome respectively.

4. Anaphylaxis **Answers: A D E**

Anaphylaxis is an example of a type 1 reaction responsible for immediate hypersensitivity. Binding of monomeric IgE alone to the antigen has no effect but binding monomeric IgE which is cell-associated cross links immunoglobulin molecules, triggering off a series of events within the cell. Clinically these are characterised by vasodilation, bronchospasm, oedema and collection of eosinophils. It may be acquired by passive administration of antibody within six hours after injection. Typical type 1 reactions may be organ specific as in asthma or atopic dermatitis. Generalised anaphylaxis may occur if the antigen is widely distributed, manifest by marked vasodilation, oedema and shock.

5. Urticaria **Answers: A B D**

Urticaria may be a feature in many of the diseases caused by nematode or flatworm infestation (e.g. strongyloidiasis, filariasis and schistosomiasis). The opiate drugs are histamine-releasers and salicylates can aggravate urticaria and asthma. SLE may present with urticarial vasculitis.

6. Delayed hypersensitivity reaction **Answers: B C**

The delayed type hypersensitivity reaction (Type IV) is a T cell mediated response that results in a mononuclear cell infiltration into the site of antigen deposition. The cutaneous response to tuberculin purified protein derivative (PPD) is a typical example. Humoral antibodies are involved in types II and III hypersensitivity. In type II hypersensitivity, autoantibodies are directed against cell surface antigens, as in autoimmune haemolytic anaemia. In type III hypersensitivity, immune complexes are deposited in tissues, either in antibody excess (e.g. farmer's lung) or in antigen excess (e.g. serum sickness). E refers to immediate (type I) hypersensitivity.

7. Specific precipitating antibodies **Answers: B C E**

Precipitating antibodies against sugar cane occur in bagassosis and similar antibodies are present in histoplasmosis and bird fancier's lung. In fibrosing alveolitis, rheumatoid factor (50%), anti-nuclear factor and other non-organ specific antibodies (30%) may be present. Antibodies have not been found in byssinosis.

8. Anti-histone antibodies **Answer: B**

Although anti-histone antibodies are found in 30–80% of sera from patients with idiopathic SLE, their presence in patients with clinical SLE who lack antibodies to native DNA is suggestive of a drug-induced syndrome. Anti-histone antibodies are found in 15–20% of patients with rheumatoid arthritis and are therefore only diagnostically valuable in the appropriate clinical setting. A refers to anti-cardiolipin antibodies. C refers to antibodies to the Ro (SS-A) antigen. D refers to antibodies to the Jo-1 antigen.

9. Non-familial hypogammaglobulinaemia **Answers: A B C D**

Lymphoid tissue hyperplasia is a typical finding amongst this group of patients who have the most frequent form of primary immunodeficiency. Recurrent pneumonia (leading to bronchiectasis), sinusitis, otitis media, and gastrointestinal infections are the most frequent infections. There is no marked predisposition to viral infections, and very few suffer from the opportunistic infections seen in patients with AIDS. Secretory and serum IgA levels are virtually absent, IgG and IgM levels being reduced. There is an association with autoimmune disorders.

10. IgM paraprotein **Answers: B C D**

No paraproteins are seen in kala-azar, but often there is a massive polyclonal rise in IgM. Cold agglutinin disease, CLL and Waldenström's disease are all B-cell lymphoproliferative disorders sometimes associated with IgM paraprotein, whilst this is not seen in any of the myeloproliferative disorders.

11. Cytokine production and function **Answers: C D E**

The cytokine family includes interleukins, TNF, IFN, colony-stimulating factors, growth factors and chemokines. TNF-alpha is mainly produced by macrophages. It regulates cell growth and stimulates leucocytes and the induction of adhesion receptors. TNF-beta is produced by T cells. IFN-alpha and IFN-beta induce biochemical adaptation in uninfected cells, increasing protection against viral invasion. IFN-gamma has little antiviral action in this way and is more important in regulating cell-mediated immunity. IL-1 and IL-2 stimulate both B and T cells; IL-1 also stimulates prostaglandin synthesis. TGF-beta promotes humoral rather than cellular immunity and appears to reduce the intensity of the acute inflammatory reaction.

12. Interleukin-1 (IL-1) Answers: A B C D

IL-1 has many biological effects including A, B, and D. IL-1 also is chemotactic for lymphocytes, increases the thrombogenicity of the endothelial luminal surface, promotes leucocyte adhesion to endothelium by an action on endothelial cells, and stimulates fibroblast proliferation. IL-1 is synthesised by many cells, of which macrophages are amongst the most important. Other sources include Langerhan's cells, dendritic cells, keratinocytes and endothelial cells.

13. Complement deficiency Answers: All true

Inherited deficiencies of all 11 classical pathway proteins have been described with deficiency in several control proteins. With the exception of C1 they are all inherited as co-dominant. There are three general patterns of clinical manifestation associated with complement deficiencies. 1) connective tissue disorders with C2 deficiency; 2) recurrent pyogenic infections with C3 deficiency; and 3) recurrent sepsis with *Mycelia* species in patients with deficiencies C5, C6, C7, C8 and C9. The genes for all complement proteins are located in the major histocompatibility complex region of chromosome 6.

14. Hypocomplementaemia Answers: A C E

Hypocomplementaemia results from immune complex formation and complement consumption in SLE, cryoglobulinaemia and post infective glomerulonephritis. Hypocomplementaemia can also result from non-immune complement activation as in severe sepsis, pancreatitis and atheroembolism. Pregnancy and chronic inflammatory states lead to an increase in serum complement levels.

15. Pneumococcal vaccination Answers: A C

Pneumococcal vaccine is a polyvalent vaccine made up of capsular polysaccharide from 23 capsular types of pneumococcus. Vaccination should be considered for all those in whom pneumococcal infection is more common and/or more serious. This includes patients with homozygous sickle cell disease, asplenia and chronic renal, cardiac, liver or respiratory disease. In HIV-positive patients serological response to vaccination, and hence benefit, decline with increasing immuno-compromise. Routine revaccination is not normally recommended.

INFECTIOUS DISEASES AND TROPICAL MEDICINE: ANSWERS AND EXPLANATIONS

1. Antibiotics **Answer: D**

Teicoplanin is a cousin of vancomycin and has the same spectrum of action, namely only against Gram-positive organisms. Cefuroxime is a second generation cephalosporin and as such has no activity against *P. aeruginosa*; ceftazidime, however, does have good activity. Ciprofloxacin has much weaker action against Gram-positives than Gram-negatives and is especially weak in its activity against *S. pneumoniae*. Benzyl penicillin is still the treatment of choice for patients with *S. pyogenes* infection. Methicillin-resistant *S. aureus* will be resistant against all beta-lactam antibiotics including flucloxacillin and the cephalosporins.

2. Ciprofloxacin **Answers: A B D**

Ciprofloxacin has good broad spectrum bactericidal and antituberculous activity. It is however inactive against anaerobes and has only moderate activity against certain Gram-positive organisms including the pneumococci. Because of widespread drug resistance it is now the treatment of choice for typhoid fever.

3. Pneumonia **Answers: A C D E**

Three types of *Chlamydia* can cause pneumonia; *C. psittaci, C. pneumoniae* and *C. trachomatis*. The latter occurs in children infected at birth, 2–6 weeks after delivery. *Legionella pneumophila* is the commonest of the legionellas to cause pneumonia but remember other legionellas can also cause pneumonia. *Mycoplasma pneumoniae*, not *Mycoplasma hominis*, causes pneumonia.

4. *Legionella pneumophila* **Answers: B C E**

Legionella pneumophila is a Gram-negative bacillus. The organism multiplies in water but infection is by inhalation. The subsequent illness varies from mild bronchitis to severe pneumonia. Pontiac fever is an acute flu-like illness without pneumonia which requires symptomatic therapy only.

5. Tuberculosis **Answers: A B C E**

Drug resistance remains low in the UK (2–3% in the non-treated Caucasian population) but is much higher in certain areas of the USA, especially New York. Large tuberculous pleural effusions respond well to a combination of chemotherapy and prednisolone.

6. Tuberculosis **Answer: E**

HIV-positive patients with tuberculosis respond well to standard combination therapy. Although multiple drug resistance (MDR TB) has been a particular problem in this group it is not host-dependent and fatal cases of MDR TB have occurred in previously healthy hospital staff. Standard treatment is now six months rifampicin and isoniazid with pyrazinamide for the first two months. In spinal disease the initial site of infection is the intervertebral disc.

7. *E. coli* gastroenteritis **Answers: A D E**

The haemolytic uraemic syndrome occurs in both enterohaemorrhagic coli and *Shigella dysenteriae* infections. Enteropathogenic strains include the subgroup of enteroadherent *E. coli* which are associated with childhood diarrhoea and probably also play an important role in chronic diarrhoea and childhood malnutrition in developing countries.

8. Hepatitis B virus **Answers: A C D**

Hepatitis is a small DNA virus consisting of genomic DNA, core protein and surface protein. The core gene encodes for both core antigen and a cleavage product e antigen, which is a good marker of active viral replication. Pre S, which is closely associated with the surface antigen viral envelope, has specific attachment sites for hepatocytes. Interferon inhibits virus replication. Hepatitis D is a defective virus that requires hepatitis B virus to supply envelope proteins and can only infect man in the presence of HBV.

9. Hepatitis C virus **Answers: A B C E**

Hepatitis C causes chronic hepatitis in at least 50% of those infected. Transmission is primarily via blood products and needle sharing. Second generation ELISA kits for hepatitis C antibodies now give reliable results. Positive results are a marker of prior exposure only and liver biopsy or PCR for hepatitis C RNA are required to establish the presence of active disease.

10. Chronic hepatitis **Answers: B C D**

Leptospira icterohaemorrhagiae is the commonest leptospira associated with Weil's disease characterised by jaundice and renal failure; chronic hepatitis does not occur. Hepatitis B, C and Delta virus are all spread by blood or contaminated body fluids and they all can result in chronic hepatitis. For acute delta co-infection (occurring simultaneously with acute hepatitis B) 5% of cases develop chronic hepatitis whereas with Delta super-infection (already hepatitis B surface-antigen carriers) 70% of cases develop chronic hepatitis. 5% of patients with hepatitis B and approximately 30% of those with hepatitis C go on to develop chronic hepatitis. Hepatitis A and hepatitis E do not lead to chronicity.

11. Leptospirosis **Answers: A B E**

The most prominent signs in the initial leptospiraemic phase of the illness are conjunctival suffusion, neck stiffness, cutaneous haemorrhages and fever. Splenomegaly may occur but is uncommon. Jaundice is common but there is only mild hepatitis. The organism can be grown in blood cultures although the diagnosis is usually made by rising serological titres.

12. Typhoid **Answers: B C E**

Bone marrow aspiration recovers *S. typhi* in 90% of patients which compares to 75% from blood cultures. The Widal test is a poor diagnostic test because of cross-reactivity with other *Salmonella* species and past immunisation. Although classically *S. typhi* is absent from the stools in the first week this is not invariable and a stool culture should always be performed when a patient with suspected typhoid is admitted to hospital.

13. Typhoid fever (rose spots) **Answers: All false**

Rose spots classically occur over the upper abdomen and lower thorax. They are erythematous macules that blanch on pressure and last only 3–4 days. The rash is more common in paratyphoid.

14. Organisms causing fever and jaundice **Answers: B C D**

Entamoeba histolytica may cause dysentery or an amoebic liver abscess, either of which may result in fever; jaundice, however, is exceptionally rare. *Fasciola hepatica* is a sheep liver-fluke whose habitat in animals or man is the biliary system. Cholangitis may occur – as it can with *Clonorchis sinensis* which is a common biliary tract fluke in the Far East. Clonorchis biliary infection may predispose to the development of cholangiocarcinoma. *Leptospira icterohaemorrhagiae* is the commonest leptospira causing Weil's disease where renal failure and jaundice are part of the syndrome. *Paragonimus westermani* is the lung fluke.

15. Amoebic liver abscess **Answer: E**

Jaundice is exceptionally rare in amoebic liver abscess unless the abscess is compressing one of the major intrahepatic bile ducts. Splenomegaly is also rarely seen and active concomitant dysentery only occurs in a minority of patients (15%) although about the same percentage will give a history of previous dysentery in the preceding two months. Only 1% of abscesses will rupture into the pericardium and these will be left lobe abscesses which only account for 1 in 5 of the total. This is the most serious complication and patients rapidly develop tamponade. A raised hemidiaphragm is commonly seen and is one of the most helpful radiological features.

16. *Neisseria meningitidis* infection **Answers: A B D E**

Clinical parameters identified as indicating poor prognosis include severe hypotension (< 75 mmHg systolic pressure), skin/rectal temperature difference of > 3°C, Glasgow coma scale of < 8, recent deterioration, absence of meningism and rapid extension of purpuric rash. Laboratory measures that are also helpful include the detection of meningococcal antigen in the serum and leucopenia.

17. Lymphocytic meningitis **Answers: A B D E**

Mycobacterium bovis is part of the mycobacterium tuberculosis complex including *M. tuberculosis, M. bovis* and *M. africanum*; all can cause clinical and extra-pulmonary tuberculosis. *Treponema pertenue* is the cause of yaws and does not result in neurological disease. Cryptococcal infection is an important cause of a lymphocytic meningitis in immunocompromised persons and those with diabetes mellitus. Brucellosis and Lyme disease are other important, but rare, causes of lymphocytic meningitis.

18. Encephalitis **Answers: C E**

Chickenpox encephalitis is an immune phenomenon occurring with the resolution of skin lesions. The clinical features are cerebellar and the process is self-limiting. Herpes simplex encephalitis predominantly affects the temporal lobes and in 90% of cases is due to HSV 1. Encephalitis as well as transverse myelitis and Guillain-Barré syndrome may complicate *Mycoplasma* infection.

19. Transmissible spongiform encephalopathies (prion diseases) **Answers: B C D**

Creutzfeldt-Jakob disease (CJD), Gerstmann-Straussler-Sheinker disease (GSSD), familial fatal insomnia and kuru are all examples of transmissible spongiform encephalopathies occurring in humans. Bovine spongiform encephalopathy (BSE) occurs in cattle and scrapie in sheep. GSSD is familial, usually of cerebellar onset and tends to have a slower progression than CJD. The spongiform encephalopathies are thought to be due to an abnormal prion protein (PrP) which does not contain nucleic acid but is transmissible. SSPE is produced by a conventional paramyxovirus and PML by a papova virus.

20. Borreliosis **Answers: A B C D E**

Lyme disease is characterised by erythema chronicum migrans, fever, arthralgia, myalgia, lymphadenopathy and neurological and cardiac complications. Louse-borne (epidemic) and tick-borne (endemic) relapsing fever are associated with hepatic and splenic tenderness and enlargement, jaundice, liver failure and DIC. Tetracycline treatment of louse and tick-borne disease can produce a sometimes fatal Jarisch–Herxheimer reaction. Steroids do not prevent the Jarisch–Herxheimer reaction in louse-borne relapsing fever unlike their effect in acute syphilis; they are however useful in helping to reduce temperature and hypotension. The reaction can also be reduced by meptazinol, an opiate antagonist, and polyclonal anti-tumour necrosis factor antibody.

21. Listeriosis **Answers: A B C D**

Listeria monocytogenes is a non-spore-forming facultative intracellular anaerobe. Meningoencephalitis can lead to progressive neurological signs. Less common local infections include peritonitis, cholecystitis, osteomyelitis and septic arthritis. It should be treated with ampicillin and gentamicin. It is mildly sensitive to cefotaxime and resistant to other cephalosporins. Mortality rates are between 20–40% with septicaemia and meningoencephalitis despite treatment.

22. Botulism **Answers: A B**

Spores of *Clostridium botulinum* are ubiquitous in soil and the distribution of types A and B is global. Types A, B and E most commonly produce disease in man; types F and G have only rarely caused human illness. *Clostridium* is a spore-forming anaerobic genus and characteristic features of botulism include the absence of fever, fixed dilated pupils and extreme dryness of the throat due to interruption of cholinergic autonomic transmission. Fatality is approximately 25% if intensive care back-up is available.

23. *Plasmodium vivax* **Answers: B E**

Plasmodium vivax causes benign tertian malaria. The hypnozoite stage is responsible for relapses and should be eradicated with primaquine in those who are not G6PD deficient. Chloroquine resistance is generally only seen in falciparum malaria but is now also being seen with *P. vivax* in Oceania.

24. Acute falciparum malaria **Answers: A D**

Falciparum malaria is the most virulent of the four types of malaria and splenomegaly is an important clinical sign. Acute renal failure is common. There is no dormant liver stage as in *P. vivax, P. ovale* or *P. malariae* and recurrence of fever after one year is rare. Tertian periodicity does occur but is far from characteristic.

25. Severe falciparum malaria **Answers: A B C D**

Hypoglycaemia complicates malaria in three clinical settings which may overlap; in patients given quinine, in pregnant women and in patients with severe disease, especially young children. Mild hyponatraemia is relatively common and is often accompanied by mildly reduced plasma osmolality. Severe hyponatraemia does occur but is rare; there is no evidence of defective ADH control. Haemoglobinuria (black-water fever) occurs in severe malaria. However, it must be remembered that some patients may be suffering from the oxidant effect of antimalarial drugs when they are G6PD deficient. Raised intracranial pressure is common in cerebral malaria and because of this the justification for doing a lumbar puncture to exclude meningitis has recently been challenged. Hepatic dysfunction is common but clinical signs of liver failure are never seen unless there is concomitant viral hepatitis.

26. Life cycles of helminths **Answers: A B C**

A. lumbricoides, S. stercoralis and *N. americanus* all have life cycles that involve spread to the lungs via the bloodstream, breakthrough into the alveoli and then migration to the pharynx to be swallowed again; during this period they mature. *A. braziliensis* is a cause of cutaneous larva migrans and *S. japonicum* a cause of intestinal schistosomiasis.

27. *Schistosoma mansoni* infection **Answers: B D E**

Schistosoma mansoni is principally found in Africa and South America. Chronic disease mainly affects the gut and liver although the brain, spinal cord and lungs may also be affected. Praziquantel and oxamniquine are the two main choices in treatment. Cercarial dermatitis (swimmer's itch) may follow exposure to water containing any schistosomes.

28. Periorbital oedema **Answers: All true**

Migrating parasitic larvae are responsible for tissue oedema in trichinosis and gnathostomiasis. Adult loa-loa worms are occasionally seen crossing the conjunctiva and in addition cause Calabar swellings which are not infrequently periorbital. Chagas disease (American trypanosomiasis) is transmitted by the contaminated faeces of infected reduviid bugs and an inflammatory lesion often occurs at the portal of entry. This may be the conjunctiva, resulting in Romana's sign.

29. *Pneumocystis carinii* infection **Answers: A B C D E**

Co-trimoxazole is the therapy of choice and is usually given in high doses intravenously. Petamidine is an alternative. Both are associated with a high incidence of side effects in AIDS patients. Bronchoalveolar lavage is diagnostic in 90% of cases.

30. Common associations **Answer: C**

Epidermolytic toxins of *S. aureus* cause scalded skin syndrome. This is indistinguishable from toxic epidermal necrolysis which has a number of additional causes. However, given the number of staphylococcal infections, the association is uncommon. Toxic shock syndrome is mediated by toxins TSST1 and enterotoxins B and C; bacteraemia is rare and treatment is mainly supportive though antibiotics are required to eradicate the focal source. A rapid onset of septicaemia is an infrequent complication of streptococcal cellulitis. Group A beta-haemolytic *Strep. pyogenes* is associated with erysipelas in the elderly. Impetigo is usually superficial, not affecting the dermis. Ecthyma is an ulcerating form of impetigo extending into the dermis. Both forms are associated with increased risk of glomerulonephritis.

31. Toxic shock syndrome **Answers: A B C D**

Toxic shock syndrome is caused by *S. aureus* producing either TSST-1 or enterotoxins B or C. TSST-1 toxin accounts for all menstrual-related cases and half of the non-menstrual-related cases. Enterotoxins B or C account for the remaining non-menstrual cases. Hypotension is one of the diagnostic criteria which need to be fulfilled, and is present in 100%. Various types of rash can be seen, classically a sunburn-erythema or maculo-papular rash with fine desquamation at day 7–10, especially around the nail-beds. Alopecia does not occur.

32. *Streptococcus pyogenes* infection **Answers: A B C**
Erythema marginatum is one of the major criteria for diagnosing rheumatic fever complicating *S. pyogenes* tonsillitis. Slapped cheek syndrome has been a label given to parvovirus infection (fifth disease) and *Haemophilus influenzae* Group B cellulitis. Ecthyma gangrenosum is seen in neutropenic patients and results from Gram-negative infection, especially *Pseudomonas aeruginosa.*

33. Urinary infection **Answers: B C**
Escherichia coli accounts for three-quarters of urinary tract infections in general practice. *Proteus mirabilis* infection is common in hospital practice and points to the possibility of renal tract abnormalities, renal calculi and previous operative intervention. Inadequate bladder emptying due to bladder neck obstruction impairs bacterial elimination, the infection arising from faecal organisms ascending from the perineum. In the absence of urinary tract abnormalities, renal calculi and analgesic abuse, urinary tract infection is rarely associated with renal failure.

34. Blood film **Answers: A B D E**
Rat-bite fever can be due to two organisms – *Spirillum minis* which is a spirochete and can be seen on blood films, and *Streptobacillus moniliformis* which is a fastidious Gram-negative rod that is grown from blood cultures. *Borrelia recurrentis* is the cause of relapsing fever and is diagnosed by blood film examination whereas Lyme disease is caused by *Borrelia burgdorferi* and is diagnosed primarily by serology. Early African and American trypanosomiasis can be diagnosed by blood film as can Oroya fever, which is a bacterial infection of red cells caused by *Bartonella bacilliformis.* Of course the major reason for performing a blood film in patients with a fever recently returned from abroad is to diagnose malaria.

35. Infections **Answers: A B C D**
Local *Pasteurella* infection of the bite wound complicated by septicaemia, hydatid disease and leptospirosis are all recognised infections that may result from contact with dogs. Dysgonic-fermenter 2 septicaemia is a rare sequelae in patients who have had a splenectomy or are otherwise immunocompromised, and it has a high mortality. Whereas *Campylobacter jejuni* may be contracted from dogs, *Campylobacter foetus* cannot.

36. Rabies **Answers: A C**
The disease is caused by an RNA virus and is invariably fatal. Corneal transplants have been recognised as a method of transmission. Rabies may be either 'furious' or 'dumb' so hydrophobia is not a universal presentation.

37. Hantavirus infection **Answers: B C E**

Hantavirus has no arthropod vector. The reservoir of infection is in wild rodents. Nephropathia epidemica is a less severe form of haemorrhagic fever with renal syndrome and occurs primarily in Scandinavia. Recent outbreaks of hantavirus in the USA have been associated with pulmonary disease.

38. Mumps virus infection **Answers: A D E**

Symptomatic meningitis occurs in 5–10% of patients but it is usually mild. CSF abnormalities (lymphocytosis and virus isolation) are more common. Pancreatitis is very rare and the amylase may be raised due to parotitis. Oophoritis is a well known complication and like orchitis is nearly always unilateral.

39. Parvovirus B19 **Answers: A C E**

The tropism for red cells is mediated through erythrocyte P antigen. Individuals who lack P antigen are immune to B19. Infection is transmitted through the respiratory route or via blood products. In the presence of chronic haemolysis and therefore reduced red cell life, B19 can cause a transient aplastic crisis by interrupting erythropoiesis over a 5 to 7 day period. Infection is otherwise usually benign though it may cause a polyarthritis. Skin rash is more commonly erythematous but may be purpuric even in the absence of thrombocytopenia. There is no evidence that B19 causes birth defects. It is associated with second trimester fetal loss and hydrops fetalis.

40. Intracellular inclusion bodies **Answers: B E**

Intracellular inclusion bodies are a histological feature of certain viral infections. In rabies the Negri bodies are accumulations of viral RNA and are seen in the hippocampus and cerebellar Purkinje cells. 'Owls eye' inclusions are seen in parotid, liver, lung and kidney in CMV infections. The Councilman bodies demonstrable in the liver in yellow fever are not inclusions but eosinophilic necrotic cells and these are present in other forms of hepatitis. Although an infectious aetiology has been postulated in Alzheimer's disease evidence suggests that non-viral agents could be implicated.

41. Fungal arthritis **Answers: A B C**

Fungal arthritis is a rare disorder but a long delay in diagnosis is usual, frequently resulting in irreversible joint destruction. In non-endemic areas infection is predominantly seen in compromised hosts. Most cases result from direct extension from a bony focus, examples include maduromycosis, coccidioidomycosis and blastomycosis.

42. *Candida albicans* **Answer: A**

Although lymphopenia, and in particular CD4 lymphocyte depletion, in HIV patients is associated with oropharyngeal and oesophageal candidiasis, candidaemia and deep infection is principally a problem in neutropenic patients. Endocarditis is usually left sided and should be considered in cases of culture-negative endocarditis.

43. Actinomycosis **Answers: B D**

Several species of *Actinomyces* can cause actinomycosis but *Actinobacillus actinomycetemcomitans* is a Gram-negative rod that is often found in association with *Actinomyces israelii*; it is not a cause. Pelvic actinomycosis may be associated with IUDs, and can present with anything from a vaginal discharge to a frozen pelvis mimicking malignancy. The disease most commonly affects the cervico-facial area and less commonly the lung or abdomen/pelvis. Disseminated actinomycosis may occur resulting in soft tissue abscesses and optional therapy is benzyl penicillin for prolonged periods. In a penicillin allergic individual, clindamycin is a suitable alternative.

METABOLIC DISEASES: ANSWERS AND EXPLANATIONS

1. Hyperuricaemia **Answers: A B C D**

Lesch-Nyhan syndrome is an X-linked disorder in which there is deficiency of hypoxanthine guanosine phosphoribosyl transferase. There is overproduction of urate, gout, neurological disease and self-mutilation. The serum uric acid is elevated in myeloproliferative disorders such as polycythaemia rubra vera. Hyperuricaemia is also associated with hyperparathyroidism and hypothyroidism but not with thyrotoxicosis. Hydroxybutyrate accumulation in fasting inhibits renal tubular urate secretion.

2. Hypouricaemic therapy **Answers: A B E**

Indications include any evidence of bone destruction, renal disease, renal stone formation and very high uric acid levels. It would not be usual to initiate hypouricaemic therapy until three or more acute attacks had occurred.

3. Acute intermittent porphyria **Answers: A B C E**

Porphobilinogen excreted in large amounts in the urine in acute attacks gives a red colour with Ehrlich's reagent which is not extractable with chloroform (cf. urobilinogen and indoles). Labile hypertension, postural hypotension, tachycardia and neuritic limb pains are attributed to autonomic and peripheral nervous system dysfunction. Classical precipitant drugs include barbiturates, anticonvulsants, oral contraceptives and sulphonamides. Glucose infusions often help to abort acute attacks but hypotonic fluid must be used with extreme caution because of the risk of inappropriate ADH secretion (SIADH) in this condition.

4. Wilson's disease **Answers: C D E**

The basic abnormality in Wilson's disease is a failure to excrete copper into the bile. Excess copper is toxic and gives rise to various forms of liver disease, a neurological disorder affecting mainly the basal ganglia, Kayser-Fleischer rings in the cornea and renal tubular defects (hence the osteomalacia). The plasma caeruloplasmin and total copper are reduced and the urinary copper excretion is high.

5. Delayed bone age **Answers: A C**

Bone age or skeletal maturity is estimated by comparing the appearance of bones on an X-ray of the left hand and wrist with those in a standard atlas, or by the more accurate bone-scoring method of Tanner and Whitehouse. Delay in bone age is found in children with growth hormone deficiency and hypothyroidism. Bone age is usually normal in familial or genetic short stature, and advanced in precocious puberty.

6. Postmenopausal osteoporosis **Answers: A D**

The density of the proximal femur is most useful for predicting fractures, while lumbar spine density is most useful for monitoring therapy. Bisphosphonates are anti-resorptive agents; however, they not only affect bone resorption but also bone formation, although the latter lags behind the former by a couple of months. With anti-resorptive therapy, bone density increases by about 5–10%, and this usually takes two to three years, after which there is little change in bone density. Fluorides increase new bone formation, and the increase in bone mineral density continues beyond two years. Despite this increase in bone density with fluorides, there is only a small effect on fracture rate. Indeed, the benefit of bisphosphonates in reducing fracture rates is greater than would be expected from the change in bone mineral density.

7. Glucocorticoid effects **Answers: B E**

Glucocorticoid-induced osteoporosis occurs as a result of increased osteoclast-mediated bone resorption and decreased osteoblast-mediated bone formation. Glucocorticoids also cause a decrease in intestinal absorption of both calcium and phosphate. In addition, renal excretion of calcium is increased probably due to a direct effect on tubular reabsorption of calcium. In addition, glucocorticoids cause a reduction in sex hormone production. There are no consistent abnormalities in vitamin D, PTH, or calcitonin levels.

8. Paget's disease of bone **Answers: A B C D E**

Hypercalcaemia may occur in patients with extensive Paget's disease when immobilised or when osteosarcoma develops. Deafness may be due to either direct Paget's involvement of the ossicles of the inner ear or to pressure on the eighth cranial nerve by Pagetic bone. Overgrowth of Pagetic bone at the base of the skull may lead to brain stem compression. Angioid streaks in the retina are found very rarely in Paget's disease and much more commonly in pseudoxanthoma elasticum. Radiologically, both lytic and sclerotic phases are recognised: the lytic phase may be well defined in the calvarium of the skull and is then called osteoporosis circumscripta

9. Avascular necrosis of bone **Answers: A B C E**

The precise aetiology is unknown and cannot be purely a problem of inadequate blood supply. There are many causes including SLE (though treatment by corticosteroids may be contributory), sickle cell disease and Cushing's syndrome (presumably high corticosteroid output). The immunosuppressive treatment including prednisolone given to renal transplant patients is also considered causative.

10. Hypocalciuric hypercalcaemia Answers: All false

Familial hypocalciuric hypercalcaemia is a relatively benign autosomal dominant disease. Although PTH levels may be elevated hypercalcaemia is not PTH-dependent. There is an abnormality of the calcium-sensing receptor resulting in a shift in the calcium set point for PTH secretion from apparently otherwise normal glands. It is not associated with other (multiple) endocrine neoplasia. Thiazide diuretics can cause hypercalcaemia in patients with borderline hyperparathyroidism and are used as a treatment to reduce urinary calcium loss in idiopathic hypercalciuria.

11. Hypercalcaemia Answers: B C E

95% of hypercalcaemia is due to hyperparathyroidism or malignancy. Serum alkaline phosphatase levels are only raised in hyperparathyroidism in severe disease. Squamous cell, renal and breast tumours may produce parathyroid hormone-related peptide (a different gene from parathyroid hormone itself) and hence 'humoral' hypercalcaemia in the absence of metastases. Suppressed parathyroid hormone (PTH) production by the remaining three parathyroid glands in parathyroid adenoma may result in temporary (days to weeks) but severe hypocalcaemia following adenoma removal. Detectable PTH levels with modern assays in the presence of hypercalcaemia do indicate hyperparathyroidism; however, surgery is only indicated if symptoms are present, there is renal impairment or serum calcium exceeds 3.0 mmol/l. Treatment of hypercalcaemia includes aggressive rehydration, calcitonin (acutely), bisphosphonates (in malignancy), surgery (in hyperparathyroidism) and dialysis in refractory cases.

12. Hypomagnesaemia Answers: A B C

Magnesium is lost from the extracellular fluid in diabetic ketoacidosis and diarrhoea. Hypomagnesaemia may also follow long-term use of loop diuretics. Magnesium is predominantly an intracellular ion and behaves in this respect like potassium. However, extracellular magnesium is predominantly protein-bound and is handled in a similar way to calcium. Magnesium has been used to prevent ventricular arrhythmias but hypomagnesaemia is not a direct consequence of acute myocardial infarction.

13. High plasma inorganic phosphate level **Answers: A B C**
Phosphate (like potassium) is predominantly an intracellular ion and this may be reflected by an increased extracellular fluid concentration in the presence of acidosis, due to cell membrane dysfunction. Hyperphosphataemia is believed to play an aetiological role in renal osteodystrophy by leading to secondary (and tertiary) hyperparathyroidism. The plasma phosphate is typically low in all vitamin D deficiency related bone disease. It is normal in uncomplicated Paget's disease.

14. Plasma bicarbonate levels **Answers: C E**
The metabolic acidosis of uraemia and diabetic ketoacidosis would make a high plasma bicarbonate an extremely unlikely occurrence. Most causes of hypokalaemia, including Conn's syndrome, are associated with a metabolic alkalosis which can be gross in pyloric stenosis. In chronic cor pulmonale, a raised bicarbonate level would indicate renal compensation of a respiratory acidosis due to CO_2 retention.

15. Anion gap **Answers: D E**
The anion gap is the sum of (Na^+ + K^+) – (Cl^- + HCO_3^-). It is normally between 10 and 18 mmol/l and represents the unmeasured negative charge on albumin, phosphate, sulphate, lactate and other organic acids. Normal anion gap acidosis occurs when there is increased bicarbonate loss (e.g. from the GI tract in ureterosigmoidostomy or in proximal renal tubular acidosis), or if there is HCl retention (e.g. distal renal tubular acidosis or ammonium chloride ingestion). In maple syrup urine disease branched chain keto acids accumulate increasing the anion gap. Similarly, in salicylate poisoning this exogenous acid contributes to the unmeasured anions resulting in an increased anion gap acidosis. In the nephrotic syndrome, serum albumin is low and, therefore, its effective negative charge is less, resulting in a lowering of the anion gap.

16. Serum K^+ 2.5 mmol/l and HCO_3^- 14 mmol/l **Answers: A D**
Causes of hypokalaemia with acidosis include renal tubular acidosis, uretero-colic fistula (spontaneous or surgical) and acetazolamide treatment. Hypokalaemic alkalosis is a feature of bulimia and Conn's syndrome. Methanol poisoning typically produces features of metabolic acidosis with hyperkalaemia and low plasma bicarbonate.

17. Apoprotein A1 **Answers: B C**

Apoprotein A1 is an apolipoprotein that is predominantly associated with HDL and is representative of HDL particle number. It is inversely related to cardiovascular disease risk. It is involved in removal of cholesterol by HDL from the tissues and facilitates transfer back to VLDL and the liver. It is not involved in intestinal transport and not present in chylomicrons. It is elevated in nephrotic syndrome, along with increased HDL particle number.

18. Apolipoprotein E **Answers: B C D**

Apoprotein E is a lipoprotein involved in the mobilisation of cholesterol for repair and growth. It is also produced by astrocytes and helps maintain myelin and neuronal membranes. The gene for Apo E is on chromosome 19 and has three common polymorphic variants – one of which, E4, is associated with Alzheimer's disease. As Apo E is found within the amyloid plaques associated with Alzheimer's disease it may be involved in the pathogenesis of this form of dementia. Amyloid precursor protein is distinct from apoprotein E.

19. LDL receptor **Answers: C D**

The LDL receptor continuously recycles from the cell surface to endosomes (or receptorsomes), internalising LDL for catabolism. HDL does not compete with LDL for receptor mediated uptake. Once internalised LDL undergoes lysosomal degradation and its cholesterol ester is hydrolysed to free cholesterol. Release of this free cholesterol from the lysosome regulates cellular cholesterol content by:

- down regulating 3-hydroxy-3-methyl glutaryl-CoA (HMG-CoA) reductase
- repressing LDL receptor synthesis
- activating acetyl CoA: cholesterol O-acetyl-transferase (ACAT) so that any cholesterol surplus to requirements is reconverted to cholesterol ester and stored as droplets in the cytoplasm. The LDL receptor is encoded on chromosome 19 and more than 100 mutations occurring in the genes encoding this receptor-mediated LDL catabolism can lead to the clinical syndrome of familial hyper-cholesterolaemia. Familial hypercholesterolaemia is autosomal, affecting males and females equally and therefore the LDL receptor could not be encoded on the X chromosome.

20. Heterozygous familial hypercholesterolaemia Answers: C E

Familial hypercholesterolaemia is an autosomal dominant condition with a gene frequency between 1:300 and 1:500 in the UK. Heterozygotes are affected later and less severely than homozygotes, but ischaemic heart disease risk is increased in all subjects. Tendon and cutaneous xanthomas are rare before the age of ten years in the heterozygote. Screening of neonates (cord blood) allows early detection and treatment when one or both parents are affected. The basic biochemical defect has been localised to the LDL receptor.

21. Pyridoxine Answers: A B E

The tryptophan loading test can be used to assess vitamin B6 status, except in patients receiving oestrogens or with increased secretion of corticosteroids. Vitamin B6 deficiency can be induced by penicillamine, and isoniazid (which increases urinary excretion). Cycloserine and hydralazine are antagonists of vitamin B6. The liver plays a major role in the metabolism of pyridoxine. Pyridoxine can be used in pregnant women, for example in patients with hyperemesis gravidarum. Pyridoxine should not be given to patients receiving L-dopa as the action of L-dopa is antagonised. However, the vitamin can be used if the preparation contains both L-dopa and the dopa decarboxylase inhibitor carbidopa. High doses of pyridoxine may lead to sensory nerve damage and be manifested as paraesthesiae; this is reversible on stopping vitamin B6.

22. Homocystinuria Answers: All false

Homocystinuria is an autosomal recessive disorder due to deficiency of beta-cystathione synthetase. It shares many phenotypic features with Marfan's syndrome but patients do not develop aortic root dilation. There is an increased arterial thrombotic risk. In approximately 50% of patients homocystine levels (and thrombotic risk) fall with pyridoxine therapy. It does not cause renal stones. Urinary cystine stones can be treated by penicillamine which increases the solubility of cystine in urine (but does not alter urinary cystine concentration).

23. Neuroleptic malignant syndrome **Answers: B D E**

The neuroleptic malignant syndrome usually complicates phenothiazine therapy and often occurs within two weeks of a change of dose. It can be a complication of tricyclic antidepressants, levodopa and amantadine, and phenytoin. The classical features are hyperthermia and rigidity with autonomic dysfunction and altered state of consciousness in many. Rhabdomyolysis, seizures, DIC and catatonia frequently occur. Treatment is largely supportive with withdrawal of the neuroleptic, but dantrolene, bromocriptine and benzodiazepines have all been used with favourable effects.

24. Secondary amyloidosis **Answers: All false**

Reactive amyloidosis occurs as a result of a prolonged acute phase response, particularly elevation of the serum amyloid A protein which in genetically predisposed individuals cannot be catabolised and so becomes deposited in tissues as fibrils. The tongue may be enlarged with amyloid but not ulcerated. It typically presents with nephrotic syndrome. It may occur in children as well as adults and is progressive and fatal despite good control of the underlying disease.

25. Hypothermia **Answers: A B C D**

Hypothermia is defined as a core temperature of 35°C or less. Shivering is usually present until the temperature falls below about 30°C. Myotonia or impaired muscle relaxation is a recognised manifestation. Pancreatitis but not hepatic necrosis commonly complicates the condition. Hypothermia also impairs tissue oxygen delivery through its effect on haemoglobin-oxygen dissociation.

MOLECULAR MEDICINE: ANSWERS AND EXPLANATIONS

1. Renin **Answers: C D**

Renal renin is synthesised, stored and released from the cells located in the afferent glomerular arteriole (juxtaglomerular cells). Renin acts on angiotensinogen to produce angiotensin I. The transcription rate of the renin gene is stimulated by cyclic AMP and inhibited by angiotensin II: treatment with ACE inhibitors stimulates transcription. Renin release is stimulated by lowered renal perfusion pressure, reduced delivery of chloride to the macula densa and renal nerve stimulation. However, circulating renin concentration is a poor predictor of renal artery stenosis.

2. Endothelium derived relaxation factor **Answers: B E**

Endothelium derived relaxation factor is nitric oxide. It is formed by endothelial cells from L-arginine and is released immediately into the microenvironment where it acts directly on guanylate cyclase to increase cyclic GMP leading to vasodilation.

3. Endothelin-1 **Answers: A C E**

Endothelin-1 is a 21 amino acid peptide, produced primarily from endothelial cells. It is secreted as a prohormone and endothelin-1 is generated by the action of endothelial membrane bound endothelin converting enzyme. Endothelin-1 is a potent long acting vasoconstrictor and bronchoconstrictor. Unlike angiotensin, it has equal effects on afferent and efferent glomerular arterioles. Endothelin-1 levels are elevated in acute myocardial infarction, chronic heart failure, acute renal failure, asthma and primary pulmonary hypertension.

4. Transforming growth factor beta **Answers: A B D**

Transforming growth factor beta is a 25 kD homodimeric peptide that can occur in at least three isoforms, each with discrete biological effects. It is released from platelets during degranulation and is able to induce its own production from monocytes. It is intimately involved in the inflammatory response promoting wound healing and modulating the immune response by suppressing lymphocyte proliferation.

5. Tumour necrosis factor-alpha **Answers: B C D**

Tumour necrosis factor-alpha is a proinflammatory cytokine, predominantly synthesised by macrophages and released in response to bacterial or inflammatory stimuli. It predominantly acts in a paracrine fashion at the site of release to promote inflammation/injury rather than repair or fibrosis. It has two receptors present on the surface of nearly all cells, except erythrocytes, and cleaved fragments of these receptors act as binding proteins in the serum.

6. Haemopoietic growth factors **Answers: A B**

Haemopoietic growth factors are glycoprotein hormones that regulate the proliferation and differentiation of haemopoietic progenitor cells and the function of mature cells. They include erythropoietin, granulocyte macrophage colony stimulating factor (GM-CSF), granulocyte colony stimulating factor (G-CSF), macrophage colony stimulating factor (M-CSF) and interleukin 3. Each growth factor is encoded by a single gene on a number of different chromosomes. These factors are unrelated to the immunoglobulin superfamily.

7. G Proteins **Answers: B C E**

Guanine nucleotide binding proteins are ubiquitous proteins located at the inner aspect of cell membranes. They include a large family of proteins, including Ras oncogene. During activation, guanosine triphosphate is bound to the subunit which promotes signal transduction. Deactivation occurs through hydrolysis of GTP to GDP.

8. Nuclear factor kB **Answers: A B C D E**

Nuclear factor kB is a transcription factor that acts on genes for pro-inflammatory cytokines (TNF, IL-1E, IL-2, IL-6), chemokines, enzymatic mediators of inflammation, immune receptors and adhesion molecules. It therefore has a pivotal role in the inflammatory response. In unstimulated cells it is found in the cytoplasm bound to a carrier. On activation it passes into the nucleus to act on specific promotor regions of target genes. Its actions are inhibited by glucocorticoids. Inducible nitric oxide synthase expression is enhanced by NF-kB.

9. Cell cycle **Answers: B D E**

The mitotic cell cycle is made up of: (a) Interphase; subdivided into G1 (the synthesis of RNA and proteins), S (replication of DNA) and G2 (synthesis of organelles); (b) Mitotic nuclear division; subdivided into protophase (chromosomes become visible and spindles are formed), metaphase (chromosomes line up at the spindle equator), anaphase (chromatids and centromeres separate) and telophase (where two new nuclear membranes are formed); (c) Cytoplasmic cleavage.

10. Apoptosis **Answers: B D E**

Apoptosis is programmed cell death and leads to the removal of 'unwanted cells' (and their potentially injurious contents) without tissue necrosis or injury. It is involved in a wide variety of important biological processes; including embryological remodelling, thymic selection of lymphocytes and tumour involution. The biochemical 'hallmark' is internucleosomal chromatin cleavage, resulting in condensation of nuclear chromatin as a result of endogenous endonuclease activation.

11. Adhesion molecules **Answers: C D**

Endothelial-leucocyte adhesions molecules control leucocyte transmigration to sites of inflammation. They include selectin-carbohydrate interaction, immunoglobulin super family member cell adhesion molecules (IgCAMs) that bind to integrins and CD31 that is capable of homophilic interaction between endothelial and leucocyte CD31.

12. Steroid hormone receptors **Answers: C E**

Steroid receptors represent a class of ligand activated transcription factors, with differing binding affinities that include vitamin D receptors and thyroid hormone receptors. They are located intracellularly and function primarily by virtue of their DNA binding activity. Certain steroid receptors are stabilised by heat shock proteins. Aminoglutethimide acts predominantly by inhibiting the conversion of androgens to oestrogens in the peripheral tissues.

13. Antisense oligonucleotides **Answer: E**

Antisense oligonucleotides have a deoxynucleotide sequence of 13 to 20 base pairs in length – not amino acids. They hybridise to a specific complementary mRNA sequence, which is then subject to RNAse degradation resulting in a translational block. They do not lead to expression of 'nonsense' proteins. Decoy oligonucleotides (not antisense oligonucleotides) mimic the DNA binding domain of certain transcription factors and thereby down regulate gene expression.

14. Cardiac sarcomere **Answers: A C D E**

The sarcomere is made of two interdigitating filaments, thick filaments of myosin and thin filaments of actin. The actin filaments have a complex structure associated with tropomyosin which maintains the structure of the actin chain and troponin complex. Contraction in the cardiac sarcomere is initiated by the binding of calcium to troponin C which then no longer causes troponin I to inhibit the interaction between actin and myosin. The myosin head contains an ATPase which breaks down ATP to provide energy for contraction but ATP is also necessary for relaxation.

15. Dystrophin **Answers: B C E**

Dystrophin is a large submembrane protein that is orientated parallel to the muscle cell membranes and provides part of the extracellular to intracellular protein chain by linking beta-dystroglycan and F-actin. It is absent in Duchenne muscular dystrophy which is an X-linked disease. Limb girdle muscular dystrophies encompass a diverse set of diseases frequently associated with mutations to dystrophin-associated proteins that interact with dystrophin (but not abnormalities of dystrophin itself).

16. The P53 gene **Answers: A D E**

P53 is a tumour suppressor gene that regulates apoptosis and can halt the cell cycle in response to cell injury. The frequency of P53 mutations is 90% in small cell and 55% in non small cell lung cancer. Retroviral mediated wild type P53 gene transfer to tumours of patients with lung cancer increases apoptosis and tumour regression. Tobacco smoke carcinogens induce a specific pattern of P53 mutations and detection of P53 mutations in sputum can precede diagnosis of lung cancer. Cytochrome P450 (not P53) is induced by alcohol and enzyme-inducing drugs.

17. Plasma proteins **Answers: A D E**

The different electrical charges of plasma proteins permit electrophoretic separation. They are mainly in the anion form, and contribute to the anion gap. Their weak ionization confers a buffering action. The main buffering action of plasma is provided by the carbon acid-bicarbonate mechanism.

18. Proto-oncogenes **Answers: C D**

Proto-oncogenes are normal cellular genes that control a variety of processes associated with cell growth and differentiation. They are transiently stimulated by growth factors. Oncogenes are altered or overexpressed versions of proto-oncogene counterparts that lack regulatory constraints and do not need external activation signals. Oncogenes are associated with the development of a wide variety of human tumours.

19. Associations of tumours and circulating markers Answers: A C

The relatively recently described CA125 antigen is a useful tumour marker in some forms of ovarian carcinoma. Alpha fetoprotein levels are increased with both hepatoma and malignant teratoma. Embryonic tumours may also secrete HCG, as in choriocarcinoma and teratoma. Medullary carcinoma of the thyroid characteristically produces calcitonin: thyroglobulin may however be a useful tumour marker for other thyroid cell carcinomas. PTH-related peptide is the main mediator of the humoral hypercalcaemia of malignancy and is most commonly produced by tumours of epithelial rather than mesenchymal origin.

20. Angiotensin converting enzyme Answers: A C D

Angiotensin converting enzyme inactivates bradykinin. Levels may be raised in sarcoid and also in tuberculosis, berylliosis, silicosis, asbestosis, carcinoma of the lung, primary biliary cirrhosis and leprosy. ACE inhibitors may increase ACE levels in active sarcoidosis but not in normals.

21. Pathological lesions Answers: A B C E

Hepatic vein thrombosis is typically responsible for severe centrilobular necrosis. The amyloid plaques characteristic of the cerebral pathology of Alzheimer's disease may contain prions (proteinaceous infectious agents). Colitis occurring in Crohn's disease is transmural, whereas it is more superficial in ulcerative colitis. Alpha-1 anti-trypsin deficiency is associated with a panacinar form of emphysema.

22. Malignant tumours Answers: A B E

In malignancy, mitoses tend to be not only abnormal, but numerous. Anaplasia is used to denote lack of resemblance of a malignant tumour to its parent organ. Invasiveness is the hallmark of malignancy. Some malignant tumours produce a marked fibrous reaction (e.g. scirrhous carcinoma of the breast), but this is exceptional.

NEPHROLOGY: ANSWERS AND EXPLANATIONS

1. Renal blood flow **Answers: A E**

More than 90% of the renal blood flow is directed to the cortex. Simulation of the renal nerves causes vasoconstriction. In contrast to most tissues, renal blood flow tends to fall with anaemia and rises with polycythaemia thus keeping plasma flow constant. Blood transfusion in chronic renal failure can sometimes lead to a serious fall in renal plasma flow. Autoregulation occurs in the kidney so that the blood flow remains constant over the range of blood pressure 90–200 mmHg.

2. Atrial natriuretic factors **Answers: All false**

Atrial natriuretic peptides are released from myocytes in response to atrial stretch rather than absolute atrial pressure. They have a variety of actions within the kidney including vasorelaxation of renal arterioles, modulatory effects on GFR, and they diminish the ADH-induced water reabsorption in the collecting ducts. Natriuretic effects are seen in the distal tubule (inhibition of aldosterone-mediated Na reabsorption) but there is no action on the loop of Henle. Massive ANF activity is observed in patients with congestive cardiac or end-stage renal failure.

3. The ureter **Answers: A D E**

The ureter and bladder are lined with transitional epithelium whereas the vas deferens is lined with columnar epithelium. The sympathetic nerve supply to the ureter is from spinal cord segments L1 and L2. Remember that there is no sympathetic outflow below L2.

4. Renal disease **Answers: B C D E**

In advanced chronic renal failure injected contrast may not be concentrated by the kidneys; IVU may also exacerbate renal damage in some forms of acute renal failure. DMSA is avidly taken-up and bound by renal tissue and provides accurate evidence of structure. DTPA and MAG3 are rapidly concentrated and excreted by the kidneys and so allow assessment of differential blood flow and function (including the excretory phase). IVU provides information from the whole of the urinary tract in the search for urothelial malignancy in patients with haematuria.

5. Microalbuminuria in a diabetic patient — Answers: B E

Microalbuminuria, defined as detectable albuminuria (30–300 mcg/min or roughly 25–250 mg/24 hour) below the clearly proteinuric range is best assessed with a timed overnight specimen as 24 hour specimens may be affected by orthostatic proteinuria. Angiotensin converting enzyme inhibitors reduce protein excretion and delay development of renal impairment even in normotensive individuals. Microalbuminuria should raise the level of suspicion for proliferative retinopathy but this is not universal. In NIDDM patients there is a strong association between the findings of microalbuminuria and development of macrovascular disease.

6. Urobilinogen in urine — Answer: D

Urobilinogen is present in the urine of normal subjects. An excess of urobilinogen can be detected by Ehrlich's aldehyde reagent. Distinction from porphobilinogen is by solubility in aqueous and non-aqueous phases. An increase of urobilinogen in the urine occurs in hepato-cellular dysfunction; urobilinogen disappears from the urine in intrahepatic obstruction. Urobilinogenuria is also found with the increased bilirubin formation of haemolysis. Mild haemolysis is a feature of pernicious anaemia.

7. Urine sodium concentration — Answers: B C

Renal sodium loss is excessive when there is damage to the medullary tissue (as in chronic pyelonephritis) and following relief of obstruction. Severe dehydration alone, without the development of acute tubular necrosis, leads to avid conservation of sodium by the kidney, with urinary sodium concentration as low as 5 mmol/l. Once acute tubular necrosis has developed, the ability to conserve sodium correctly is lost. In cranial diabetes insipidus, the urine is very dilute, with conservation of sodium to maintain plasma volume (via activation of the renin angiotensin aldosterone axis).

8. Hypokalaemic states — Answers: A C D E

Pathological changes occurring in severe hypokalaemia are predominantly in the tubular cells and interstitium. Alkalosis is usually present in those cases of hypokalaemia not due to intrinsic renal disease (Conn's and Cushing's syndromes, pyloric stenosis, diuretic or exogenous steroid excess), but acidosis is observed with severe diarrhoea because of excessive bicarbonate loss. In Bartter's syndrome there is considerable salt wasting, and untreated cases are hypotensive due to hypovolaemia; renin secretion is over-stimulated with consequent hypertrophy of the juxta-glomerular apparatus.

9. Serum osmolality **Answers: B C D**

The osmolality is a direct measure of the osmolar concentration of 1 kg of plasma whereas the osmolarity is an estimation derived from the measured Na, K, urea and glucose concentrations. The osmolarity will thus be unreliable in conditions where pseudo-hyponatraemia is present, such as that due to hyperlipidaemia (which will occur in severe nephrotic syndrome) or hyperproteinaemia. The osmolality will also take account of plasma constituents that are not normally present (e.g. alcohol).

10. Metabolic acidosis **Answers: A B C**

The anion-gap is calculated by subtracting the measured plasma anionic concentration (bicarbonate and chloride) from the added serum sodium and potassium value, and should be in the range 10–16 mmol/l. In the presence of metabolic acidosis a normal or low anion gap would indicate hyperchloraemic acidosis (such as with diarrhoea or renal tubular acidosis), whereas an enlarged gap would signify the presence in plasma of a normally undetected anion/acid that might be contributing to the acidosis (e.g. lactic, salicylic or ketoacids, unmeasured uraemic toxins). Acetazolamide inhibits bicarbonate reabsorption in the renal tubule.

11. Renal tubular acidosis **Answers: A C E**

Aminoaciduria is found as an associated proximal tubular defect in proximal (type II) RTA. In distal RTA there is failure of hydrogen-ion excretion; this abnormality can be primary, or far more commonly occurs as a result of conditions which predominantly affect the renal medulla and interstitium, such as chronic reflux uropathy, hypercalcaemia, hypokalaemia, obstructive uropathy, Sjögren's syndrome and other interstitial nephritides. Considering the primary form, the polyuria is due to impaired osmotic concentrating ability, in part due to hypokalaemia, which also gives muscle weakness. Nephrocalcinosis and urinary stones form due to hypercalciuria, alkaline urine and low urinary citrate excretion. They may contribute to glomerular failure in some cases, but uraemia is not a typical early feature. The other major problems arise from osteomalacia.

12. An increase in the ratio of plasma urea to creatinine
Answers: A C D E

In addition to glomerular filtration, the major determinant of plasma creatinine concentration is the rate of production which depends on skeletal muscle mass. Urea production, however, rapidly rises in catabolic states (with injury, heart failure, infection and corticosteroid therapy) and with increased gastrointestinal absorption of nitrogen (GI haemorrhage, uretero-colic anastomosis, and high protein diet). Urea production falls in severe liver disease. Urea excretion falls in dehydration due to increased renal tubular re-absorption, hence increasing the plasma urea/creatinine ratio.

13. Acute renal failure **Answer: D**

Acute renal failure is most commonly the result of circulatory stress such as hypovolaemic, cardiogenic or septic shock (acute tubular necrosis). If the patients are adequately supported renal function usually returns, but as many are severely ill with multi-organ failure overall mortality remains high. Paracetamol can directly cause tubular necrosis.

14. Renal failure **Answers: A B C**

ARF may follow ACE inhibitor treatment in patients with pre-existent renovascular disease or renal hypoperfusion; renal size is normal or kidneys may be swollen in ARF. Haemolytic anaemia occurs in haemolytic-uraemic syndrome and certain vasculitides (e.g. SLE). Reflux uropathy accounts for 30% of cases of CRF, but a history of urinary infection is only documented in 25% of cases. An aortic aneurysm may involve the renal arteries, resulting in either CRF or ARF if acute thrombosis of the vessels occurs or the aneurysm ruptures.

15. Uraemic osteodystrophy **Answers: A B C D**

The major metabolic abnormalities in uraemic osteodystrophy include hyperparathyroidism (resulting in increased bony resorption), hyperphosphataemia and decreased 1-alpha hydroxylation of vitamin D (such that calcium absorption from the gut is attenuated).

16. Anaemia in chronic renal failure — Answers: A C D

Anaemia in CRF is largely due to lack of erythropoietin, is least marked in polycystic renal disease, and is only consistently reversed by successful renal transplantation. The degree of anaemia is broadly related to the serum creatinine, becoming manifest when the GFR falls below 30 ml/min. Increased red cell 2,3 DPG shifts the oxygen dissociation curve to the right, increasing tissue oxygenation. Iron utilisation is disordered in CRF and iron deficiency is recognised by lack of stainable iron in the bone marrow or by a low serum ferritin.

17. End-stage renal failure — Answer: D

Subcutaneous administration of erythropoietin (EPO) is more efficacious than intravenous administration as the latter reduces bioavailability of the product. Initiation phase treatment may last 3–4 months before target haemoglobin is achieved, and response is enhanced by parenteral iron supplementation. The mean haemoglobin concentration of a haemodialysis population is usually less than that of a corresponding CAPD programme, perhaps due to increased blood losses, red cell fragmentation or comorbidity in the former group. Hyperparathyroidism and chronic infection also diminish response to EPO.

18. Chronic renal failure — Answers: A C

Progression of moderate chronic renal failure can be attenuated by optimising hypertensive control especially with ACE inhibitors; protein restriction has little effect. Reducing sodium intake may also improve blood pressure control but diuretics have no effect on outcome.

19. Drugs — Answer: E

Digoxin undergoes renal elimination and toxic concentrations develop if given in normal doses in patients with chronic renal failure. The other agents largely undergo hepatic excretion and standard doses can be used safely in renal impairment.

20. Dialysis-related amyloidosis — Answers: A D

Dialysis-related amyloidosis is due to deposition of beta 2 microglobulin as amyloid fibrils predominantly in and around joints classically resulting in carpal tunnel syndrome or shoulder girdle arthropathy. It can affect patients treated by all forms of dialysis. Transplantation results in increased beta 2 microglobulin excretion and improvement of the condition. There is no increase in renal transplant failure. It is not associated with any particular primary renal disease – diabetics are less likely to survive the long time on dialysis necessary for the condition to manifest itself.

21. Renal transplantation **Answers: C E**

If lymphocytotoxic antibodies directed against HLA antigens are present in the recipient's serum then the chances of a successful transplant may be reduced; immuno-absorption has been used to remove the antibodies in selected cases. The most important loci for the purposes of donor/recipient matching are HLA-B and HLA-DR. Mesangiocapillary glomerulonephritis can re-occur in a renal transplant (as can focal segmental sclerosis, IgA nephropathy, Goodpasture's and the vasculitides, although in the latter examples a rise in auto-antibody titre will herald disease recurrence) but as in the case of previous hepatitis B infection this should not preclude transplantation. Marked aortic and iliac vessel atheroma may render the patient unsuitable for transplantation..

22. Renal transplantation **Answers: A B D E**

Currently immunosuppressive regimes, in most transplant units, include corticosteroids. Complications attributed to steroid therapy include avascular necrosis of bone, most commonly to the hip, cataracts producing visual impairment and growth retardation. Hirsutism is a common complication of cyclosporin A therapy which is invariably a component of the immunosuppressive drug regime. There is an increased incidence of malignancy particularly malignant lymphoma and skin cancer.

23. Nephrotic syndrome **Answers: A B D E**

The commonest lesion in children is minimal-change nephropathy which responds well to corticosteroids; cyclosporin A has been used successfully to treat relapses in adults. Chronic hepatitis B surface antigenaemia may cause a membranous glomerulonephritis, and this lesion can also result from *Plasmodium malariae* infection (quartan nephropathy) which is the most frequent cause of nephrotic syndrome world-wide. Levels of clotting factors are increased and fibrinolytic components reduced in nephrotic states, and as the intravascular fluid volume is also contracted thrombosis is a frequent complication (e.g. renal vein thrombosis).

24. Rapidly progressive glomerulonephritis **Answers: A B**

The characteristic histology of extensive glomerular epithelial cell proliferation (hence 'crescentic glomerulonephritis') may be associated with infection (SBE, post-streptococcal disease) and occurs in other acute systemic disorders such as SLE and Henoch-Schönlein purpura. ANCA may be present in vasculitides (microscopic polyarteritis, Wegener's granulomatosis) and anti-GBM antibodies seen in Goodpasture's syndrome are IgG. Patients usually develop oligo-anuria and early treatment with immunosuppressive drugs with or without plasma exchange may considerably influence outcome.

25. Goodpasture's syndrome **Answers: B E**

Two-thirds of patients with anti-GBM disease have pulmonary haemorrhage and plasma exchange in addition to immunosuppressive therapy may be required for life-saving control. Transplantation is an effective treatment for end-stage renal failure where anti-GBM titres are low; in patients where titres are elevated intercurrent infection frequently triggers clinical relapse.

26. Serum complement **Answers: B C**

A low serum complement level is seen in disorders in which there is complement fixation and deposition within glomeruli. This pattern occurs in glomerulonephritis associated with SLE, infected ventriculo-atrial shunts and in post-streptococcal disease. One variety of mesangio-capillary glomerulonephritis is characterised by the presence of a protein in the serum (C_3 nephritic factor) that can induce C_3 cleavage *in vitro*.

27. Membranous glomerulonephritis **Answers: B E**

One-third of patients with idiopathic membranous glomerulonephritis (GN) progress to end-stage renal failure. The condition may recur in renal transplants, but less frequently than focal segmental glomerulosclerosis, IgA nephropathy and mesangiocapillary glomerulonephritis. Although an immune aetiology is established, circulating immune complexes do not play a major role. Secondary membranous GN is linked to solid malignancies (breast, stomach, colon) and non-Hodgkin's lymphoma; Hodgkin's disease is associated with minimal change GN. Gold and penicillamine therapy in rheumatoid arthritis may also induce a reversible secondary membranous GN.

28. Incontinence of urine **Answers: A B C D**

Inflammatory changes in the bladder mucosa due to infection, catheters, stones etc. may give urgency incontinence. In a patient whose control of micturition is tenuous, the use of diuretics will often precipitate incontinence. Any obstruction to bladder outflow such as chronic prostatic enlargement may lead to chronic retention and overflow incontinence. Diabetes insipidus must be incredibly rare as a cause of incontinence. Far more important are the above, and gynaecological stress incontinence, with faecal impaction often playing a role in the elderly.

29. Urinary stones **Answers: A C D E**

There is a marked tendency for idiopathic hypercalciuria, which is a predominantly male disease and the commonest single cause of calcium stones, to run in families. Persistently acid urine is a feature of uric acid stone formers. Calcium phosphate tends to precipitate in alkaline urine whereas calcium oxalate stones do not depend on urine pH. Factors that predispose to oxalate stones include hyperuricosuria, either dietary or due to gout, and increased absorption of oxalate from the bowel in malabsorption states.

30. Ureteric obstruction **Answers: A B C D E**

Intestinal by-pass operations may result in secondary hyperoxaluria with formation of calcium oxalate stones. Ureteric obstruction occurs in analgesic nephropathy due to sloughed papillae. In schistosomiasis (due to *S. haematobium*), fibrosis occurs in the bladder and ureters, stones are common, and in Egypt, carcinoma of the bladder develops. Ureteric necrosis, due to disturbance of the vascular supply, is a not uncommon complication of transplantation. Leakage from an abdominal aortic aneurysm may be important in the pathogenesis of some cases of retroperitoneal fibrosis.

31. Haemolytic-uraemic syndrome **Answers: B C D**

Haemolytic-uraemic syndrome occurs either sporadically or in minor epidemics, the latter often associated with infective diarrhoea (including that due to verocytotoxin-producing coliforms) and having a better prognosis. The resulting oliguric acute renal failure is best treated by either haemodialysis or haemofiltration as hypercatabolism is often a feature.

32. Unilateral renal artery stenosis **Answer: A**

Accelerated hypertension due to renal artery stenosis is caused by hyper-reninaemia and consequent hyperaldosteronism, the latter resulting in hypokalaemic alkalosis. Until significant hypertensive damage occurs in the contralateral kidney, renal function, both tubular and glomerular, is maintained even when the blood pressure is lowered by the angiotensin convertase inhibitor, captopril. Increased pyelographic concentration may occur in the affected kidney.

33. Renal amyloid deposition **Answers: A C E**

Deposition of amyloid protein within the kidneys may occur in primary amyloidosis or as a result of conditions involving chronic suppuration or inflammation, disorders of plasma cell function and with hereditary amyloid (familial Mediterranean fever). A nephrotic presentation is common and the classical histological staining is with Congo red (apple-green birefringence is seen under polarised light). The recently developed SAP scan utilises serum amyloid P component, a normal plasma constituent, which binds to amyloid fibrils – I^{123} radiolabelled SAP is injected and localises to amyloid present in any region of the body. The amyloid protein that accumulates in dialysis patients is β_2-microglobin and this is deposited within connective tissues and not in major organs.

34. Polycystic disease of the kidneys **Answers: A B C**

Berry aneurysms and urinary stones occur in about 10% of cases. Although liver cysts are found in perhaps a third of cases, they rarely give rise to symptoms and probably never to liver failure. This is in contrast to the much rarer polycystic disease of childhood, where liver failure and portal hypertension due to hepatic fibrosis may be the dominant clinical features.

35. Polycystic kidney disease **Answers: B D E**

Autosomal dominant polycystic kidney disease is common with a gene frequency of approximately 1 in 1000. Cysts can be present from birth and enlarge over time. End-stage renal disease is unusual before age 40 (< 5%). The renal cysts produce excessive amounts of erythropoietin that can result in polycythaemia. Other common features are haematuria, hypertension, mitral valve prolapse and ruptured berry aneurysms. The commonest form of APCKD – type I – which accounts for 90% of cases results from an abnormality in the gene for polycystin on chromosome 16, a protein that has a role in epithelial cell differentiation. Liver cysts are more numerous and larger in women than in men, presumably as a consequence of hormonal differences.

36. Alport's syndrome **Answer: A**

Alport's syndrome is usually transmitted as an X-linked dominant trait. It is due to an abnormality of type IV collagen resulting in weakness of the basement membranes. These are glomerulopathy, sensorineural deafness and anterior lenticonus and retinitis pigmentosa. Cardiac conduction defects are not a feature of Alport's syndrome. Post-transplant anti-glomerular basement membrane disease complicates less than 5% of Alport syndrome renal transplants.

37. Renal disease **Answers: All false**

ACE inhibitors are relatively contraindicated in bilateral renovascular disease but they may be necessary for control of resulting hypertension; they may be useful in cases of unilateral renal artery stenosis. In IDDM, untreated renal failure is the commonest cause of death, whereas in NIDDM the majority of patients die from cardiovascular complications. Episodes of macroscopic haematuria in IgA nephropathy tend to occur at the same time as, or shortly after, an upper respiratory tract infection, and the majority of patients with reflux nephropathy have no relevant antecedent history. Although renal transplant function may be satisfactory after a period of cold ischaemia of up to 30 hours, donor organ warm ischaemia should be minimised and certainly should not exceed 45 minutes.

NEUROLOGY: ANSWERS AND EXPLANATIONS

1. Thrombosis of posterior inferior cerebellar artery

Answers: All false

Thrombosis of the posterior inferior cerebellar artery or vertebral artery may cause infarction of the lateral medulla oblongata (Wallenberg's syndrome). It gives rise to ipsilateral Horner's syndrome, palatal paralysis and ataxia. Sensory loss is dissociated, with ipsilateral loss of pain and temperature sensation in the face and contralateral loss in the limbs. Contralateral hemiplegia may occur if the entire half of the medulla is affected but should not be considered a feature of this discrete syndrome. Cranial nerve nuclei concerned with eye movement lie within the pons and midbrain.

2. Occlusion of the left middle cerebral artery **Answers: D E**

The motor and sensory abnormalities affect predominantly the face and arm. The cortical representation for the leg is parasagittal and is supplied by the anterior cerebral artery. Both the motor area for speech in the frontal lobe and the language areas in the temporal and parietal lobes are affected producing a global aphasia, including difficulties with reading and calculation. Conjugate gaze to the opposite side of the lesion is affected. Anosognosia describes the loss of ability to recognise or to acknowledge bodily defect and is a non-dominant parietal lobe disorder.

3. Stroke **Answers: A B C D E**

Mitral annular calcification is an independent risk factor for embolic stroke (relative risk x2), as is atrial fibrillation in non-rheumatic (x6) and rheumatic (x17) heart disease. Coarctation of the aorta is associated with upper body hypertension and berry aneurysms, which predispose to intracranial haemorrhage. Rarely, a patent foramen ovale may allow passage of a paradoxical embolus (i.e. from right to left atrium).

4. Anterior cerebral artery territory infarction Answers: B C D

Anterior cerebral artery territory infarction is very uncommon in primary occlusive cerebrovascular disease and is almost always caused by secondary vasospasm following subarachnoid haemorrhage. Infarction in this territory causes predominant weakness of the lower limb and the proximal upper limb (the shoulder). The hand may be weakened by damage to the underlying fibres of the internal capsule but is less severely affected. Language function may be involved if the dominant hemisphere is damaged and this aphasia is characterised by a non-fluent aphasia (reduced word output) with good understanding and preserved ability to repeat words (transcortical motor aphasia). Damage to the anterior cerebral artery territory due to cerebral embolism is almost unheard of.

5. Lacunar syndromes Answers: A B C E

Lacunar syndromes are predictive of small deep lesions in the motor (50%) and sensory (5%) pathways (mixed 35%). Most are due to small infarcts seen best on MRI. Higher cortical function loss is not a feature of lacunar syndromes. Ataxic hemiparesis occurs in about 10% and is the combination of corticospinal and ipsilateral cerebellar signs.

6. Aneurysmal subarachnoid haemorrhage Answers: A C D E

Over 90% of aneurysms lie on the anterior part of the circle of Willis and multiple aneurysms are detected in 20% of patients. Vasospasm is common between the fourth and tenth days post haemorrhage and may be worsened by angiography and surgery, causing stroke, ST segment elevation on ECG is thought to be due to sympathetic hyperactivity caused by intracranial haemorrhage, however, the most characteristic changes are deep symmetrical inverted T waves. Normal pressure hydrocephalus due to arachnoid granulation blockage causing dementia, gait disturbance and incontinence is a late complication.

7. Complex partial seizures Answers: A C D

Complex partial seizures of temporal lobe onset may be accompanied by an aura of fear, dread, visceral sensation and dysmnesic phenomena such as jamais vu and déjà vu. Primitive visual aura suggests an occipital focus. Versive seizures with turning of the eyes and/or head to the contralateral side suggest a frontal focus.

8. Periodic complexes **Answers: B C D**

Periodic complexes are typically detected in Creutzfeldt-Jakob disease, SSPE, herpes simplex encephalitis and hepatic coma. In the latter the complexes often have a triphasic appearance. In Pick's disease the EEG is invariably normal whereas in PML the recording shows a diffuse slowing of rhythms.

9. Juvenile myoclonic epilepsy **Answer: C**

Juvenile myoclonic epilepsy typically presents around puberty with myoclonic jerks and generalised tonic-clonic seizures on waking. The interictal EEG shows polyspike wave complexes and photosensitivity is common. There is a family history of seizures in about a quarter of patients. The treatment of choice is sodium valproate on which about half of patients will become seizure-free.

10. Seizures **Answers: A D E**

The patient but not his or her doctor is obliged to contact the DVLC, although it is sensible practice to record in the case notes that a patient has been counselled about driving. Patients must be free from any attack for two years or have had only attacks whilst asleep for three years before driving is permitted. A diagnosis of primary malignant cerebral tumour, cerebral metastasis or even bronchogenic carcinoma without cerebral metastasis is associated with such a high risk of a seizure that driving is prohibited.

11. HIV-1 virus related dementia **Answers: A C E**

HIV-1 virus related dementia eventually affects 70–90% of patients with AIDS and may be the presenting feature. Patients present with apathy, depression and irritability. Features of cortical dysfunction, such as aphasia and visuoconstructive difficulties, are late manifestations. Toxoplasmosis is the most common opportunistic cause of dementia.

12. Alzheimer's disease **Answers: C E**

Alzheimer's disease causes an early degeneration of the limbic system and temporo-parietal neocortex. Decreased brain activity in these areas appears to predate degeneration and may be detected by positron or single photon emission tomography. In the late stages patients develop extrapyramidal features (rigidity, hypokinesia and stooped posture) and myoclonus. The cortico-spinal tracts are not affected. Neurofibrillary tangles are also found in other degenerative diseases including progressive supra-nuclear palsy and dementia pugilistica. Features of frontal lobe dysfunction suggest an alternative diagnosis such as lobar atrophy or Pick's disease.

13. Creutzfeldt-Jakob disease — Answers: B D E

Creutzfeldt-Jakob disease is a transmissible spongiform encephalopathy which is thought to be due to an abnormal prion protein (PrP). It is rapidly progressive with death usually within 12–18 months of onset. The EEG is markedly abnormal with repetitive triphasic discharges on a flat background.

14. Subcortical dementia — Answers: A C E

Alzheimer's disease and Pick's disease are associated with a cortical distribution of pathology. Binswanger's disease is due to multiple small infarcts within the subcortical white matter. Normal pressure hydrocephalus, Parkinson's disease and Wilson's disease are also associated with subcortical dementia.

15. Pick's disease — Answers: A B

Pick's disease is a primary degenerative condition with a fronto-temporal distribution of cerebral pathology which is quite distinct from that in Alzheimer's disease. Behavioural disturbance and frontal lobe release signs are typical early clinical features. Extrapyramidal rigidity may be a late clinical feature. The EEG is usually normal. It is familial in approximately 20% of cases.

16. Benign intracranial hypertension — Answers: A E

In benign intracranial hypertension most investigations including CSF protein levels are normal. The lateral ventricles are usually normal or 'slit-like'. Signs reflect the raised intracranial pressure (sixth nerve palsy) and papilloedema (enlarged blind spots). Acuity is not normally affected unless papilloedema extends to affect the macula. The combination of a blurred optic disc and reduced visual acuity suggest papillitis. BIH usually occurs in overweight young females and is associated with pregnancy, oral contraceptives, tetracyclines and nalidixic acid. Presentation in the puerperium, after infection or dehydration, suggests venous sinus thrombosis and urgent consideration of anticoagulation.

17. Normal pressure hydrocephalus (NPH) Answers: B E

Normal pressure hydrocephalus is associated with the clinical triad of subcortical dementia, gait disturbance and urinary incontinence. The gait disturbance is usually postural and broad based. The term 'gait apraxia' has been applied but it is not due to primary cerebral cortical dysfunction. The lateral ventricles are enlarged, resulting in greater deviation of fibres from the medial cerebral cortex (leg and sphincter motor fibres). CSF pressure studies demonstrate an intermittent rise in CSF pressure. Good prognostic factors for improvement following a CSF shunting procedure are: known aetiology (e.g. subarachnoid haemorrhage), short duration of symptoms, motor signs and transient improvement following CSF drainage (lumbar puncture).

18. Transient global amnesia (TGA) Answers: A B C D E

TGA is an ill understood disorder in which there is an abrupt onset of anterograde amnesia with repetitive questioning. It is associated with precipitating factors such as vigorous exercise, sexual intercourse, sudden temperature change and may follow vertebral angiography. It tends to last only a few hours. It is due to transient bilateral medial temporal lobe dysfunction and may have an underlying vasospastic basis. Repetitive episodes of memory disturbance with associated reduction of conscious level in an individual less than 40 years old are more suggestive of complex partial seizures of temporal lobe onset. Repetitive episodes of memory disturbance with vertigo, unsteadiness and visual disturbance are more suggestive of transient ischaemic episodes in the vertebrobasilar territory. Loss of memory and personal identity usually has an underlying psychiatric basis.

19. Lesion of the cerebral cortex Answers: C D

Dysphasia is due to a lesion in the dominant cerebral cortex. Hemianopia indicates a lesion of the optic tract, radiation or occipital cortex. Dysarthria is most likely to be due to subcortical, midbrain or brain stem pathology. Upper motor neurone signs may be produced by cerebral, midbrain, brain stem or cord pathology.

20. Associations **Answers: A B C**

Pineal tumours may be of many different cell types, the minority (25%) originating from pineal cells. Clinical features are from local pressure effects on the midbrain, aqueduct blockage of CSF and spread of cells through the 3rd ventricle causing hypothalamic damage (diabetes insipidus, hyper/hypophagia, precocious puberty and hypopituitarism) or optic chiasmal damage. Localisation of brain function is a common topic for MCQ questions. Broca's area is frontal, Wernicke's (receptive dysphasia) is temporal. Cortical sensation is a parietal lobe function (postcentral gyrus). Apraxia and agnosia are usually non-dominant parietal lobe functions.

21. Speech **Answers: B C E**

Aphonia refers to noise production which may still be present with a parietal lesion. Spastic dysarthria is caused by upper motor neurone lesions which are commonly due to stroke, tumour or motor neurone disease. Extrapyramidal disease (Parkinson's/Huntington's chorea) may cause fast speech although hypokinetic speech is more common. Polio causes a lower motor neurone, therefore bulbar, dysarthria.

22. Unilateral ptosis **Answers: A B D E**

Causes of Horner's syndrome include damage to the sympathetic pathways of the medulla, such as in syringobulbia, lesions of the first thoracic root in the thoracic outlet syndrome and external carotid artery dilatation in cluster headache. The IIIrd nerve runs in the lateral wall of the cavernous sinus and may be damaged in cavernous sinus thrombosis.

23. Lesion of the III cranial nerve **Answers: B C**

A lesion of the III cranial nerve causes an efferent pupillary defect, mydriasis and divergent strabismus. A midbrain lesion may produce a III cranial nerve palsy and contralateral hemiplegia (Weber's syndrome).

24. Horner's syndrome **Answers: B D**

Horner's syndrome consists of mild ptosis, miosis and variable loss of sweating over the affected side of the face. The lesion may be central, preganglionic or postganglionic according to its site with respect to the superior cervical ganglion. Hydroxyamphetamine drops release noradrenaline from the terminal axon if this is functioning and therefore dilate the pupil of central or preganglionic Horner's but not of postganglionic Horner's (because the axon is no longer functioning). Phenylephrine dilates the normal and abnormal pupil equally in both central and preganglionic peripheral types of Horner's. However, in postganglionic Horner's denervation hypersensitivity causes the affected pupil to dilate more widely than the normal side. Cocaine blocks the re-uptake of noradrenaline from the neuromuscular junction of the dilator muscle of the pupil, dilating the normal pupil. In any type of Horner's cocaine drops will not dilate the pupil of the affected eye, because noradrenaline is not being liberated into the nerve-muscle junction. The outflow of sympathetic innervation to the pupils is at T1 level and therefore Horner's syndrome may follow damage to the lower trunks of the brachial plexus.

25. Internuclear ophthalmoplegia **Answers: B D E**

The diagnosis of multiple sclerosis depends on the demonstration of central nervous system lesions disseminated in time and place. An internuclear ophthalmoplegia is a sign of an intrinsic brain stem lesion affecting the median longitudinal fasciculus. If the spinal fluid is shown to contain gammaglobulin in an oligoclonal pattern it is very likely that multiple sclerosis is the cause. However, oligoclonal bands are present in many other intrathecal inflammatory diseases and do not make multiple sclerosis certain. If delayed latency in the visual evoked response is demonstrated in a patient with an internuclear ophthalmoplegia, then more than one lesion is present and multiple sclerosis is probable. If there is a past history of optic neuritis the diagnosis is confirmed. In acute central nervous system demyelination due to multiple sclerosis, high dose intravenous steroids have been shown to shorten the duration of relapses though they probably have no effect on long-term disability.

26. Bilateral facial weakness **Answers: All true**

Other causes of bilateral facial weakness include fascioscapular humeral dystrophy and polymyositis. A unilateral basal pontine lesion may produce an ipsilateral lower motor neurone seventh cranial nerve palsy due to involvement of the upper motor neurone fibres which subsequently cross to the contralateral seventh cranial nerve nucleus. An associated contralateral hemiplegia will usually be evident (Millard-Gubler syndrome). Bilateral lesions above the pons can produce bilateral upper motor neurone facial weakness, pseudobulbar palsy and associated long tract signs.

27. VIII nerve schwannoma **Answers: A C**

There are at least two genetically distinct forms of neuro-fibromatosis (NF). Patients with NF-2 are at risk of bilateral VIII nerve schwannomas and other brain tumours, including meningiomas. Cutaneous manifestations are rare. Patients with NF-1 have prominent cutaneous manifestations including café-au-lait macules, neurofibromas, axillary freckles and Lisch nodules but brain tumours, apart from optic pathway gliomas, are rare. Phaeochromocytomas occur in NF-1. Ash-leaf spots are hypopigmented macules which occur in tuberous sclerosis.

28. Unilateral pontine lesion **Answer: B**

A unilateral dorsolateral pontine lesion will produce an ipsilateral Horner's syndrome, ataxia and contralateral loss of pain and temperature sensation in the limbs. A unilateral paramedian pontine lesion will produce ipsilateral VI and lower motor neurone VII cranial nerve palsies and contralateral loss of touch and proprioception in the limbs. A unilateral basal pontine lesion will produce ipsilateral VI and lower motor neurone VII nerve palsies and contralateral hemiplegia (Millard Gubler syndrome). In addition, upper motor neurone fibres to the contralateral seventh cranial nerve nucleus may produce a contralateral upper motor neurone seventh cranial nerve palsy. A contralateral hemiplegia occurs since the pyramidal tract decussates in the medulla. The III cranial nerve nucleus lies within the midbrain. Bilateral lesions above the medulla are required to produce a pseudobulbar palsy.

29. Unilateral lesion **Answers: A B**

Ipsilateral XII cranial nerve palsy, contralateral hemiplegia and contralateral loss of touch and joint position sense are typical of a medial medullary lesion. Ipsilateral Horner's syndrome and ataxia are features of a lateral medullary lesion.

30. Pseudobulbar palsy **Answers: B D**

Pseudobulbar palsy is caused by bilateral lesions of the cortico-bulbar tracts. Typical causes are small vessel cerebral vascular disease, multiple sclerosis and cerebral trauma. Examination reveals upper motor neurone signs affecting the bulbar structures. Nasal speech is caused by palatal weakness and may be found in both bulbar and pseudobulbar palsy.

31. A right-sided cord lesion **Answers: A B C E**

A right-sided cord lesion will produce ipsilateral pyramidal and dorsal column signs and contralateral spinothalamic signs – the Brown-Séquard syndrome. Hoffman's sign indicates a pyramidal lesion above the eight cervical segment.

32. Extensor plantar responses **Answers: B D**

Deficiency of vitamin B12 causes degeneration of large fibre sensory neurones in the peripheral nerves and their central connections in the dorsal columns of the spinal cord, causing loss of tendon jerks and sensory ataxia. With more prolonged deficiency the pyramidal tracts degenerate causing an extensor plantar response. At the conus medullaris, the spinal root entry zones and the pyramidal tracts are in close proximity and may be damaged by a small lesion such as a neurofibroma. Taboparesis and Friedreich's ataxia are other causes of an extensor plantar response and absent ankle jerks.

33. Abdominal aortic aneurysm **Answers: A B**

The artery of Adamkiewicz, the major abdominal tributary of the anterior spinal artery is occasionally damaged by aortic aneurysms and their repair. The anterior spinal cord at the lower thoracic level is typically infarcted, producing pyramidal and spinothalamic signs below the level of the lesion and sphincter dysfunction. Prognosis for recovery is poor.

34. Syringomyelia **Answers: A C E**

Syringomyelic cavities typically involve the anterior aspect of the cervical and upper thoracic cord. Involvement of the spinothalamic tract produces a dissociated sensory loss in the upper limbs. The posterior columns are typically spared. Involvement of anterior horn cells produces lower motor neurone signs in the upper limbs and corticospinal tract involvement leads to upper motor neurone signs in the lower limbs. The syrinx may extend into the medulla to produce a (true) bulbar palsy (syringobulbia) and occasionally into the thoracolumbar cord. Associated anomalies at the craniovertebral junction (Arnold-Chiari malformation) can produce nystagmus.

35. Guillain-Barré syndrome — Answers: A B D E

Post-infective polyradiculopathy or the Guillain-Barré syndrome usually presents with sensory symptoms in the limbs followed by an ascending sensorimotor deficit. Severely affected cases show quite marked ataxia which cannot be entirely explained by joint-position loss and may be related to defective functioning of muscle spindle afferents. In the initial few days of symptoms the CSF cell count may be raised but later the classical pattern of high protein with a normal cell count appears. Ventilation may be impaired in severe cases in which the bulbar musculature is denervated and it is essential to monitor this. The test to use is the vital capacity, not the peak flow which is mainly a measure of airway size rather than ventilation volume. Uncommonly the Guillain-Barré syndrome may be the presenting feature of an underlying lymphoma.

36. Normal autonomic nervous system — Answers: C E

2.5% methacholine causes pupillary constriction in denervated pupils (e.g. Holmes Adie). The superior colliculus is involved in gaze, the Edinger Westphal nucleus supplies the ciliary muscle. Heart rate changes in response to the Valsalva manoeuvre, deep breathing and posture are also used to assess autonomic innervation of the heart. The bladder, along with the genitalia and rectum, is innervated via the S2–4 parasympathetic nerves (S2, 3, 4 keep the wee off the floor!!). Preganglionic sympathetic and pre- and post-ganglionic parasympathetic nerves use acetylcholine as their neurotransmitter.

37. The median nerve — Answer: C

The median nerve enters the palm by passing underneath the flexor retinaculum and supplies the muscles of the thenar eminence and the 1st and 2nd lumbricals. The muscles of the hypothenar eminence, the interossei, the adductor pollicis and the 3rd and 4th lumbricals are supplied by the ulnar nerve, which enters the palm superficial to the flexor retinaculum.

38. Anterior interosseous nerve — Answer: B

The anterior interosseous nerve is a branch of the median nerve (C6, 7, 8, T1). Abductor pollicis brevis and the first and second lumbricals are supplied by the median nerve. Extensor pollicis longus is supplied by the posterior interosseous nerve.

39. Carpal tunnel syndrome **Answers: A B D**

The common causes of carpal tunnel syndrome are pregnancy, hypothyroidism, acromegaly and rheumatoid arthritis. Diabetes is associated with problems in the hand – cheiroarthropathy, not of carpal tunnel syndrome. Delayed median nerve conduction is the hallmark and abductor pollicis brevis wasting largely contributes to the thenar eminence wasting. It is difficult to explain how the pain often radiates as proximally as the elbow, but it is a common symptom.

40. C7 nerve root lesion and a radial nerve palsy **Answers: A B C**

Weakness of triceps is unusual in a radial nerve palsy as the lesion is typically distal to the triceps branch. The radial nerve (C5, 6, 7, 8) supplies triceps (C7), brachioradialis (C5, 6), supinator (C6, 7) and wrist, finger and thumb extensors (C7, 8). Flexor carpi radialis (C6, 7) is supplied by the median nerve (C6, 7, 8, T1). A C7 nerve root lesion is associated with sensory loss affecting the middle finger. A radial nerve palsy causes an absent brachioradialis reflex (C5, 6), and only if the lesion is very proximal will the triceps reflex (C7) be lost.

41. Peripheral innervation **Answers: A B D E**

Peripheral innervation is another common MRCP topic. Brachioradialis is supplied by the musculocutaneous nerve. Supination is the movement of moving the hand from palm down to palm up; supinator, C6, radial nerve. Pronation is the opposite; pronator teres/pronator quadratis, C6, median. The anterior interosseous nerve is a branch of the median nerve given off just below the elbow. A lesion will give rise to weakness of the long flexors of the thumb and index finger.

42. Diabetic amyotrophy **Answer: B**

Diabetic amyotrophy is thought to be caused by occlusion of the vasa nervorum of the proximal lumbar plexus and/or the femoral nerve, causing infarction. Pain in the thigh followed by weakness and wasting of the quadriceps and loss of the knee jerk are typical clinical features. Recovery over a period of months is the rule. The CSF protein is raised in two-thirds of patients with diabetes mellitus but does not correlate with the presence or the severity of neuropathy.

43. The sciatic nerve **Answers: A B**

The obturator nerve (L2, 3, 4) supplies gracilis and adductor brevis, longus and magnus. The femoral nerve (L2, 3, 4) supplies quadriceps femoris. The inferior gluteal nerve (L5, S1, 2) supplies gluteus maximus.

44. A lesion of the common peroneal nerve Answer: A

The common peroneal nerve and tibial nerve are branches of the sciatic nerve. A common peroneal nerve palsy causes weakness of foot eversion and dorsiflexion (foot-drop). Foot inversion is not completely lost as tibialis posterior is supplied by the tibial nerve. Skin over the medial aspect of the lower leg is supplied by the saphenous branch of the femoral nerve and that over the lateral aspect of the lower leg by the superficial branch of the common peroneal nerve. A sciatic nerve lesion causes loss of the ankle reflex.

45. Neuralgia Answers: D E

A-delta fibres signal sharp pain. C fibres, the slowest conducting fibres, give rise to dull or burning pain; some carry the sensation of itch. Trigeminal neuralgia is usually treated successfully by carbamazepine. Causalgia usually occurs after partial nerve injury and along with other chronic pains may benefit from sympathetic blockade. This may be achieved by lesioning sympathetic ganglia (surgery or phenol) or by noradrenaline depletion of sympathetic nerve terminals by regional intravenous guanethidine.

46. Essential tremor Answers: B D

Essential tremor is most pronounced with outstretched arms (sustained posture) and is typically relieved by alcohol. A Parkinson's disease tremor is most pronounced at rest and a cerebellar tremor with movement (intention). Anxiety may exacerbate both an essential and Parkinson's disease tremor.

47. Extrapyramidal rigidity Answers: A C D E

Phenothiazine and butyrophenone tranquillisers block the D2 dopamine receptors in the corpus striatum and are the principal causes of iatrogenic Parkinsonism. In the early 1980s, a severe Parkinsonian syndrome appeared in Californian drug addicts caused principally by 1-methyl-4-phenyl-1,2,5,6-tetrahydropyridine (MPTP), a by-product of synthetic opiate manufacture. This has provided experimental opportunities to understand the pathogenesis of idiopathic Parkinson's disease. In particular the possible role of monoamine oxidase B inhibitors in preventing the conversion of MPTP to MPP+, which is responsible for the substantia nigra neuronal damage, raises the possibility of new treatments to prevent progress of the disease. The neuroleptic malignant syndrome is a rare, life-threatening complication of neuroleptic therapy which may also follow withdrawal from amantidine. Features include hyperpyrexia, severe extrapyramidal rigidity and autonomic disturbances. Treatment is by withdrawal of the neuroleptic drug and administration of dantrolene and/or bromocriptine.

48. Myotonia **Answers: B C D E**

Myotonia is typically relieved by exercise and exacerbated by cold. Myotonia congenita can be dominantly (Thomsen's) or recessively (Becker's) inherited. Thomsen's myotonia congenita is associated with muscle hypertrophy. Myotonic dystrophy (autosomal dominant) can be distinguished by the occurrence of cataracts, ptosis, muscle wasting, gonadal atrophy and cardiomyopathy. The EMG invariably shows typical myotonic (dive bomber) discharges.

49. Chorea **Answers: All true**

Pregnancy (chorea gravidarum) and oral contraceptive medication may precipitate chorea. Amphetamines, tricyclic antidepressants, lithium, phenytoin, carbamazepine and cimetidine may also induce chorea. Tardive dyskinesia may follow long-term neuroleptic medication. Systemic lupus erythematosus, Huntington's disease, Wilson's disease and hyperthyroidism also cause chorea.

50. Huntington's chorea **Answers: B D**

Huntington's chorea is inherited as an autosomal dominant characteristic with near complete penetrance. However the age of onset varies and may be delayed until the fifth or sixth decade of life. In younger patients there may be marked extrapyramidal rigidity, such juvenile onset cases having usually inherited the Huntington's gene from their father rather than their mother. The volume of caudate nucleus can be reduced on CT scan but this is not a reliable test particularly early in the course of the disorder.
L-dopa will worsen the choreic movements of patients with Huntington's, the therapy for which is tetrabenazine. Major tranquillisers in the phenothiazine and butyrophenone classes may be necessary in more severely hyperkinetic patients.

51. Parkinson's disease **Answers: B E**

Parkinson's disease is typically associated with bradykinesia, cogwheel or 'lead pipe' rigidity and resting tremor. The voice may be monotonous and hypophonic. Upward gaze is typically restricted. Supranuclear gaze palsy, pseudobulbar palsy and axial rigidity are characteristic of Steele-Richardson-Olszewski syndrome, a condition which may superficially mimic Parkinson's disease.

52. Parkinsonian syndrome **Answers: B D E**

Manganese and carbon monoxide poisoning may produce a Parkinsonian syndrome. N-methyl-4-phenyl-1,2,3,6-tetrahydropyridine (MPTP) is a synthetic opiate drug which is metabolised to the neurotoxic MPP+ to produce a Parkinsonian syndrome very similar to Parkinson's disease. In Huntington's disease of juvenile onset, extrapyramidal involvement can predominate to give a rigid-akinetic syndrome with little or no chorea.

53. Muscle fasciculations **Answers: A B C E**

Fasciculations consist of spontaneous contractions of single motor units visible to the naked eye. They are frequently seen in the quadriceps and calf muscles of healthy individuals and by themselves are not diagnostic of MND. In the latter disease the fasciculations are seen in many more muscles and are associated with wasting, weakness and other features of MND. Fasciculations may occur pathologically in many situations where there is partial denervation (e.g. root lesions). The origin is probably in the electrical instability of the reinervation (and excessive sensitivity to acetylcholine) that occurs in chronic partial denervation. Though not frequently seen in spinal muscular atrophy, fasciculations may occasionally be found in adult onset cases.

54. Muscular dystrophies **Answers: A B D**

DMD and Becker dystrophy are X-linked recessive, therefore males suffer the disease and females carry it unless the good X chromosome is missing (Turner's 45XO) or turned off (lyonisation) when the phenotype will be expressed. Becker dystrophy usually starts later, is less common and progresses slower than the other dystrophies. Cardiac muscle is spared and therefore there is not even subclinical involvement! Pseudo-hypertrophy results from fatty infiltration, the gastrocnemius, quadriceps, deltoid and tongue being most affected. Mean IQ is 10–20 points lower in Duchenne but normal in Becker; Duchenne and Becker are allelic variants. EMG is not helpful in detecting female carriers but creatine kinase estimation is.

55. Myasthenia gravis **Answers: D E**

Myasthenia gravis is associated with anti-nicotinic acetylcholine receptor antibodies in around 90% of patients. Anti-striated muscle antibodies suggest the presence of thymoma. Around 30% of patients are rendered symptom-free by thymectomy – mostly those with thymic hyperplasia. Corticosteroids cause decreased acetylcholine release from the presynaptic terminal which may cause a temporary worsening of weakness before the immunosuppressive actions take effect.

56. Myoclonus **Answers: B C D E**

Myoclonus is not a feature of Pick's disease but may be a late clinical manifestation of Alzheimer's disease. Myoclonus is a prominent and relatively early clinical feature of subacute sclerosing panencephalitis and Creutzfeldt-Jakob disease. Primary generalised epilepsy is associated with three main seizure types: generalised absence seizures (petit-mal), generalised tonic-clonic seizures (grand-mal) and myoclonic seizures. Juvenile myoclonic epilepsy is generally considered to be a sub-type of primary generalised epilepsy in which myoclonic seizures are a particularly prominent feature. Post anoxic brain damage causes myoclonus which is most marked on intention (action myoclonus).

57. CSF pleocytosis **Answer: C**

Increased white cells and low glucose are seen in combination in TB meningitis, chronic infections and malignant meningitis. Be careful to read the question carefully to avoid making silly mistakes and losing marks!

58. Chronic fatigue syndrome **Answers: A C D E**

Few risk factors have been identified for the chronic fatigue syndrome apart from previous psychiatric illness. More than 75% of affected patients have a concurrent psychiatric illness, depression being present in more than half. No relationship has been demonstrated between clinical status and any laboratory findings. The treatment of choice appears to be a gentle return to physical activity and treatment of the associated depression, usually with a tricyclic antidepressant.

59. Chronic alcoholism **Answers: A B C D**

Alcohol abuse is a well recognised cause of an acute painful myopathy. Auditory hallucinations are a prominent feature of delirium tremens. Hypoglycaemia is believed to result from the blockage of gluconeogenesis when there are depleted liver glycogen stores. Children are particularly prone to alcohol-induced hypoglycaemia. Downbeating nystagmus is a sign of a lesion at the foramen magnum.

60. Multiple sclerosis **Answer: E**

The only treatment proven to reduce the severity of relapse in MS is dietary supplementation with linoleic acid. Recent trials have shown both azathioprine and hyperbaric oxygen to be ineffective and potentially dangerous. Corticosteroids and ACTH bring forward remission following relapse but do not modify the overall course of the disease.

61. Multiple sclerosis **Answers: B C E**

Demyelination typically affects white matter of the brain and spinal cord. It may occasionally affect grey matter of the cerebral cortex but only rarely affects the grey matter of the spinal cord.

62. Motor neurone disease **Answers: A B D E**

Sensory disturbance is not a feature of motor neurone disease. Familial cases may exhibit extrapyramidal signs and dementia.

63. Neurological imaging **Answers: A B**

In T1 weighted images the CSF is black. Demyelinating plaques are easily seen. A T1 nerve root lesion due to an apical lung tumour or a cervical rib may show on a plain X-ray. However, most T1 lesions have other causes. PET scans need changes in blood flow for several tens of seconds for accurate localisation. Angiography remains the 'gold standard' for investigating carotid stenosis.

OPHTHALMOLOGY: ANSWERS AND EXPLANATIONS

1. Painful red eye **Answers: A C D**

Other causes of 'red eye' are subconjunctival haemorrhage, which is not painful, and acute closed-angle glaucoma and keratitis which are. With conjunctival injection, the vessels fade from fornix to limbus, and move with the conjunctiva. Ciliary vessel injection with intraocular inflammation gives the reverse findings.

2. Primary open-angle (simple) glaucoma **Answers: A B D**

By far the commonest variety of primary glaucoma, this disease is one of insidious onset and progression. There are arcuate scotomata, peripheral field loss and excavated pale optic discs. Central vision is preserved until late, which tends to delay presentation. Treatment is essentially medical and based on parasympathomimetic and beta blocker eyedrops. Carbonic anhydrase inhibitor drugs are also used.

3. Anterior uveitis **Answers: B D E**

Keratoconjunctivitis sicca is common and episcleritis and scleritis are important manifestations of rheumatoid disease. In sarcoidosis the eye is involved in 10–25% of cases, the usual lesion being acute or chronic uveitis; occasionally choroido-retinitis, sicca syndrome and optic nerve lesions are seen. Although SLE can produce inflammatory changes anywhere in the eye, the most frequent sign of ocular involvement is retinal exudates (cytoid bodies). Recurrent anterior uveitis is the most commonly disabling complication of Behçet's disease.

4. Abnormalities of the optic lens **Answers: A B C D E**

Downward dislocation of the lens is characteristic of homocystinuria and cataracts may form at a later stage. Cataracts can develop as a result of chronic hypocalcaemia, which is also associated with papilloedema, and are also the main optic manifestation of myotonic dystrophy. Maternal rubella infection in the first trimester of pregnancy may result in a host of congenital abnormalities including cataracts. Kayser-Fleischer rings are the corneal copper deposits characteristic of Wilson's disease but 'sunflower' cataracts that do not disable vision are also recognised in this condition.

5. Unilateral exophthalmos **Answers: A B E**

Unilateral exophthalmos should raise the suspicion of an orbital tumour and is invariably an indication for CT scanning of the orbit, even in the presence of Graves' disease (where eye signs may be asymmetrical or unilateral). Wegener's more typically causes destruction of bone in the midline but may rarely lead to exophthalmos. Cigarette smoking exacerbates Graves' ophthalmopathy but does not itself cause exophthalmos. Exophthalmos means protrusion of the orbital contents and though there may be enophthalmos in Horner's syndrome, this does not imply contralateral exophthalmos.

6. The orbit **Answers: B C E**

The abductor muscle (the lateral rectus) is supplied by the abducent (6th cranial) nerve and the superior oblique muscle is supplied by the trochlear (4th cranial) nerve. All the other muscles are supplied by the oculomotor (3rd cranial) nerve. The levator palpebrae superioris is supplied by the 3rd cranial and cervical sympathetic nerves and hence, paralysis may be due to lesions of either. The superior ophthalmic vein is one route by which infection can reach intracranial structures. The ophthalmic artery is one of the anastomotic links between the external carotid artery (via the facial artery) and the internal carotid artery from which it arises. Its branch to the retina is an end artery.

7. Diabetic maculopathy **Answer: A**

Maculopathy is certainly more common in the older patient with NIDDM but may occur in young patients as well. The patient may be registered blind because of the damage to the very sensitive macular area. However, even though the patient may be unable to read, they may retain excellent peripheral (navigational) vision. Treatment of maculopathy is usually with small, focal laser burns to the macular area, avoiding the fovea, in contrast to treatment for proliferative retinopathy which usually involves several thousand burns to the peripheral retina. Drusen are a normal feature in some patients. Hard exudates, often in rings (circinates) are characteristic of diabetic maculopathy. Painful visual loss is not a feature of maculopathy and suggests glaucoma, uveitis or corneal ulcer.

8. Visual field defects **Answers: A B**

Bitemporal hemianopia can result from optic chiasmal compression by a craniopharyngioma. Retrobulbar neuritis, which most frequently accompanies multiple sclerosis, can lead to central scotoma which may also result from optic atrophy, optic nerve compression and choroido-retinitis. Posterior uveitis may also occur rarely in tertiary syphilis but the characteristic ocular abnormality is the Argyll-Robertson pupil. Weber's syndrome refers to infarction of one half of the midbrain, resulting in ipsilateral oculomotor nerve palsy, contralateral hemiplegia and paralysis of upward gaze. Conjunctival pingueculae may be associated with Gaucher's disease.

9. Macular sparing hemianopia **Answers: C D E**

The macular region of the visual cortex is at the tip of the occipital lobe on its medial aspect and is supplied with blood by both the middle and posterior cerebral arteries. The result is that an infarction in the posterior cerebral artery territory causes a homonymous hemianopia which spares the macular region. Patients can usually read with this deficit since the ability to scan is retained. Lesions which interrupt the optic radiation in the parietal lobe cause a hemianopia which involves the macula and there are often visuoperceptual deficits which interfere with the ability to read. A patient with a visual field defect below the horizon of vision is not permitted to hold a driving licence.

PSYCHIATRY: ANSWERS AND EXPLANATIONS

1. Schizophrenia **Answer: D**

Onset of schizophrenia, usually between 15 and 45 years of age, occurs on average five years earlier in males (median onset 28 years). One-third of patients have a good or fair outcome and 10–20% a severe chronic illness. Deterioration in function usually plateaus after 3–5 years and florid symptoms often reduce with increasing age. Outcome is worse in developed countries, although incidence and symptomatology is similar worldwide. Increased prevalence within socio-economically deprived areas is due to downward 'social drift' after illness onset. High 'expressed emotion' in family members, particularly those with more than 35 hours per week contact with the patient, is highly predictive of relapse.

2. Schizophrenia **Answers: B C E**

The most frequent occurring symptoms of acute schizophrenia are lack of insight, auditory hallucinations, ideas of reference, suspiciousness, flatness of mood, voices speaking to the patient, persecutory delusions, and hearing one's own thoughts spoken aloud. The commonest forms of hallucinations are auditory, but visual, tactile olfactory and somatic are recognised. The patient is usually fully orientated. Perseveration is the persistent and inappropriate repetition of the same word and thoughts, and is a recognised feature of dementia. There are three common changes in mood: patients can be irritable, anxious, depressed or elated; they can show a flattening of mood; they can display incongruity of affect (an inappropriate mood state).

3. Schneiderian first rank symptoms of schizophrenia
Answers: A D E

In the absence of coarse brain disease the presence of Schneider's first rank symptoms point to a diagnosis of schizophrenia. They are:

(1) Specific types of auditory hallucination (audible thoughts, voices talking about the patient in the third person, voices commenting on actions (running commentary)).
(2) Passivity phenomena (breakdown of ego-boundaries), thought insertion, withdrawal and broadcast, made acts and feelings (somatic passivity).
(3) Delusions (primary delusions or delusional perceptions).

4. Schizophrenia **Answers: A B D E**

Factors predictive of a poor outcome and chronic course in schizophrenia include an early age of onset, low socio-economic status, irregular occupational record, social adversity, a family history of schizophrenia, schizoid or asocial premorbid personality traits, low intelligence, lack of a lasting heterosexual relationship, absence of precipitating factors, insidious onset, longer duration of untreated psychosis, lack of clouding of consciousness or confusion, absence of a family history of affective disorder or an affective component to the illness, presence of primary negative symptoms, neurological signs and symptoms and a history of perinatal trauma.

5. Delusions **Answers: B E**

Delusions are morbid false beliefs, which occur in a wide range of psychoses including schizophrenia. Classically they are firmly held out of keeping with the patient's subculture and cannot be altered by reason or demonstration of their falsity. They often occur secondary to hallucinations, which are false percepts apparently in the external world. Obsessions are recurrent thoughts, images or impulses resisted by the patient who finds them both senseless and distressing, but recognises them as their own mental products.

6. Affective disorders **Answer: E**

Whilst depressive symptoms are very common, lifetime prevalence of unipolar depression is about 6% and bipolar disorder 1%. The male: female ratio of unipolar depression is 1:2 whilst the sex ratio for bipolar disorder is approximately equal. Only 1:5 patients with major depression receive treatment, 1:50 enter hospital and 1:200 commit suicide. There are no consistent social class differences in the prevalence of unipolar depression although bipolar disorder may be slightly increased in social class I. There are no racial or cultural differences in the prevalence of depression although somatic symptoms are often prominent in third world settings and guilt in Judeo-Christian cultures.

7. Depression in the elderly **Answers: A B D E**

Agitation and retardation both occur in a significant number of elderly depressives. When delusions are present, they usually have a depressive flavour (e.g. poverty or physical illness). A certain proportion have apparent cognitive deficits, which improve in parallel with the symptoms of depression: this is the commonest variety of 'pseudo-dementia'. Severe life events can precipitate depression in the elderly, but bereavement is less important as a cause of mental illness than in younger age groups.

8. Normal bereavement reaction **Answers: A B D**

Bereavement reactions are normal, but share features in common with depression such as misery, tearfulness, insomnia, poor concentration and anorexia. Other features of depression such as psychomotor retardation, delusions, suicidal thinking and generalised loss of self-esteem only rarely occur in bereavement. Physical symptoms are more commonly reported by the bereaved. Most typically, three stages of grieving can be distinguished: an initial phase of emotional numbness and unreality; secondly a mourning phase of variable length which may include experiences of the presence or voice of the deceased and searching behaviour; finally there is gradual acceptance and resolution.

9. Depressive pseudodementia **Answers: A B D E**

The differential diagnosis of dementia and depression can be troublesome when cognitive symptoms complicate the latter. In depression, careful questioning will typically elicit more recent onset and more rapid progression of symptoms and possibly a past history or family history of depression. Features of the mental state suggesting depression include complaints about memory loss, 'don't know' rather than 'near miss' answers to specific questions and concurrent depressive symptoms. All these features are less common in dementia. In depression there is morning worsening of mood while in dementia there is evening worsening of confusion.

10. Hypomania **Answers: A C E**

Flight of ideas, where there is an excessively fluent flow of thoughts and ideas, but with some thread of connection between them, is characteristic of hypomania. Thought insertion is a first rank symptom of schizophrenia. Overactivity and a sense of grandiosity can lead to sexually promiscuous behaviour. Delusions of bodily illness are a feature of depression, not mania. The manic patient is so active they tend to have very little sleep and can become ill through exhaustion.

11. Puerperal psychosis **Answers: A B C D**

The majority of puerperal psychoses begin within the first two weeks after childbirth, and rarely in the first two days. The illness usually starts with a period of delirium. The outlook is favourable. Auditory hallucinations are frequently experienced, but obsessional ruminations are not part of the clinical picture.

12. Anxiety states **Answers: A E**

Many physical symptoms are associated with anxiety states: dyspnoea, difficulty inhaling, overbreathing, dry mouth, difficulty swallowing, palpitations, chest pain, frequency and urgency of micturition, tinnitus, blurred vision, paraesthesia, dizziness and sweating. Difficulty concentrating and complaints of poor memory occur. Persistent and objective memory loss is not present and raises the possibility of an organic cause. Depressive illnesses may present with anxiety symptoms; low mood and early morning wakening would be indicative of this. Problems getting to sleep are more usual with anxiety disorders.

13. Agoraphobia **Answers: B C D**

Agoraphobia generally commences suddenly in adult life following a recent traumatic event. There is a large preponderance of women patients, and a worsening of symptoms can occur as a result of other emotional changes such as a period of depression. Treatment is very difficult, but the condition can respond to desensitisation by systematically introducing the patient to the feared situation.

14. Obsessive-compulsive disorder **Answers: A E**

Obsessive-compulsive disorders are characterised by obsessional thinking and compulsive behaviour. Obsessional thoughts are words, ideas or beliefs that intrude into the patient's mind. They are recognised as the patient's own thoughts, are alien to their personality and are seen as nonsensical. They are usually unpleasant, are resisted and are associated with anxiety. Obsessional thoughts lead to obsessional actions which may reduce anxiety. Obsessional ruminations are endless internal debates, sometimes about insignificant details. In a minority of patients this may lead to obsessional slowness. Obsessional impulses are urges to perform acts which are often embarrassing or violent; they are seldom acted upon. Anxiety and depression are commonly associated. Men and women are equally affected. Two-thirds improve by the end of a year, cases of more than one year run a fluctuating course.

15. Somatization disorder **Answers: C D E**

Somatization disorder is a chronic syndrome of multiple somatic symptoms that cannot be explained medically. It is associated with psychosocial distress and medical help-seeking. Diagnosis requires a history of several years' duration. The onset occurs in early adulthood and rarely after 30 years of age. The belief that a person has been sickly most of their life is common. It is more common in women affecting 1–2% of all females. Interpersonal problems are prominent with anxiety and depression being the most prevalent psychiatric conditions. Menstrual symptoms, sexual indifference and frigidity, alcohol and drug abuse and antisocial personality disorder all occur more frequently. Whilst the disorder fluctuates, patients are rarely symptom-free.

16. Post-traumatic stress disorder **Answers: C D**

Whilst a vulnerable personality increases risk of PTSD, 50–80% of survivors of a disaster may develop the syndrome. Other risk factors include prior psychiatric disorder, extremes of age, concurrent physical disabilities and social depravation. PTSD usually develops sometime, possibly years, after the trauma and may mimic affective, anxiety or personality disorders. Features include reliving the trauma, dissociative flashbacks, illusions and hallucinations in full consciousness. Recurrent nightmares, intrusive recollections and avoidance of reminders of the trauma occur with intense distress if exposed to these and persistently increased autonomic arousal. Secondary problems include alcohol or drug dependence and marital discord. Psychodynamic theories invoke regression, repression, denial and undoing but child-like behaviour is not characteristic.

17. Hysterical amnesia **Answers: A B D E**

When amnesia is of hysterical origin, rather than due to some organic cause, emotionally charged events may be forgotten, whilst memory for other events taking place at the same time may be retained. The majority of such states resolve quickly as the situation which produced them alters. The symptoms are of unconscious, rather than conscious origin. The reaction can follow traumatic events, in particular head injury, and can be provoked by physical or psychological stress. If no stress can be found even after interviewing an informant, the diagnosis of hysterical amnesia should be doubted.

18. 'Hysteria' Answers: B C

A hysterical symptom is one that suggests physical illness but occurs in the absence of physical disease and is not produced deliberately. Hysterical symptoms occur in association with several psychiatric disorders: depression, anxiety and organic mental disorder. 'La belle indifference' is a characteristic, but is not always present. Hysterical symptoms developing for the first time in middle or old age should raise a high suspicion of organic disease. There are usually obvious discrepancies between signs and symptoms of hysteria and those of organic disease, although this depends on the patient's medical knowledge.

19. Compensation neurosis Answers: B E

The incidence of compensation neurosis has an inverse relationship with the severity of the injury. It is twice as common after industrial injuries as after road traffic accidents. Little recovery is found in patients with severe symptoms even after settlement of the compensation claim. The main symptoms are headaches, dizziness, poor concentration and irritability. Malingering is not a common occurrence, and the mechanisms involved in producing these symptoms are subconscious ones.

20. Anorexia nervosa Answers: B D E

The anorectic patient is typically alert and active in spite of severe emaciation. There may be episodes of hyperactivity. Nonetheless, there is a high incidence of depression and, terminally, weakness and apathy predominate. Hypokalaemia is commonly found, often due to self-induced vomiting or purgation. Amenorrhoea, primary and secondary, is a characteristic feature, and may occur before significant weight loss. The typical endocrine findings are low FSH, LH and oestrogen levels; evidence suggests that the fault lies in hypothalamic control of the anterior pituitary.

21. Bulimia nervosa Answers: B C D E

The central clinical features of bulimia nervosa are an intractable urge to overeat, self-induced vomiting and laxative abuse. Patients are usually of normal weight. Most patients are female and usually menstruate normally. Patients have distorted body image. Depressive symptoms are common.

22. Suicide **Answers: A C D**

Tactful enquiry about suicidal intent may decrease the risk of suicide. The following factors are associated with an increased risk of suicide: male sex, old age, alcohol abuse, drug dependence, epilepsy, chronic physical illness (especially chronically painful conditions), bereavement, social isolation, psychiatric disorder (apart from obsessional illness), family history of suicide or depression, previous suicide attempts, unemployment.

23. Suicide **Answers: All true**

Suicide is commonest amongst elderly men, although rates amongst young men have been rising dramatically in recent years. Rates increase progressively through the married, never married, widowers and widows and the divorced. Suicide is increased amongst social classes I and V, individuals with a past history of suicide attempts, history of depression, alcohol abuse, drug abuse, schizophrenia or antisocial or borderline personality disorders. Feelings of hopelessness are an important predictor of immediate and long-term suicide risk. In most cases a warning is given before committing suicide with two-thirds expressing suicidal ideas to relatives and one-third expressing clear suicidal intent. 40% of suicide completers had consulted their GP in the previous week.

24. Delirium **Answers: A B C E**

Delirium is an acute onset syndrome characterised by inattention and an impaired level of consciousness. Thinking is often disorganised and perseverative. Perceptual disturbances include misinterpretations, illusions and hallucinations. There is disturbance of the sleep-wake cycle with insomnia and daytime sleepiness. Psychomotor-activity may be increased or decreased. Disorientation and memory impairment are common. The patient has no insight during episodes of confusion and amnesia for the episode once it has resolved. A catastrophic reaction has been described in dementing patients which is characterised by marked agitation secondary to the subjective awareness of intellectual deficits under stressful circumstances.

25. Acute confusional state **Answers: C D E**

Almost every disease, bodily insult and drug has been credited with precipitating acute confusion. Commonly implicated factors are trauma, surgery, heart failure, infection, anoxia and sedative drugs. Confusion is not, however, a characteristic feature of myxoedema. Senile dementia is a very common predisposing condition and tricyclics may precipitate a confusional state. Phenothiazines such as thioridazine may be used therapeutically but dealing with the precipitating factor is most important.

26. Dementia **Answers: A B C D E**

In dementia, there is a selective impairment of memory for recent events in the early stages. Later, this generalises and eventually extends to loss of memory for distant events too. There is difficulty in adapting to new situations, so the patient persists or perseverates with old themes. The memory loss is accompanied by disorientation, which may be in time, place or person. Depression is quite common in early dementia. The dementing process is a result of slowly progressive cortical disease resulting in cortical atrophy.

27. Alzheimer's disease **Answers: A D E**

With the exception of the very elderly, risk of Alzheimer's disease (AD) increases with age. Other well confirmed risk factors include family history of Alzheimer's disease (particularly with early onset AD) and Down's syndrome. Recent findings have also implicated past inanition (later onset and sporadic AD), nervous breakdown (early onset AD), head injury (sporadic AD) and curiously nose picking (later onset AD). Alcohol is related to a small increase and smoking a small decrease in risk. At present evidence for aluminium in the aetiology and pathology of AD is considered circumstantial.

28. Alcohol dependence **Answer: A**

Dependent alcoholics suffer withdrawal symptoms as their blood alcohol level falls. The commonest feature is acute tremulousness in the morning, often with agitation, nausea, retching and sweating. These and more severe features such as fleeting hallucinations, fits and clouding of consciousness can be reduced by inpatient detoxification with chlormethiazole or benzodiazepine cover. Disulfiram (*Antabuse*) is used as an aid to willpower as it blocks oxidation of alcohol and produces unpleasant flushing, nausea and headache. Liver cirrhosis occurs in 10% of alcoholics. Intensive programmes of counselling are probably no more effective than brief advice.

29. Alcohol withdrawal **Answers: A B D**

Delirium tremens on withdrawal from alcohol includes a coarse, persistent tremor of the hands. Often, the patient experiences visual hallucinations such as seeing animals crawling on the floor or the bedclothes. There is free perspiration, oliguria and dehydration. Passivity feelings are features of schizophrenia. Confabulation, part of Korsakoff's syndrome is a result of chronic alcohol abuse, not of acute withdrawal.

30. Korsakoff's syndrome **Answers: A D E**

Korsakoff's syndrome is characterised by a severe memory defect both retrograde and antegrade, i.e. an inability to retain new information. Other mental functions may be more or less intact. Confabulation is common, but not invariable. With Korsakoff's syndrome in chronic alcoholism, beriberi and prolonged vomiting, Wernicke's encephalopathy is frequently associated giving nystagmus, ocular palsies and ataxia. Vitamin B1 (thiamine) deficiency is the major aetiological factor. Korsakoff's syndrome also occurs after head injuries and cerebral anoxia and with cerebral tumours.

31. Paranoid psychoses **Answers: A D E**

Hallucinogens including cannabis, mescaline, ecstasy, phencyclidine, psilocybin (magic mushrooms) and volatile solvents may induce a paranoid psychosis characterised by paranoid delusions and hallucinations without significant impairment of consciousness. CNS stimulants including amphetamines and cocaine and CNS depressants including alcohol, barbiturates and some high potency benzodiazepines have also been implicated. Temazepam withdrawal will rarely cause hallucinations but not a full blown paranoid psychosis. Heroin does not induce psychotic symptoms either in chronic use or during withdrawal.

32. Morbid jealousy **Answers: B C E**

Pathological jealousy occurs in a wide range of psychiatric conditions notably personality disorder, paranoid psychosis and schizophrenia, depression and alcoholism. It is commoner in men, and is associated with erectile impotence. Freud believed it was caused by repression and reaction formation of homosexual drives. Morbid jealousy can be highly dangerous and is the cause of 10–20% of homicides in special hospitals (both male and female). Treatment of the primary disorder can be helpful but in most cases the symptom persists and marital separation may be the only solution.

33. Sleep disturbance **Answer: D**

Most (85%) insomnias are secondary to psychological factors, psychiatric or physical illness or drug-induced states; caffeine abuse is often associated. Alcohol decreases total sleep time but decreases the time required to fall asleep. Neuroleptics cause akathisia. Unlike narcolepsy, hypersomnia is not associated with an irresistible urge to sleep but consists of 'hangover' symptoms caused by excessive sleep, which leads to the need for more sleep.

34. Psychiatric sequelae to head injury Answers: B C

Retrograde amnesia is not a good prognostic factor. The duration of post-traumatic amnesia is more variable and is predictive of time to return to work, psychiatric disablement and personality change. Complete recall of the injury, particularly in an emotionally loaded setting, is predictive of neurotic disabilities. A personal or family history of mental disorder predicts later psychiatric incapacity. An increase in post-traumatic neurotic symptoms, intellectual and memory impairments and mortality is seen with increasing age. Compensation and litigation increase psychiatric sequelae, such symptoms being rare after injuries at sport or in the home where compensation is not payable. However settlement of compensation rarely leads to a significant resolution of psychiatric symptoms.

35. Heritability Answers: A B D E

Heritability of schizophrenia is between 63% and 80%, with no common environmental effect. It is also substantial in bipolar disorder, and to a lesser extent unipolar depression. With decreasing severity of illness the genetic effect in 'neurotic' disorders decreases, whilst a common environmental component becomes more important. Proneness to 'life events' also has a genetic component and implicated life events are those felt to have been influenced by 'hazard prone' individuals. Male homosexuality has a heritability of between 31% and 74%. Genetic factors significantly influence adult criminality, with pairwise concordance rates of 51% in monozygous twins and 22% in dizygous twins, contrasting with rates for juvenile delinquency (monozygous 87% and dizygous 72%), which suggest an insignificant genetic effect.

36. Psychogenic pain Answers: A C D E

The core clinical features are severe and prolonged pain which is inconsistent with anatomical patterns of innervation, and the absence of an organic cause. Patients have usually been extensively investigated. The onset of pain may be related to emotionally difficult events. The pain may allow the patient to avoid certain activities and result in attention from relatives and friends. However the patient does not intentionally produce the pain. The pain may be associated with a depressive illness, and may respond to antidepressants (response may also occur in the absence of overt depression). Response to standard analgesics is poor. The course of psychogenic pain is variable and may persist for years.

37. Mental Health Act **Answer: B**

Section 5(2) is an emergency holding order allowing detention of a patient, suspected of having a mental illness and of being a risk to themselves or others, for up to 72 hours. Recommendation is by the Responsible Medical Officer of the patient, or their nominated deputy. Only a consultant psychiatrist may nominate a deputy. Section 5(2) gives no rights to treatment without consent. No part of the MHA allows for non-psychiatric treatments without consent except when such treatment is for a physical disorder which is directly causing a psychiatric disorder. Where necessary treatment must be given under common law or section 62 of the MHA. Section 2 allows commencement of treatment. Section 3 is a 6 month treatment order. Neither the patient nor the next of kin have the right to appeal against section 5(2).

RESPIRATORY MEDICINE: ANSWERS AND EXPLANATIONS

1. Haemoglobin-oxygen dissociation curve **Answers: A C D**

The oxygen dissociation curve is usually plotted as the percentage saturation of haemoglobin with oxygen against oxygen tension. A shift to the right means that for a given oxygen tension there is reduced saturation of haemoglobin with oxygen. This shift can be brought about by increases in hydrogen ion concentration, in pCO_2 and 2,3 diphosphoglycerate (2,3 DPG). The dissociation curve applies in anaemia even though the oxygen capacity is low.

2. Transfer factor **Answers: A B E**

Transfer factor (TLCO) is a measure of gas exchange which substitutes carbon dioxide for oxygen and depends on alveolar ventilation (oxygen to lungs), blood flow (oxygen to body), Hb (oxygen carriage) and lung volume (surface area for gas exchange). Matching of ventilation and blood flow is much more important than the membrane diffusion characteristics. Its elevation in IPH is due to uptake by Hb in the alveoli.

3. Basic pulmonary anatomy **Answers: A B E**

The cholinergic activity of the vagus nerve maintains normal bronchial tone. There are 5 lobes, divided into 18 bronchopulmonary segments (10 right, 8 left). At birth there are some 25 million alveoli which increase in the adult to 300 million per lung. The right middle lobe extends from the 5th rib in the axilla to the 4th costochondral junction superiorly (horizontal fissure), and to the 6th costochondral junction inferiorly (oblique fissure). Surfactant is a mixture of phospholipids, with dipalmitoyl lecithin predominating.

4. Lung compliance **Answers: A B D**

Lung compliance is a static measure of lung and chest recoil and is expressed as a change in lung volume per unit change in airway pressure. Since it is a static measure, it cannot be determined by using a peak flow meter. It is approximately half of normal in a person with one lung, as the lung volume is approximately half.

5. Cryptogenic fibrosing alveolitis **Answers: C D E**

The characteristic symptoms and signs are dyspnoea, cyanosis, clubbing and basal crepitations. Honeycombing is a non-specific X-ray appearance of many diffuse lung diseases in an advanced stage. Rheumatoid factor is found in an appreciable percentage of cases; frank rheumatoid arthritis sometimes is associated. There is also an association with chronic active hepatitis, Hashimoto's disease and renal tubular acidosis.

6. Alpha$_1$-antitrypsin deficiency **Answers: A E**

Alpha$_1$-antitrypsin deficiency is associated with severe panacinar emphysema and is an autosomal co-dominant condition with incomplete penetrance. Patients present in early adult life, usually before the age of 40, and the emphysema is more severe in cigarette smokers. Children with alpha$_1$-antitrypsin deficiency are prone to severe liver disease such as neonatal hepatitis and cirrhosis.

7. Heart-lung transplantation **Answers: A C D**

Both pleurectomy and pleurodesis are contraindications to HLT at present. Retransplantation of the recipient's heart is a standard procedure (the 'domino operation'). Azathioprine and cyclosporin form routine maintenance immunosuppressive therapy. As for HLT in general, obliterative bronchiolitis is a major long term problem. The increased potential difference across the respiratory mucosa, typical of cystic fibrosis, has remained normal in transplanted lungs up to two years after the procedure.

8. Dusts **Answers: A C D**

Not all inhaled inorganic dusts cause fibrosis of the lung. It is not a feature of simple coal miner's pneumoconiosis, siderosis from pure iron oxide inhalation (e.g. in welding) or stannosis (in tin smelting workers). Silica, tungsten carbide and aluminium are fibrogenic dusts.

9. Asbestosis **Answers: A C**

Pleural plaques only indicate asbestos exposure and are not premalignant. Diffuse fibrosis, not pulmonary nodules are found, and bronchial carcinoma is a recognised complication of pulmonary involvement.

10. Farmers' lung **Answers: A B**

Farmers' lung is usually caused by *Micropolyspora faeni* which flourishes in hay which has been harvested without drying. Breathlessness, rigors, fever and a dry cough occur 2–6 hours after exposure. Marked eosinophilia is not a feature.

11. Diffuse interstitial fibrosis **Answers: B D E**

The PO_2 may fall on exercise but not at rest. Lung function studies indicate a restrictive defect with reduced FVC but normal FEV_1/FVC ratio, and a reduced diffusing capacity.

12. Bronchoalveolar lavage **Answers: A C D E**

Extrinsic allergic alveolitis characteristically produces a high lymphocyte percentage consisting of T8 suppressor cells in contrast to sarcoid in which T4 helper cells predominate. A normal lavage consists of 90% alveolar macrophages, 10% lymphocytes and 1% neutrophils.

13. Surgical resection of carcinoma of the bronchus **Answers: A B**

Resection is contraindicated if mediastinal nodes are involved, signs of which are pressure on the SVC or recurrent laryngeal nerve. CT cannot confirm malignant involvement by size alone. Hypercalcaemia may be due to tumour PTH production rather than metastatic bone deposits. Unlike phrenic nerve palsy, the raised hemi-diaphragm of a collapsed lung caused by proximal tumour compression is mobile, and does not contraindicate resection.

14. Bronchial carcinoma **Answers: A B C D**

Bronchial carcinoma is now the most common malignant disease in western Europe. Occupational risk factors include exposure to asbestos, nickel, arsenic, haematite, chromates and coal/radioactive gases.

15. Pancoast tumour **Answers: A B C D**

An apical lung tumour can invade the ipsilateral sympathetic fibres (Horner's syndrome), eighth cervical and first thoracic ventral rami (pain in fourth and fifth digits: paralysis of forearm and hand muscles) and the first rib.

16. Hypertrophic osteoarthropathy **Answers: B C D**

Hypertrophic osteoarthropathy is characterised by clubbing, gynaecomastia, sub-periosteal new bone formation and symmetrical arthropathy, the pain of the latter being helped by vagotomy below the origin of the recurrent laryngeal nerve. Squamous cell carcinoma of the bronchus is the commonest cause. It should be distinguished from 'thyroid acropachy' of which pretibial myxoedema forms a part.

17. Asthma **Answer: D**

Asthma mortality has not improved significantly over the past 50 years. Long-acting inhaled bronchodilators are currently only recommended when inhaled steroids have proved inadequate control. Viral infections commonly precipitate attacks. Virtually all symptomatic asthmatics have hyperreactive airways, as do a significant number of the normal population. There is no direct adrenergic innervation of the airways by beta-2 agonists acting on adrenergic receptors.

18. Asthma **Answers: A B C**

Isocyanates are used in polyurethane foam manufacture and platinum in the electronics and chemical industries. An increasing number of organic dusts are being recognised as causes of occupational asthma. Asbestosis gives diffuse lung fibrosis and berylliosis is a granulomatous disease resembling sarcoidosis.

19. Acquired immunodeficiency syndrome **Answers: A D E**

The lung is affected in more than 70% of AIDS patients. The symptoms of pneumocystis pneumonia (dyspnoea, dry cough and fever) usually develop insidiously over several weeks. Non-tuberculous mycobacterial infection is found in 12–20% of AIDS patients during life, the commonest being *M. avium-intracellulare*. The combined diagnostic yield of BAL and TBB in PCP is greater than 90%. Tuberculosis occurs earlier in the natural history of HIV infection than PCP, with a better preserved CD4 count.

20. Tuberculosis of the respiratory tract **Answers: All true**

Wheezing may result from endobronchial tuberculosis and this may be steroid responsive. In patients with disseminated/miliary tuberculosis, adult respiratory distress syndrome may occur and this tends to happen between 1 and 3 weeks after commencing antituberculous agents. Both pleural effusion and unilateral hilar lymphadenopathy are complications of primary tuberculosis. Remember that pleural effusion is a lymphocytic exudate with a low glucose ratio compared to blood, and a high adenosine deaminase level. Significant haemoptysis occurs in about 8%; massive haemoptysis (> 1000 ml/24 hr) can occur when there is erosion of a major blood vessel, either bronchial or pulmonary, and is a medical emergency. It is more common when there are cavities or bronchiectasis.

21. Cavitating lung lesions **Answers: B C D**

Other causes of cavitating lung lesions include tuberculosis, staphylococcal and *Klebsiella* pneumonia, fungal infections such as aspergillosis, septic and non-septic pulmonary infarction, rheumatoid nodules, and progressive massive fibrosis in silicosis and coal-miners' pneumoconiosis.

22. Pulmonary nodules **Answers: A D E**

Rheumatoid nodules, up to 1 cm in diameter, may appear in the lung. Very large nodules may be associated with coal workers' pneumoconiosis (Caplan's syndrome). Systemic sclerosis gives rise to pulmonary fibrosis and inhalation pneumonia. Pulmonary manifestations of SLE include recurrent infections, pleural effusions, atelectasis and shrinking lung syndrome.

23. Pleural calcification **Answers: B C D**

Silicosis causes calcification of intra-thoracic lymph glands producing an 'egg-shell' appearance. The extensive pleural plaques of asbestosis with interlobar, diaphragmatic and pericardial location is often diagnostic. Haemosiderosis gives intra-pulmonary calcification.

24. Chest X-ray **Answers: B D**

Pulmonary fibrosis of silicosis and ankylosing spondylitis affects predominantly the upper zones whereas that of asbestosis, fibrosing alveolitis and systemic sclerosis occurs predominantly in the lower zones. In systemic sclerosis there may be a combination of diffuse fibrosis and basal aspiration pneumonia.

25. Pulmonary eosinophilia **Answers: A D**

Perhaps the most important cause of pulmonary eosinophilia in the UK is allergic bronchopulmonary aspergillosis. Other causes include allergic reactions to a variety of parasites such as filaria, (tropical eosinophilia) or drugs (nitrofurantoin, sulphonamides, chlorpropamide, and others). Löffler's syndrome is a term used to describe mild transient illnesses with pulmonary eosinophilia for which no cause is found.

26. Stridor **Answers: B C E**

A foreign body in a main bronchus may cause initial spluttering and coughing when first inhaled, but will then probably be silent until infection or lung collapse occur. *Haemophilus influenzae* is a frequent secondary invader in acute laryngotracheitis, which causes marked stridor. A vascular ring round the trachea may cause definite, though rather faint stridor, and *C. diphtheriae* will cause stridor by infection of fauces or larynx.

27. Haemoptysis **Answers: B C D**
Haemoptysis is an important part of the clinical picture of idiopathic pulmonary haemosiderosis, aspergilloma and Goodpasture's syndrome (pulmonary haemorrhage and glomerulonephritis with anti-basement membrane antibody). It would be atypical in byssinosis, which is due to inhalation of dusts of cotton, flax or hemp, or in asbestosis, unless complicated by lung cancer.

28. Cheyne-Stokes breathing **Answers: A B C E**
Cheyne-Stokes respiration (periods of apnoea alternating with a series of breaths of increasing then decreasing amplitude) is usually due to brain stem compression with raised intracranial pressure. It may also occur as a result of metabolic upsets (such as cardiac, respiratory or renal failure) and as a result of CNS depressant drug poisoning. In diabetic ketoacidotic coma, the respirations are deep and sighing (Kussmaul).

29. Bilateral basal crackles **Answers: B C D**
Crackles are heard in bronchiectasis, pulmonary oedema, left ventricular failure and pulmonary fibrosis as in extrinsic allergic alveolitis and sarcoidosis.

30. Obstructive sleep apnoea syndrome **Answers: B C E**
Muscle tone is at its lowest during REM sleep when complete obstruction tends to occur. Oximetry alone will show recurrent and persistent falls in oxygen saturation during periods of obstruction and is probably the best first-line approach. A number of cardio-respiratory complications occur, including pulmonary arterial hypertension and cor pulmonale. Tracheostomy completely bypasses the obstruction and is almost 100% effective.

31. Associations **Answers: All true**
'Crunching sounds' or 'systolic clicks' can be heard synchronously with the cardiac cycle at the apex with a small left pneumothorax (with or without mediastinal emphysema). Enzymes released in acute pancreatitis damage, amongst other tissues, the lung surfactant and capillaries. Bronchial obstruction in sarcoidosis can be due to endobronchial disease or external compression by enlarged lymph nodes. Dressler's syndrome has amongst its other features, fever, pericarditis, pneumonitis and arthralgia. Pulmonary fibrosis is a recognised complication of chronic nitrofurantoin therapy. An acute lung reaction can occur within hours of taking the drug; there are chest X-ray changes and often a blood eosinophilia.

32. Pulmonary hypertension **Answers: B C D**

The ECG changes might include right axis deviation, dominant R waves over the right sided precordial leads and evidence of right atrial hypertrophy. Exertional dyspnoea in pulmonary hypertension without lung or left sided heart disease, has been attributed to ischaemia of the muscles of respiration. Finger clubbing is likely if the cause of the pulmonary hypertension is destructive lung disease or cyanotic heart disease, but is not a sign of pulmonary hypertension itself.

33. Pulmonary disease **Answers: B C E**

Ankylosing spondylitis is associated with fibro-bullous disease of the apices. Pleurisy with or without effusion can complicate any collagen vascular disorder. Basal pneumonia in systemic sclerosis results from oesophageal dysfunction and aspiration. Yellow nails demonstrate a deficiency of lymphatics and the effusion is not chylous. The most frequent primaries to cause lymphangitis are stomach, pancreas, breast and prostate.

34. Treatments of choice **Answers: A B**

Lung lavage is the single most useful therapy in alveolar proteinosis. Symptomatic bronchopulmonary aspergillosis requires steroids in the therapy regimen. Parenteral pentamidine or cotrimoxazole should be given in PCP if the PaO_2 is less than 8.0 kPa (60 mmHg). Tetracycline is the treatment of choice in psittacosis. Several recent studies have confirmed the lack of benefit with methylprednisolone in ARDS due to sepsis.

35. Pleural effusion **Answers: B D E**

Pleural effusions are very unusual in PCP. In asbestos-related disease, effusions are frequently benign. Blood staining may be due to a PE or malignancy.

RHEUMATOLOGY: ANSWERS AND EXPLANATIONS

1. D-Penicillamine therapy **Answers: A B C D**

Penicillamine can lower rheumatoid factor titres. The recorded side-effects are legion: commonly rash and pruritus, ageusia (blunting of taste perception which is not dose-related), leucopenia, thrombocytopenia and proteinuria secondary to an immune complex nephritis. Rarer penicillamine-induced syndromes include myasthenia gravis, SLE, polymyositis, thyroiditis, haemolytic anaemia and Goodpasture's syndrome.

2. Rheumatoid arthritis **Answers: C D E**

Episcleritis is a benign, relatively common manifestation of rheumatoid arthritis. Scleritis is rarer and more serious, being a manifestation of vasculitis, as is digital gangrene. Amyloidosis is a complication of many chronic inflammatory conditions.

3. Rheumatoid arthritis **Answers: D E**

Recent literature suggests azapropazone to have the highest and ibuprofen the lowest risk of adverse events. Gold produces a rash, leucopenia and thrombocytopenia; proteinuria tends to be reversible on stopping the drug. D-penicillamine has an association with myasthenic syndrome; hydroxychloroquine requires ophthalmic review. Methotrexate is an antifolate drug and its effect is increased by other antifolates, except sulphasalazine. Methotrexate can cause a pneumonitis and hepatitis. Cyclosporin A may also be therapeutic; it inhibits the production of interleukin 2 (IL-2) by activated T-cells and reduces IL-2 receptor expression.

4. Anti-nuclear factors **Answers: A B C**

Antibodies to ds-DNA are very specific for SLE but are only seen in 60% of patients. They may be detected either by radio-immunoassay or by use of the haemoflagellate *Crithidia luciliae*. Single stranded antibodies to single stranded DNA are much less specific and are found in a very wide variety of disorders. They may have some pathogenic role. Patterns of nuclear immunofluorescence may be of some limited use. Homogeneous and speckled patterns are very non-specific. The peripheral pattern is almost exclusively seen in SLE and a nucleolar pattern and centromere pattern predominantly in systemic sclerosis, the latter being associated with a CREST syndrome. Titres of antinuclear factors are not helpful in monitoring disease activity.

5. Drug-induced systemic lupus erythematosus Answers: A C D

Drug-induced SLE is equally common in men and women whereas 'idiopathic' SLE has a 9:1 female to male preponderance. The list of drugs that may precipitate lupus includes sulphonamides, isoniazid, griseofulvin, hydralazine, penicillamine procainamide and carbamazepine. Slow acetylators are more prone and slower metabolism of the drugs is important. Drug-induced SLE is virtually never complicated by renal disease. Withdrawal of the offending drug leads to disappearance of the disease, but complete reversal has been recorded as taking up to two years in some cases of hydralazine-induced SLE.

6. Systemic lupus erythematosus Answers: All false

Joint deformities are uncommon in SLE, their presence would favour rheumatoid arthritis. A lung cavity and anti-neutrophil cytoplasmic antibodies suggest Wegener's disease; peripheral neuropathy (especially if mononeuritis multiplex), polyarteritis nodosa; RNP antibodies would indicate mixed connective tissue disease and severe Raynaud's, systemic sclerosis or mixed connective tissue disease.

7. Anti-phospholipid antibodies Answers: B D E

Antiphospholipid antibodies are associated with widespread arterial and venous thrombosis. They are a common cause of recurrent spontaneous abortion, due to placental vessel thrombosis and ischaemia. Rarely Addison's disease can result from adrenal thrombosis. Antibodies are neither specific nor sensitive for SLE but cause the laboratory phenomenon of lupus anticoagulants. The bleeding time is normal. Valvular heart disease is common in the antiphospholipid syndrome and can manifest as culture negative endocarditis.

8. Extractable nuclear antigens Answers: B E

Extractable nuclear antigens are antibodies directed against various cytoplasmic antigens. The commonest are Ro, La, RNP, Scl 70 and Sm. Ro and La are usually present in patients with primary Sjögren's syndrome and RNP typically present in mixed connective tissue disease. Sm is present in only 10% of patients with SLE.

9. Systemic sclerosis **Answers: A C E**

The CREST syndrome (Calcinosis, Raynaud's, Oesophageal involvement, Sclerodactyly, Telangiectasia) is generally a benign disorder not associated with the systemic involvement seen in scleroderma. Whereas the feature of myopathy runs throughout the spectrum of connective tissue diseases, CNS complications are not a feature of systemic sclerosis and are more characteristic of SLE. However, systemic sclerosis can cause resistant malignant (accelerated-phase) hypertension which could, in turn, cause cerebrovascular disease. Polymyositis and dermatomyositis in adults are associated with underlying malignancy.

10. Mixed connective tissue disease **Answers: A B D**

Mixed connective tissue disease is a clinical syndrome with Raynaud's myositis and swollen digits as common abnormalities. It is typified by the presence of antibodies to ribonucleoprotein. Some cases progress to systemic sclerosis. Renal involvement is uncommon.

11. Vasculitides **Answer: A**

A positive cANCA is sensitive for Wegener's granulomatosis. Both Wegener's granulomatosis and microscopic polyangiitis are more common in men and associated with pulmonary–renal disease. ENT symptoms are an important feature of Wegener's granulomatosis. Churg–Strauss patients rarely have neurological complications. Biopsy in HSP shows IgA deposits. Polyarteritis nodosa is associated with renal disease due to thrombosis, infarction or aneurysms and necrotising arteritis.

12. Polymyalgia rheumatica **Answers: All false**

The muscles involved are painful and stiff but not generally wasted, though wasting can occur due to disuse atrophy. It is now appreciated that the disease can remain active and need steroid therapy for many years in an appreciable percentage of cases. Muscle enzymes, as well as EMG and muscle biopsy are generally normal and unhelpful in diagnosis. The ESR is characteristically 80 mm/hr or more, but by no means invariably so.

13. Synovial fluid **Answers: A D**

Synovial inflammation is associated with release of proteolytic enzymes which degrade the hyaluronate making the fluid less viscous. A turbid fluid indicates the presence of white cells, not necessarily infection. Raised lactate levels are found in septic arthritis. Crystals of pyrophosphate and urate can be seen using polarised light microscopy. They are not visible to the naked eye.

14. Reactive arthritis **Answers: C E**

Reactive arthritis may occur following enteric or urethral infections typically with *Yersinia, Salmonella, Shigella, Campylobacter* or *Chlamydia*. The joint is 'non-infective', enthesitis is common, hence the occurrence of tendonitis. Eye involvement is in the form of conjunctivitis or anterior uveitis.

15. Radiological bone erosions **Answers: A C E**

Gout and psoriatic arthritis can both cause relatively coarse erosion of bone adjacent to affected joints. A finer bony destruction, especially subperiosteal, is typical of the osteitis fibrosis cystica of hyper-parathyroidism. Important sites to examine are the middle phalanges, the symphysis pubis and skull. Erosions have been reported in SLE but are rare and are not typical. Wegener's granulomatosis is typified by necrotising lesions of nasal mucosa, lung, kidney, joints, skin and nervous system.

16. Joint pain **Answers: B D E**

Christmas disease is indistinguishable clinically from haemophilia, and haemarthrosis is a major clinical problem. Arthritis is not a feature of thrombocytopenia, although prominent in Henoch-Schönlein purpura. Arthralgia and arthritis occur in sarcoidosis with erythema nodosum and, more chronically, in more indolent disease. Amyloid arthropathy, which is seen especially in multiple myeloma, can mimic rheumatoid arthritis.

17. Pseudo-gout (chondrocalcinosis) **Answers: A C D**

Calcium pyrophosphate dihydrate crystals, which are weakly positively birefringent, are deposited in cartilage and can be seen in joint fluid. Chronic forms of the disease without acute attacks may mimic osteoarthritis, chronic gout, or rheumatoid arthritis. There is no effective prophylactic drug for acute attacks, although nonsteroidal anti-inflammatory drugs can be used.

18. Sacroiliitis **Answers: A B D E**

Sacroiliitis is invariably present in patients with ankylosing spondylitis; HLA-B27 antigen occurs in excess of 95% of these patients. Sacroiliitis is also a feature of inflammatory bowel disease, reactive arthritis, and some types of psoriatic arthritis, especially if the patient possesses the B27 antigen.

19. Behçet's disease **Answers: A C**

Arthritis, anterior uveitis and CNS involvement are other characteristic features. Skin lesions, pustules, papules and erythema nodosum are common.

20. Patterns of arthropathy **Answers: B C**

Sacroiliitis is characteristically bilateral and symmetrical in ankylosing spondylitis. Unilateral, asymmetrical involvement is more common in other forms of seronegative spondarthritis such as psoriasis and Reiter's syndrome. Fluffy periostitis often occurs in conjunction with erosions in psoriatic arthropathy, so-called proliferative erosions. SLE is a non-erosive arthropathy and although there may be considerable hand deformity, this is due to tendon involvement rather than joint destruction. Gouty tophi do not calcify as a rule and are therefore radiolucent. The bone density around gouty erosions is usually normal although during an acute attack of gout there may be osteoporosis in the affected joint.

21. Patterns of arthropathy **Answers: B E**

There are several characteristic patterns of joint involvement in psoriasis: 1. DIP joint disease in association with nail dystrophy (10%); 2. asymmetrical oligoarticular involvement of the small distal joints (70%); 3. symmetrical polyarthritis (15%); 4. axial with spondylitis as a major feature (5%); 5. arthritis mutilans (rare). Generally, a seronegative oligoarthritis with DIP and PIP involvement with relative sparing of the MCP joints suggests a diagnosis of psoriatic arthritis. Extraspinal joint involvement occurs in 40% of patients with ankylosing spondylitis, the hip and knee being the commonest sites. Pyrophosphate deposition occurs mainly in the large joints, particularly the knees, wrists and shoulders. The joints involved in haemophilia (in order of frequency) are the knee, elbow, ankle, shoulder, wrist and sternoclavicular joint. Acute pain and swelling of a digit or a whole extremity is characteristic of multiple bone infarction in children during a sickle crisis.

STATISTICS: ANSWERS AND EXPLANATIONS

1. Clinical trial of a new drug — Answers: A B D E

A number of conditions are desirable when carrying out a clinical trial of a new drug. Firstly, the drug should be safe and have been thoroughly tested in experimental animals. A pilot study is useful to help the design of the proper study, in particular to predict the number of observations required to attain a result of statistical significance. A double-blind cross-over method is a well-tried and effective design, but is not uniformly applicable and can give rise to problems in certain circumstances. It is usually best to administer the drug to patients who are not undergoing treatment with other drugs as these may interfere with the results.

2. Clinical trial of a new treatment — Answers: B C D

The null hypothesis is rejected if there is a significant difference between the groups. A type I error occurs when the null hypothesis is wrongly rejected (i.e. concluding that a significant difference exists when in reality it does not). A type II error occurs when the null hypothesis is accepted when in reality a genuine difference exists between the two groups. The power of a trial is the probability of rejecting the null hypothesis when it is false i.e. of concluding a difference or result of a given size is statistically significant. The power of a trial generally is increased when the number of participants is large and is decreased if the difference to be detected is small.

3. Clinical trial — Answers: C E

Statistical significance does not imply clinical significance. In addition to assessing the clinical improvement produced by a therapy, account must also be taken of side-effects. Chi-squared is a calculated statistic used to compare proportions and has no immediate intuitive meaning unlike a p value or a mean. Any bias or confounding element (e.g. differences in the severity of disease between the two groups) may invalidate a trial.

4. Characteristics of normal distribution **Answers: C D**

The prevalence of a condition reflects the total number of cases in a population at a given time. Cohort studies may be used to study a defined group through time; e.g. a group of subjects exposed to a suspected cause of a disease at a particular time are then followed up to see whether they develop the disease. The mode is the value which occurs most frequently i.e. the maximum value on the frequency distribution curve. If a distribution is positively skewed (long tail on the right side, more large values) it will be less than the mean, if the distribution is negatively skewed (long tail on the left, more small values) it will be greater than the mean. The standard error of the mean of a sample (SEM) is a measure of how accurately the true population mean has been estimated. It may be calculated by dividing the standard deviation of the sample by the square root of the sample size (SD/ n).

5. Normal distribution **Answers: B D**

The median value is the value which occurs in the middle when the values are arranged in order of magnitude. For a normal (Gaussian) distribution approximately 68% of the values lie within one standard deviation of the mean and 95.5% within two standard deviations. 1.96 is the 5% percentage point of the normal distribution as 95% of the values lie within 1.96 standard deviations of the mean (2.5% in each tail). The standard deviation is a measure of the spread of a set of values; the EM measures how accurately the calculated mean approaches the true population mean.

6. Median and mean **Answer: C**

The median and mode are used in preference to the arithmetic mean when a set of values are from a population with a skewed distribution. In such situations values from the long tail of the skew distribution disproportionately affect the value of the arithmetic mean (average) which may be misleading.

7. Normal distributions **Answers: B C D**

Many other symmetrical distributions exist. The standard error, and not the standard deviation, is a measure of the reliability of the mean value.

8. Significance tests **Answers: B D**

Two normal distributions are best compared by use of a parametric test. Student's paired t-test requires knowledge of the mean difference between the pairs of observations.

9. Significance tests **Answers: B C**

An unpaired t-test would be appropriate since a between group analysis is required. The paired t-test is used for within-group comparisons. A significance value (p) is the probability that a particular result arose by chance. In small samples the estimate of the mean and standard deviation, etc. are inaccurate. To account for this uncertainty when significance values are calculated we use the number of degrees of freedom (df). The df is the number of independent values which contribute to the calculation of the t-statistic and therefore the significance value. The larger the df the smaller the t-statistic necessary to achieve conventional levels of significance. For a paired t-test this value is the number of observations minus one; in an unpaired t-test it equals the degrees of freedom of both groups which added together equals the total number of observations (in both groups) minus two.

10. Assay for serum sodium **Answers: C E**

The coefficient of variation of the assay is a measure of how often repeated measurements conform to each other; i.e. it reflects the reproducibility of the assay. The accuracy of an assay reflects the closeness which each measurement has to its true value. If the assay is specific then it measures sodium and nothing else. The precision of an assay determines how small a change the assay detects.

11. Correlation methods **Answers: A C**

Correlation methods are used to examine whether there is a linear relationship between two continuous variables; the strength of the association is reflected in the value of r (–1 to +1). If the correlation is strong r has values of less than –0.5 or greater than +0.5. The statistical significance of a particular r is calculated separately (NB even if a correlation is poor, it may still be statistically significant). Although two variables may be correlated, this does not allow a value for one variable to be calculated from a value of the second. Regression analysis and the derivation of a regression equation may be used to calculate the value of one (dependent) variable from a second (independent) variable. Mortality is not a continuous variable.

12. Concerning clinical trials **Answers: C D**

The American FDA divides trials into 4 phases: I - first exposure in man, usually healthy volunteers; II - small comparative trials; III - large scale clinical trials; IV - post marketing surveillance. Placebos are pharmacologically inert (but physiologically active in up to 50% of subjects).

Most trials compare 2 groups but large numbers are required. Where this is not possible half the number of patients required are needed in a cross-over trial, the patients acting as their own 'control'. Cross-over studies produce order effects and carry-over effects and are only applicable if therapy modifies and does not cure the condition being treated. Reassessment should be objective if at all possible but subjective visual analogue scales are reliable. Type I errors (false positive) are less common than type II errors (false negative) as the main difficulty with many trials is inadequate numbers.

PRACTICE PAPER 1

Practice Paper 1: Time allowed: 2.5 hours
Please indicate the correct answer(s) by ticking the appropriate box(es).

1. Systemic blood pressure is increased

❏ A on the assumption of the upright from the supine position
❏ B on sudden exposure to cold
❏ C always when heart rate increases
❏ D by brain stem asphyxia
❏ E in response to stimulation of peripheral chemoreceptors

2. In the management of a narrow complex tachycardia

❏ A intravenous adenosine may be used to restore sinus rhythm in atrial flutter
❏ B a Valsalva manoeuvre may cardiovert an AV nodal re-entrant tachycardia
❏ C the use of disopyramide is contraindicated in patients with impaired left ventricular function
❏ D atrial overdrive pacing may restore sinus rhythm in atrial fibrillation
❏ E a synchronised DC shock is contraindicated in patients in left ventricular failure

3. In aortic valve disease

❏ A severe aortic stenosis with a history of left ventricular failure is associated with a median survival of approximately 2 years
❏ B severe aortic stenosis is excluded by an echo gradient of < 20 mmHg
❏ C mild aortic stenosis in young people is associated with a negligible risk of endocarditis
❏ D long-term treatment with nifedipine in aortic regurgitation is associated with an improved outcome
❏ E the systolic blood pressure may be normal or elevated in patients with severe aortic stenosis

4. The following indicate a high risk of cardiac events on exercise testing in patients with chronic ischaemic heart disease without a history of myocardial infarction:

- ❏ A exercise-induced hypotension
- ❏ B exercise-induced hypertension
- ❏ C high grade ventricular ectopy
- ❏ D silent rather than symptomatic ischaemia
- ❏ E claudication

5. In acute massive pulmonary embolism

- ❏ A clinical evidence of deep venous thrombosis is characteristically present
- ❏ B pulmonary embolectomy is the treatment of choice
- ❏ C the arterial pCO_2 is characteristically raised
- ❏ D the chest X-ray shows oligaemia in the lung fields in the majority of cases
- ❏ E subcutaneous heparin should be started immediately the diagnosis is suspected

6. In pregnancy, cardiovascular changes include

- ❏ A an increase in pulmonary vascular resistance
- ❏ B an increase in blood volume of about 40%
- ❏ C tachycardia
- ❏ D an increase in cardiac output by about 45%
- ❏ E no change in stroke volume

7. Concerning calcium channel blockers

- ❏ A they inhibit slow calcium efflux during stage 2 of the cardiac action potential
- ❏ B diltiazem increases AV nodal refractoriness
- ❏ C nifedipine is safe in pregnancy
- ❏ D i.v. verapamil can safely be given to patients in ventricular tachycardia
- ❏ E gum hypertrophy is a side-effect of the dihydropyridines

8. The following are associated with cannabis abuse:

- ❑ A irreversible reduction in academic performance
- ❑ B persistent bradycardia
- ❑ C hypotension
- ❑ D hypertension
- ❑ E status epilepticus

9. The following can act as both enzyme inducers and enzyme inhibitors:

- ❑ A alcohol
- ❑ B isoniazid
- ❑ C cimetidine
- ❑ D omeprazole
- ❑ E erythromycin

10. Cyclosporin A

- ❑ A causes afferent arteriolar vasoconstriction
- ❑ B interferes with interleukin-2 gene transcription
- ❑ C toxicity can be due to allopurinol co-administration
- ❑ D causes glucose intolerance
- ❑ E causes gingival hyperplasia

11. The long-acting somatostatin analogue octreotide

- ❑ A delays gastric emptying
- ❑ B reduces splanchnic arterial blood flow
- ❑ C constricts coronary arterioles
- ❑ D can only be given intravenously
- ❑ E may cause diarrhoea

12. Crohn's colitis has a recognised association with

- ❑ A generalised plane xanthomas
- ❑ B cutaneous amyloid
- ❑ C macroglossia
- ❑ D perianal ulceration
- ❑ E granulomatous cheilitis

13. In the treatment of non insulin dependent diabetes (NIDDM)

❑ A insulin resistance contributes to the hyperglycaemia
❑ B glibenclamide is safer than glipizide in the elderly
❑ C metformin frequently causes hypoglycaemia
❑ D chlorpropamide may cause facial flushing
❑ E the metabolic abnormalities of patients with hyper-osmolar coma respond promptly to insulin therapy

14. In phaeochromocytoma

❑ A 50% of tumours are extra-adrenal
❑ B diarrhoea is common
❑ C IVP offers the best tumour localisation
❑ D medullary thyroid cancer may be associated
❑ E urgent beta blockade is essential

15. In females with hirsutism

❑ A circulating free testosterone levels are usually increased
❑ B endometriosis is a common cause
❑ C cliteromegaly is common
❑ D late-onset congenital adrenal hyperplasia may be a cause
❑ E there may be associated insulin resistance

16. Chronic pancreatitis

❑ A is associated with hypercalcaemia
❑ B may cause portal hypertension
❑ C is best diagnosed early by CT scan
❑ D produces steatorrhoea when exocrine function falls to 30% or less
❑ E is associated with peripheral vascular disease

17. In Crohn's disease

❑ A approximately one third of patients will require surgery
❑ B azathioprine's main role is steroid sparing
❑ C acute phase protein concentrations are more likely to be elevated in small bowel disease
❑ D the most important long-term adverse effect of continued corticosteroid therapy is diabetes
❑ E peri-anal involvement often responds to metronidazole

18. The irritable bowel syndrome is associated with

- ❑ A dysuria
- ❑ B a characteristic pattern of abnormal colonic motility
- ❑ C recent salmonella gastro-enteritis
- ❑ D non-ulcer dyspepsia
- ❑ E headache

19. The following are autosomal dominant:

- ❑ A Wilson's disease
- ❑ B arachnodactyly
- ❑ C familial polyposis coli
- ❑ D tuberous sclerosis
- ❑ E limb girdle muscular dystrophy (Erb's)

20. In the diagnosis of syphilis a negative VDRL and a positive TPHA are indicative of

- ❑ A past treated secondary syphilis
- ❑ B early primary syphilis
- ❑ C untreated tertiary syphilis
- ❑ D secondary syphilis
- ❑ E infectious mononucleosis

21. Thalassemia major

- ❑ A is a cause of neonatal jaundice
- ❑ B is a cause of short stature
- ❑ C results in a shortened life-span
- ❑ D is an autosomal recessive condition
- ❑ E results in a bossed forehead

22. In multiple myeloma

- ❑ A radiotherapy is a useful means of controlling hypercalcaemia
- ❑ B the prognosis is closely correlated with renal function
- ❑ C hyperviscosity is more common in IgA than IgG types
- ❑ D peripheral neuropathy is a recognised complication
- ❑ E the serum alkaline phosphatase is characteristically normal

23. In the differential diagnosis of a raised haematocrit, the following suggest polycythaemia rubra vera:

- ❑ A low serum B12
- ❑ B high serum iron
- ❑ C normal white cell count
- ❑ D splenomegaly
- ❑ E reduced number of bone marrow megakaryocytes

24. Paroxysmal nocturnal haemoglobinuria

- ❑ A is exacerbated by alkalosis
- ❑ B is due to a deficiency of red cell membrane bound decay accelerating factor
- ❑ C is an inherited haemoglobinopathy
- ❑ D can present as the Budd–Chiari syndrome
- ❑ E is associated with leukaemia

25. Secretory IgA antibody

- ❑ A is resistant to the digestive processes of the G.I.T
- ❑ B is predominantly monomeric form
- ❑ C occurs in substantial amounts in colostrum
- ❑ D binds readily to mast cells + basophils
- ❑ E requires the action of mucosal epithelium in order to assume its final form

26. The following disorders produce impairment of humoral immunity:

- ❑ A ataxia telangiectasia
- ❑ B Chediak-Higashi syndrome
- ❑ C Chronic lymphatic leukaemia
- ❑ D common variable immunodeficiency
- ❑ E sarcoidosis

27. Di George syndrome

- ❑ A produces an excess of lymphoid malignancy
- ❑ B may present as convulsions
- ❑ C produces severe impairment of B cell function
- ❑ D is inherited as X-linked recessive
- ❑ E is an indication for BCG in the neonatal period

28. Hepatitis C

❑ A is a DNA virus of the herpes type
❑ B is less likely to result in liver cirrhosis than hepatitis B
❑ C is associated with hepatocellular carcinoma
❑ D infection may be complicated by superadded hepatitis D
❑ E is less likely to produce jaundice than hepatitis B

29. In *Plasmodium falciparum* malaria

❑ A relapse from persistent liver infection is a feature
❑ B parasites can synthesise pyrimidines *de novo*
❑ C parasite specific G6PD may be found in host red blood cells
❑ D primaquine is the drug of choice
❑ E patients rarely present later than four weeks after returning from travel

30. *Escherichia coli* 0157:H7

❑ A is a cause of pseudomembranous colitis
❑ B has an incubation period of 12 hours
❑ C is usually spread by the faecal–oral route
❑ D produces a shigella-like toxin
❑ E is associated with haemolytic uraemic syndrome

31. Concerning botulism

❑ A the causative organism is a Gram-negative rod
❑ B the toxin is usually detected in patient sera
❑ C it interferes with acetylcholine release
❑ D post-tetanic compound muscle action potentials are enhanced
❑ E it rarely causes ophthalmoplegia

32. The human parvovirus (B19)

❑ A is the causative agent for roseola infantum
❑ B causes a desquamative rash
❑ C is known to cause aplastic crisis in children with haemolytic disease
❑ D is know to cause polyarthralgia in children
❑ E is known to cause the haemolytic-uraemic syndrome (HUS) in 15% of affected children

33. A serum bicarbonate concentration of 34 mmol/l is consistent with

❑ A cor pulmonale
❑ B 21-hydroxylase deficiency
❑ C the observation of carpopedal spasm
❑ D ureterosigmoidostomy
❑ E primary hyperparathyroidism

34. The following are causes of secondary hyperlipidaemia:

❑ A anorexia nervosa
❑ B chronic renal failure
❑ C hypothyroidism
❑ D steroid therapy
❑ E high alcohol intake

35. Hyperuricaemia is a recognised consequence of

❑ A hypercalcaemia
❑ B cyanotic heart disease
❑ C hypoxanthine-guanine-phosphoribosyl transferase (HGPRT) deficiency
❑ D inhibition of xanthine oxidase
❑ E glucose-6-phosphatase deficiency (Type I glycogen storage disease)

36. In osteoporosis

❑ A thyrotoxicosis may be a cause
❑ B serum alkaline phosphatase may be raised above normal levels
❑ C serum osteocalcin is a marker of bone formation
❑ D treatment with bisphosphonates may prevent vertebral fractures
❑ E bone density should be monitored at 6 monthly intervals in severe disease

37. Endothelin–I

- ❑ A acts as a local paracrine factor
- ❑ B vasodilates the pulmonary vasculature
- ❑ C is elevated in heart failure
- ❑ D is generated by a converting enzyme
- ❑ E acts on endothelial type B receptors to promote nitric oxide production

38. Adhesion molecule interactions

- ❑ A can be homophilic
- ❑ B are present at adherens junctions
- ❑ C require beta 2 microglobulin
- ❑ D can occur via the RGD motif
- ❑ E rarely result in signal transduction

39. Diabetic microalbuminuria

- ❑ A occurs within 10 years of diabetes
- ❑ B is a predictor of early cardiovascular mortality in type II diabetes
- ❑ C is best assessed by a timed collection during the day
- ❑ D is not affected by improved glycaemic control
- ❑ E when accompanied by hypertension is best treated with ACE inhibitors

40. Nephrotic syndrome is associated with

- ❑ A cholesterol emboli
- ❑ B acute renal failure
- ❑ C venous thrombosis
- ❑ D hypokalaemia
- ❑ E pneumococcal infection

41. In adult polycystic kidney disease

- ❑ A patients are always hypertensive
- ❑ B there may be cysts in the pancreas and the liver
- ❑ C haematuria is a recognised feature
- ❑ D transplantation is contraindicated
- ❑ E there is an association with medullary sponge kidney

42. The following are recognised complications in dialysis patients:

❑ A carpal tunnel syndrome
❑ B encephalopathy
❑ C cardiac arrest
❑ D high incidence of cardiovascular disease
❑ E skin tumours

43. Lewy body dementia

❑ A is a rare cause of dementia in patients over 70 years
❑ B may present with typical idiopathic Parkinson's disease
❑ C may present with cognitive change without extrapyramidal features
❑ D is rarely associated with hallucinosis
❑ E is typically associated with fluctuating cognitive impairment

44. In a patient with diplopia

❑ A the paretic eye carries the most peripheral of the two images
❑ B retained capacity of the eye to intort indicates a superior oblique palsy
❑ C if the eye is deviated down and out the third cranial nerve is involved
❑ D failure of the eye to abduct indicates a fourth cranial nerve palsy
❑ E the lateral rectus is weak if the adducted eye cannot be depressed

45. The following are true of pseudobulbar palsy:

❑ A the gag reflex is usually absent
❑ B the tongue is wasted
❑ C the jaw jerk is usually brisk
❑ D it may be caused by a syrinx extending from the cord into the medulla oblongata
❑ E it is usually due to cerebrovascular disease

46. In the lower limbs

- ❑ A the femoral nerve arises from L2,3,4 nerve roots
- ❑ B the sciatic nerve forms the tibial and common peroneal nerves
- ❑ C the tibial nerve supplies the gastrocnemius and soleus muscles
- ❑ D a complete sciatic nerve lesion will cause sensory loss over the hamstrings
- ❑ E a common peroneal nerve lesion will cause weakness of eversion of the foot

47. In Parkinson's disease

- ❑ A the onset of symptoms is typically before the age of 40
- ❑ B tremor is most pronounced on sustained posture
- ❑ C rigidity in the upper limbs is most pronounced in the flexor muscles
- ❑ D gait is typically broad based
- ❑ E urinary incontinence is an early clinical feature

48. In dystrophia myotonica (myotonic dystrophy)

- ❑ A the abnormal gene lies on chromosome 17
- ❑ B the clinical manifestations are usually more severe if the affected parent is male
- ❑ C weakness is initially marked in distal limb musculature
- ❑ D myotonia is most pronounced in the cold
- ❑ E cardiomyopathy is a recognised feature

49. The foramen magnum transmits the

- ❑ A basilar artery
- ❑ B hypoglossal nerves
- ❑ C pons
- ❑ D all of the spinal accessory nerve XI
- ❑ E posterior vertebral venous plexus

50. The following Schneiderian 'first rank' symptoms are suggestive of a diagnosis of schizophrenia:

- ❑ A voices repeating the subjects thought out loud
- ❑ B thought broadcasting
- ❑ C Knight's move thinking
- ❑ D emotional blunting
- ❑ E emotional passivity

51. Puerperal psychosis

- ❑ A is more frequent in primiparous women
- ❑ B usually begins in the first two days after delivery
- ❑ C recurrence in subsequent pregnancies is the rule
- ❑ D usually has an insidious onset
- ❑ E normally has a good prognosis

52. Factors indicating an increased risk of suicide in a depressed patient include

- ❑ A a direct statement of intent to commit suicide
- ❑ B hopelessness
- ❑ C pressure of serious physical illness
- ❑ D living alone
- ❑ E presence of paranoid delusions

53. The following are associated with dementia:

- ❑ A pernicious anaemia
- ❑ B hypervitaminosis A
- ❑ C pellagra
- ❑ D porphyria
- ❑ E Wilson's disease

54. Oxygen debt

- ❑ A may be six times the basal oxygen consumption
- ❑ B in trained athletes is greater than in an untrained person for a given amount of exertion
- ❑ C is limited by an increase in pH
- ❑ D is incurred because blood cannot be delivered to the muscle at a high enough rate
- ❑ E is possible because muscle is capable of anaerobic metabolism

55. In sarcoidosis

- ❑ A T cells accumulate in active lesions
- ❑ B granulomas caseate
- ❑ C CD4 +ve helper T cells are increased in peripheral blood
- ❑ D there is B cell overactivity
- ❑ E activated pulmonary macrophages produce calcitriol

56. In respiratory function tests

- ❑ A residual volume is reduced in chronic bronchitis
- ❑ B total lung capacity is reduced in farmer's lung
- ❑ C arterial pO_2 is a good predictor of respiratory failure in Guillain–Barré syndrome
- ❑ D transfer factor is normal in lymphangitis carcinomatosis
- ❑ E inspiratory flow is more affected than expiratory flow if large airway obstruction is intrathoracic

57. The antiphospholipid syndrome

- ❑ A is associated with arterial thrombosis
- ❑ B may cause a chorea
- ❑ C is treated with high dose warfarin
- ❑ D only occurs in association with SLE
- ❑ E can cause sudden wide spread organ failure

58. The following statements are true:

- ❑ A occipital headaches can occur in temporal arteritis
- ❑ B corneal reflex loss may be an early sign of rheumatoid cervical myelopathy
- ❑ C the nail-fold infarcts of rheumatoid vasculitis represent evidence of a life-threatening complication
- ❑ D iron therapy is effective in correcting the anaemia of rheumatoid arthritis
- ❑ E gold injections are usually given intra-articularly

59. With inflammatory myopathies

- ❑ A muscles are tender in the majority of cases
- ❑ B dermatomyositis usually has a more acute onset than polymyositis
- ❑ C in dermatomyositis, excessive discoloration of the skin implies an underlying malignancy
- ❑ D cardiac muscle may be involved
- ❑ E extraocular muscles may be involved

60. In a clinical trial of a new drug, the following results were obtained:

	Drug	Placebo
Improved	46 patients	34 patients
Not improved	14 patients	26 patients

- ❑ A the superiority of the drug over the placebo is so obvious that formal statistical testing is unnecessary
- ❑ B if a test of significance were required, computation of the Pearson coefficient of linear correlation would be appropriate
- ❑ C the data could be evaluated by computing a chi-squared statistic
- ❑ D the data could be evaluated by computing Student's t-test
- ❑ E the data could not be submitted to sequential analysis

PRACTICE PAPER 2

Practice Paper 2: Time allowed: 2.5 hours
Please indicate the correct answer(s) by ticking the appropriate box(es).

1. Tall R waves in ECG lead V1 are seen in

❑ A posterior myocardial infarction
❑ B acute pulmonary embolism
❑ C right bundle branch block
❑ D uncomplicated tricuspid atresia
❑ E Wolff-Parkinson-White syndrome

2. In the sick sinus syndrome

❑ A a degree of AV block is present in two-thirds of cases presenting with a sinus bradycardia
❑ B permanent pacing with a DDDR system improves life expectancy
❑ C cases after myocardial infarction are particularly likely to occur after occlusion of the left anterior descending artery
❑ D pacing is indicated in all patients with documented pauses of > 2 seconds
❑ E cardioversion from atrial fibrillation may be associated with asystole

3. In a patient with an atrial septal defect

❑ A left axis deviation on the electrocardiogram suggests a secundum defect
❑ B the presence of anomalous right pulmonary venous drainage into the right atrium suggests a sinus venosus defect
❑ C a tricuspid diastolic murmur suggests a large left to right shunt
❑ D sinus arrhythmia is present if the shunt is large
❑ E symptoms may only develop in middle age

4. Thrombolytic treatment with streptokinase

- ❏ A reduces overall mortality from myocardial infarction by approximately 50%
- ❏ B is not indicated in patients presenting with left bundle branch block
- ❏ C is indicated in patients with unstable angina and resting ST depression on the ECG
- ❏ D may only be given once to a given patient
- ❏ E improves outcome only in patients with myocardial infarction under the age of 70

5. Pericarditis is a recognised complication of

- ❏ A chronic renal failure
- ❏ B hypothyroidism
- ❏ C reflux oesophagitis
- ❏ D acute rheumatic fever
- ❏ E subarachnoid haemorrhage

6. Adverse effects of sulphasalazine include

- ❏ A diarrhoea
- ❏ B haemolytic anaemia
- ❏ C folate deficiency
- ❏ D male erectile impotence
- ❏ E headaches

7. Recognised side-effects of benzodiazepines include

- ❏ A confusion
- ❏ B impaired driving skills
- ❏ C potentiation of the effects of alcohol
- ❏ D ataxia
- ❏ E aplastic anaemia

8. Recognised features of digoxin toxicity include

- ❏ A weight loss
- ❏ B unilateral gynaecomastia
- ❏ C diplopia
- ❏ D ventricular fibrillation
- ❏ E delirium

9. Beta interferon in multiple sclerosis

- ❑ A reduces relapse rate by 70%
- ❑ B inhibits MHC class II expression
- ❑ C improves blood–brain barrier integrity in active disease
- ❑ D short term use can exacerbate disease
- ❑ E increases suppressor T cell activity

10. Recognised side-effects of treatment with omeprazole include

- ❑ A gynaecomastia
- ❑ B erythema multiforme
- ❑ C headache
- ❑ D bradycardia
- ❑ E pancreatitis

11. The possibility of a systemic disease should be considered in

- ❑ A pityriasis rosea
- ❑ B pompholyx
- ❑ C seborrhoeic dermatitis
- ❑ D kerion
- ❑ E alopecia areata

12. The ocular manifestations of Graves' disease

- ❑ A are nearly always seen when there is pretibial myxoedema
- ❑ B include unilateral exophthalmos
- ❑ C may occur in the absence of hyperthyroidism
- ❑ D are due to thyroid stimulating immunoglobulins
- ❑ E include severe pain in the eye

13. Cranial diabetes insipidus is a feature of

- ❑ A craniopharyngioma
- ❑ B histiocytosis X
- ❑ C sarcoidosis
- ❑ D non-secreting pituitary adenoma
- ❑ E head injury

14. *Helicobacter pylori*

- ❑ A is a Gram-positive Campylobacter-like organism
- ❑ B produces the enzyme urease
- ❑ C induces erosive antral gastritis
- ❑ D can be found in 75% of patients with a duodenal ulcer
- ❑ E can be diagnosed by a hydrogen breath test

15. Ulcerative colitis is classically characterised by

- ❑ A fistula formation
- ❑ B diarrhoea
- ❑ C cobblestoning of mucosa
- ❑ D pseudopolyps
- ❑ E rectal involvement

16. Complications of total parenteral nutrition (TPN) include

- ❑ A cholestasis
- ❑ B hyperlipidaemia
- ❑ C pancreatitis
- ❑ D aspiration pneumonia
- ❑ E acute renal failure

17. The following are features of tuberose sclerosis:

- ❑ A café-au-lait patches of pigmentation
- ❑ B ocular telangiectasias
- ❑ C cardiac rhabdomyomas
- ❑ D cerebral gliomas
- ❑ E cerebral aqueduct stenosis

18. In Down's syndrome

- ❑ A there is an increased incidence of hypothyroidism compared with normal subjects
- ❑ B there is an increased risk of atlanto-axial instability
- ❑ C hypertonia is a characteristic feature in the new-born
- ❑ D ileal atresia is the commonest gastrointestinal malformation
- ❑ E survival to adulthood is complicated by premature senility

19. The following would be against the diagnosis of *Pneumocystis carinii* pneumonia in a patient known to be HIV antibody positive:

- ❑ A normal serum lactate dehydrogenase level
- ❑ B absence of clinical signs
- ❑ C pleural effusion
- ❑ D cavities on chest X-ray
- ❑ E normal arterial gases after exercise

20. In chronic myeloid (granulocytic) leukaemia (CML)

- ❑ A the predominant white cell in the blood is the neutrophil
- ❑ B absolute basophilia and eosinophilia is usual
- ❑ C the low neutrophil alkaline phosphatase (NAP) score helps distinguish this condition from neutrophilia reactive to infection
- ❑ D interferon prolongs the chronic phase of the disease
- ❑ E priapism may be a presenting symptom

21. The following are useful in monitoring the status of multiple myeloma on chemotherapy treatment:

- ❑ A quantitation of paraprotein level
- ❑ B white cell count
- ❑ C haemoglobin level
- ❑ D 24 hour urinary protein measurement
- ❑ E serum immunoglobulin levels

22. In polycythaemia rubra vera

- ❑ A generalised pruritus is typically worse after a hot bath
- ❑ B a low MCV is a recognised complication
- ❑ C gout is a recognised complication
- ❑ D the diagnostic value of raised leucocyte alkaline phosphatase is limited
- ❑ E splenomegaly is found in 75% of cases

23. Sézary syndrome

- ❑ A has an excellent prognosis
- ❑ B is a B cell malignancy
- ❑ C frequently evolves into a non-Hodgkin's lymphoma
- ❑ D often presents with generalised erythroderma
- ❑ E lymphocytes have a typical hairy appearance

24. The following are associated with high circulating levels of IgE:

- ❑ A ataxia telangiectasia
- ❑ B HIV-1 infection
- ❑ C schistosomiasis
- ❑ D primary biliary cirrhosis
- ❑ E pemphigoid

25. Class II molecules of the major histocompatibility complex:

- ❑ A are present on the surface of virtually all cells
- ❑ B are important in antigen presentation to T-helper cells
- ❑ C are transmembrane heterodimers containing β2-microglobulin
- ❑ D are coded for by genes on chromosome 6
- ❑ E do not form haplotypes

26. Hypogammaglobulinaemia may be caused by:

- ❑ A phenytoin
- ❑ B myeloma
- ❑ C cyclosporin
- ❑ D sodium aurothiomalate
- ❑ E nephrotic syndrome

27. The following helminths may cause respiratory symptoms:

- ❑ A *Ascaris lumbricoides*
- ❑ B *Necator americanus*
- ❑ C *Paragonimus westermani*
- ❑ D *Strongyloides stercoralis*
- ❑ E *Ancylostoma braziliensis*

28. Rabies virus

- ❑ A transmission may be reduced by washing bite wounds
- ❑ B infection is diagnosed by positive serology during the incubation period
- ❑ C infection survival has improved with modern intensive care
- ❑ D infection may be diagnosed by skin punch biopsy from the neck
- ❑ E post-exposure prophylaxis is by simultaneous active and passive immunisation

29. Vancomycin resistant enterococci

- ❑ A remain sensitive to aminoglycosides
- ❑ B spread by the faecal–oral route
- ❑ C renal failure is a risk factor
- ❑ D are always invasive
- ❑ E rapidly break down vancomycin

30. Pneumococci

- ❑ A adhere to type II pneumocytes
- ❑ B serotyping is determined by cell wall antigens
- ❑ C induce tumour necrosis factor release
- ❑ D cell wall components are chemotaxic
- ❑ E are readily phagocytosed by polymorphonuclear cells

31. The syndrome of inappropriate antidiuretic hormone (SIADH) production

- ❑ A is a recognised complication of Guillain–Barré syndrome
- ❑ B can occur with lithium therapy
- ❑ C urine osmolality is typically less than 300 mosmol/l
- ❑ D aldosterone levels are suppressed
- ❑ E responds to demeclocycline

32. Hypophosphataemic ('vitamin D resistant') rickets is characterised by

- ❑ A an autosomal recessive inheritance
- ❑ B excessive renal tubular loss of phosphate
- ❑ C short stature
- ❑ D calcification of inter-spinous ligaments
- ❑ E complete resistance to treatment by vitamin D

33. Features of acute intermittent porphyria include

- ❑ A more women than men affected
- ❑ B increased urinary porphobilinogen
- ❑ C photosensitive rash in 25%
- ❑ D radial nerve palsy
- ❑ E hypernatraemia

34. Idiopathic infantile hypercalcaemia (William's syndrome)

- ❑ A is attributed to increased renal calcium reabsorption
- ❑ B has an association with patent ductus arteriosus
- ❑ C the affected infant may have distinctive facial features
- ❑ D hypercalcaemia may be related with a low calcium and vitamin D diet
- ❑ E is often associated with raised plasma cholesterol concentration

35. Constitutive nitric oxide synthase

- ❑ A is present in endothelial cells
- ❑ B is calcium independent
- ❑ C produces higher concentrations of nitric oxide than inducible nitric oxide synthase
- ❑ D is not active under normal physiological conditions
- ❑ E acts on citrulline to produce nitric oxide

36. *p53*

- ❑ A suppresses cell division
- ❑ B is a viral protein
- ❑ C mutation promotes tumorigenesis
- ❑ D controls normal development
- ❑ E is required for apoptosis

37. Causes of hypokalaemia with increased plasma renin activity include

- ❑ A psychogenic vomiting
- ❑ B laxative abuse
- ❑ C Conn's syndrome
- ❑ D diuretic abuse
- ❑ E syndrome of apparent mineralocorticoid excess (11-betahydroxysteroid dehydrogenase deficiency)

38. Rapidly progressive glomerulonephritis

- ❑ A may be precipitated by exposure to hydrocarbons
- ❑ B is always associated with antibodies to the glomerular basement membrane
- ❑ C is associated with haemoptysis most commonly in smokers
- ❑ D has a worse prognosis if the patient is anuric
- ❑ E may present with the nephrotic syndrome

39. In a patient found to be severely uraemic, the following would indicate chronic renal disease:

- ❑ A pericarditis
- ❑ B hyperphosphataemia
- ❑ C skin pigmentation
- ❑ D urinary osmolality 300 mosmol/kg
- ❑ E radiological osteodystrophy

40. A low plasma sodium (as measured by the auto-analyser) may be a consequence of

- ❑ A alcoholic cirrhosis
- ❑ B salt depletion
- ❑ C hyperlipidaemia
- ❑ D Cushing's syndrome
- ❑ E hyperglycaemia

41. The following are true of Alzheimer's disease:

- ❑ A behavioural disturbance is an early clinical manifestation
- ❑ B extensor plantar responses and myoclonus are early clinical features
- ❑ C the EEG is usually normal
- ❑ D it is associated with a predominantly frontal cortical distribution of pathology
- ❑ E it is usually familial

42. The following statements are true in internuclear ophthalmoplegia (INO):

❑ A there is often nystagmus greatest in the abducting eye
❑ B adduction is slow or restricted
❑ C bilateral INO is diagnostic of multiple sclerosis (MS)
❑ D INO may be a feature of myasthenia gravis
❑ E E-INO is associated with retraction nystagmus

43. The following statements are true:

❑ A the ulnar nerve supplies the first and second lumbricals
❑ B the ulnar nerve supplies the majority of the intrinsic muscles of the hand
❑ C the median nerve supplies flexor carpi radialis
❑ D the radial nerve supplies the dorsal interossei
❑ E the radial nerve supplies adductor pollicis

44. Carpal tunnel syndrome

❑ A may present with pain in the forearm
❑ B is associated with fasciculation of the small muscles of the hand
❑ C is exacerbated by coughing and sneezing
❑ D an underlying medical condition is usually present
❑ E is common in diffuse eosinophilic fascitis

45. The following are typical clinical manifestations of myasthenia gravis:

❑ A diplopia
❑ B dysphasia
❑ C absent tendon reflexes
❑ D distal limb weakness
❑ E fatiguability

46. In the leg

❑ A spasticity in a patient with hemiplegia is most pronounced in the extensor muscles
❑ B weakness in a patient with hemiplegia is most pronounced in the flexor muscles
❑ C sensory loss affecting skin over the lateral aspect of the lower leg may be due to a femoral nerve palsy
❑ D weakness of knee extension may be due to a sciatic nerve palsy
❑ E foot drop may be due to a common peroneal nerve palsy

47. Progressive supranuclear palsy

❑ A is linked with apolipoprotein E polymorphism
❑ B responds to levodopa
❑ C is characterised by neurofibrillar tangles in the basal ganglia
❑ D is associated with dysphagia
❑ E is due to a primary mitochondrial DNA defect

48. A radial nerve lesion above the elbow leads to

❑ A weakness of brachialis
❑ B weakness of abductor pollicis longus
❑ C weakness of extensor pollicis brevis
❑ D weakness of first lumbrical
❑ E sensory loss affecting skin over medial aspect of dorsal hand surface

49. Eaton–Lambert syndrome

❑ A is due to autoantibodies that bind to voltage-gated calcium channels
❑ B plasma exchange is an effective treatment
❑ C is associated with ventricular tachycardia
❑ D typically complicates pancreatic carcinoma
❑ E is associated with cerebellar degeneration

50. Scleritis is seen in

❑ A rheumatoid arthritis
❑ B SLE
❑ C Wegener's granulomatosis
❑ D ankylosing spondylitis
❑ E giant cell arteritis

51. Good prognostic signs of schizophrenia include

❑ A early onset
❑ B depressive features
❑ C echolalia
❑ D preservation of affect
❑ E visual hallucinations

52. Typical features of obsessive-compulsive neurosis include

❑ A ruminations
❑ B family history of neurosis
❑ C rituals
❑ D progression to schizophrenia
❑ E resistance

53. The following factors are significantly associated with episodes of deliberate self-harm:

❑ A male unemployment
❑ B recent alcohol consumption
❑ C male sex
❑ D age over 40 years
❑ E epilepsy

54. Recognised features of Korsakov's syndrome include

❑ A denial of amnesia
❑ B impaired registration rather than retention
❑ C obsession with time
❑ D dysphasia
❑ E echopraxia

55. In extrinsic allergic alveolitis

❑ A the most common sign of fine crackles
❑ B precipitating antibodies are diagnostic
❑ C there may be asymptomatic pulmonary insufficiency for several years
❑ D rheumatoid factor is positive in 30%
❑ E systemic symptoms typically occur within 20 minutes of exposure to organic dusts

56. Calcified extra cardiac lesions on chest X-ray have a recognised association with

❑ A asbestosis
❑ B farmers' lung
❑ C mitral stenosis
❑ D silicosis
❑ E chickenpox

57. In community acquired pneumonia

❑ A the most common causative organism is *S. pneumoniae*
❑ B mycoplasma occurs in five yearly epidemics
❑ C a definite pathogen is unusual
❑ D serum urea greater than 7 mmol/l is a bad prognostic sign
❑ E type II respiratory failure is common

58. In systemic lupus erythematosus

❑ A the C reactive protein (CRP) is raised
❑ B the lymphocyte count is raised
❑ C the platelet count can be low
❑ D marrow hypoplasia is seen
❑ E there is no increase risk of thrombosis

59. In scleroderma

❑ A vascular fibrosis is mediated by transforming growth factor-beta (TGF-b)
❑ B anti-RNA polymerase antibodies are associated with renal involvement
❑ C males and females are affected to the same extent
❑ D microangiopathic haemolytic anaemia can occur
❑ E hypertension should be treated with ACE inhibitors

60. An article in a medical journal states that in a study of gestational age at birth and neurological development at 12 months of age, r was found to be + 0.56 and p < 0.001

- ❑ A r is the correlation coefficient of probability
- ❑ B there is a negative association between gestational age and neurological development
- ❑ C there is a significant relationship between gestational age and neurological development
- ❑ D pre-term birth causes an inhibition in neurological development
- ❑ E the small value of p means that too few infants were studied

PRACTICE PAPER 3

Practice Paper 3: Time allowed: 2.5 hours
Please indicate the correct answer(s) by ticking the appropriate box(es).

1. The following statements are correct:

❑ A complete heart block is associated with a poor prognosis in anterior myocardial infarction
❑ B complete heart block complicating myocardial infarction characteristically resolves if the patient survives
❑ C the A-V node is supplied by the circumflex coronary artery in 90% of patients
❑ D acute mitral regurgitation associated with myocardial infarction can be easily distinguished from rheumatic mitral regurgitation by the site of the murmur
❑ E the commonest cause of chronic complete heart block is ischaemic heart disease

2. In mitral regurgitation

❑ A the systolic murmur characteristically obscures the second heart sound
❑ B the mitral valve gradient on echocardiography is a good criterion for deciding on the timing of surgery
❑ C the presence of mitral leaflet prolapse excludes severe regurgitation
❑ D treatment with vasodilators is contraindicated in severe cases due to the presence of pulmonary hypertension
❑ E balloon valvuloplasty is used in treatment

3. Infective endocarditis

❑ A is a recognised cause of glomerulonephritis
❑ B when due to *Streptococcus faecalis* should be treated with intravenous benzyl penicillin alone
❑ C is commonly seen in patients with an atrial septal defect and no other cardiac lesion
❑ D is confirmed or excluded by a normal echocardiograph
❑ E may follow sigmoidoscopy

4. In hypertrophic cardiomyopathy

- ❑ A approximately 20% of cases are familial
- ❑ B antibiotic prophylaxis is required
- ❑ C syncope occurs in 15% of patients and is associated with a poor prognosis
- ❑ D treatment with beta blockade is helpful
- ❑ E 48 hour Holter monitoring does not help in assessing the risk of sudden death

5. Recognised complications of vincristine therapy include the following:

- ❑ A diffuse pulmonary fibrosis
- ❑ B peripheral neuropathy
- ❑ C inappropriate ADH secretion
- ❑ D generalised pigmentation of the skin
- ❑ E paralytic ileus

6. In severe paracetamol poisoning

- ❑ A the hepatotoxin is a metabolite rather than paracetamol itself
- ❑ B plasma paracetamol concentrations give a useful guide to prognosis
- ❑ C the earliest evidence of liver damage is a rise in plasma transaminase concentration
- ❑ D acetylcysteine is effective only if given intravenously
- ❑ E hepatic coma responds to treatment with neomycin and lactulose

7. The following drugs are safe to use in combination with warfarin:

- ❑ A ranitidine
- ❑ B co-trimoxazole
- ❑ C carbamazepine
- ❑ D ibuprofen
- ❑ E salbutamol

8. Side-effects of non steroidal anti inflammatory drugs (NSAIDs) include

- ❑ A nephrotic syndrome
- ❑ B hypokalaemia
- ❑ C *H. pylori*-related gastric ulceration
- ❑ D heart failure
- ❑ E hyponatraemia

9. The following information may reasonably be given to patients starting a course of tricyclic antidepressants:

- ❑ A they should expect the drug to take effect within 24 hours
- ❑ B they should avoid cheese
- ❑ C they may experience a dry mouth at first
- ❑ D their skin may become sensitive to sunlight
- ❑ E it may help them to lose weight

10. The following drugs are ototoxic:

- ❑ A minocycline
- ❑ B gentamicin
- ❑ C bendrofluazide
- ❑ D aspirin
- ❑ E vancomycin

11. Skin and gut lesions occur in

- ❑ A Fabry disease
- ❑ B Albright's syndrome
- ❑ C Refsum's disease
- ❑ D Peutz-Jeghers syndrome
- ❑ E tungiasis

12. Hyperprolactinaemia is a recognised feature of

- ❑ A thyrotoxicosis
- ❑ B acromegaly
- ❑ C treatment with clozapine
- ❑ D pseudoseizures
- ❑ E hypothyroidism

13. The following suggest a diagnosis of gluten sensitivity:

❑ A Howell-Jolly bodies in the peripheral blood
❑ B a positive C14 breath test
❑ C aphthous ulceration of the mouth
❑ D osteoporosis
❑ E focal biliary cirrhosis

14. Concerning pseudomembranous colitis

❑ A it is caused by colonisation of mucosa by *Clostridium difficile* bacteria
❑ B rectal biopsy is rarely helpful in diagnosis
❑ C it requires intravenous vancomycin treatment
❑ D it can lead to toxic dilatation of the colon
❑ E it is associated with a very low recurrence rate

15. Primary sclerosing cholangitis

❑ A is associated with antineutrophil cytoplasmic antibodies
❑ B about two-thirds of patients are female
❑ C ursodeoxycholic acid improves survival
❑ D more frequently complicates ulcerative colitis than Crohn's disease
❑ E can recur following liver transplantation

16. Gastric secretion

❑ A is inhibited by sympathetic nervous activation
❑ B is approximately 1 litre/day
❑ C is inhibited by low gastric pH
❑ D has a potassium concentration of 4 mmol/l
❑ E has a chloride concentration of 140 mmol/l

17. Neurofibromatosis

❑ A may be complicated by carotid artery occlusion
❑ B is associated with an increased incidence of cerebral microgliomas
❑ C is suggested by the presence of more than five café-au-lait spots
❑ D may be complicated by bilateral sensorineural deafness
❑ E is inherited as an autosomal dominant characteristic

18. Treatment of HIV and opportunistic infection

- ❑ A zidovudine (AZT) is a proteinase inhibitor
- ❑ B ganciclovir inhibits viral DNA polymerisation
- ❑ C ganciclovir causes azoospermia
- ❑ D toxoplasmosis can be treated with clindamycin
- ❑ E clarithromycin is a suitable prophylaxis against cryptosporidia

19. In chronic granulocytic leukaemia (CGL)

- ❑ A a 9:22 chromosome translocation is necessary to establish the diagnosis
- ❑ B transformation into myelofibrosis may occur
- ❑ C development of further chromosome abnormalities heralds a change in the character of the disease
- ❑ D busulphan therapy delays the onset of blast transformation
- ❑ E bone marrow transplantation in the chronic phase may be curative

20. Idiopathic thrombocytopenic purpura (ITP)

- ❑ A in adults frequently follows a viral infection
- ❑ B in childhood is characteristically complicated by extensive haemorrhages and a fulminant course
- ❑ C is characteristically associated with moderate splenomegaly
- ❑ D is known to occur in children born to a mother previously cured of ITP by splenectomy
- ❑ E is associated with a reduction of megakaryocytes on bone marrow examination

21. Cold autoimmune haemolytic anaemia

- ❑ A has a peak incidence above 60 years
- ❑ B antibodies are typically IgG
- ❑ C causes intravascular haemolysis
- ❑ D antibodies are directed to the I-antigen
- ❑ E is secondary to cryoglobulinaemia

22. Anaphylaxis:

- ❑ A is by definition IgE mediated
- ❑ B fatalities are due to bronchoconstriction and/or arrhythmias
- ❑ C IV adrenalin is the first choice treatment
- ❑ D complement activation can induce a similar 'anaphylactoid' reaction
- ❑ E urticaria, angioedema and hypotension are cardinal signs

23. The following conditions predominantly cause cell mediated immunodeficiency:

- ❑ A Di George syndrome
- ❑ B protein-calorie malnutrition
- ❑ C chronic lymphatic leukaemia
- ❑ D sarcoidosis
- ❑ E nephrotic syndrome

24. Which of the following are associated with HLA B27 antigen:

- ❑ A rheumatoid arthritis
- ❑ B Yersinia arthritis
- ❑ C ankylosing spondylitis
- ❑ D uveitis
- ❑ E dermatitis herpetiformis

25. Cryptococcal meningitis is characterised by

- ❑ A an abrupt onset
- ❑ B a lymphocytic CSF
- ❑ C negative CSF cryptococcal antigen in 30% of cases
- ❑ D non-communicating hydrocephalus on CT scanning
- ❑ E a tendency to relapses after therapy

26. In a patient with a fever a neutrophil leucocytosis ($> 10 \times 10^9/l$) makes the following more likely:

- ❑ A brucellosis
- ❑ B amoebic liver abscess
- ❑ C malaria
- ❑ D dengue fever
- ❑ E typhoid fever

27. The following are causes of fever and pulmonary infiltrate in the immunocompromised:

❑ A Chlamydia
❑ B Herpes simplex
❑ C cryptococcus
❑ D nocardia
❑ E candida

28. *Legionella pneumophila*

❑ A has been isolated from the sea and most other types of water
❑ B grows optimally at temperatures of 10–20ºC
❑ C can be identified by culture on selective media and by guinea-pig inoculation
❑ D causes Pontiac fever
❑ E is highly infectious and case to case transmission is important during epidemics

29. In disorders of phosphate metabolism

❑ A the most common cause of hypophosphataemia is chronic renal failure
❑ B hyperphosphataemia complicates hypoparathyroidism
❑ C hypophosphataemia is a feature of Fanconi syndrome
❑ D hypoxia is associated with severe hypophosphataemia
❑ E tetany is a feature of hyperphosphataemia

30. Osteopenia is associated with

❑ A early menopause
❑ B cigarette smoking
❑ C reflex sympathetic dystrophy
❑ D testosterone deficiency
❑ E precocious puberty

31. Hypothermia

❑ A is defined as a body (core) temperature of 30ºC or below
❑ B causes involuntary shivering of the muscles
❑ C may give rise to delta waves in the ECG
❑ D is a recognised complication of alcoholism
❑ E typically produces a systemic alkalosis

32. Tumour necrosis factor

❑ A causes cachexia
❑ B is produced by bronchogenic carcinoma
❑ C enhances insulin sensitivity
❑ D is elevated in septic shock
❑ E circulates bound to alpha-2 macroglobulin

33. The following mechanisms are involved in the production of the fluid exudate in acute inflammation:

❑ A increased capillary hydrostatic pressure
❑ B increased vascular permeability to protein
❑ C breakdown of large molecular tissue proteins
❑ D diapedesis
❑ E complement activation

34. The following drugs may cause impairment of renal function:

❑ A captopril
❑ B verapamil
❑ C glyceryl trinitrate
❑ D gentamicin
❑ E indomethacin

35. The following are characteristic of renal vasculitis:

❑ A macroscopic renal infarction
❑ B inactive urinary sediment
❑ C eosinophilia
❑ D prodrome of systemic illness
❑ E progression to end-stage renal failure in over 75%

36. von Hippel–Lindau disease

❑ A is associated with multifocal renal cell cancer
❑ B is autosomal recessive
❑ C is due to the loss of a tumour suppressor gene
❑ D is associated with phaeochromocytomas
❑ E is associated with retinoblastoma

37. The following factors in a patient with acute renal failure would favour the use of peritoneal dialysis (PD) rather than haemodialysis:

- ❑ A myocardial infarction
- ❑ B chronic bronchitis
- ❑ C advanced age
- ❑ D hypotension
- ❑ E hypercatabolic renal failure

38. The following can cause a ptosis:

- ❑ A medial medullary lesion
- ❑ B pontine lesion
- ❑ C lower motor neurone seventh cranial nerve palsy
- ❑ D myotonia congenita
- ❑ E syringobulbia

39. A unilateral lesion in the midbrain can produce

- ❑ A ipsilateral sixth cranial nerve palsy
- ❑ B contralateral hemiplegia
- ❑ C contralateral ataxia
- ❑ D ipsilateral Horner's syndrome
- ❑ E pseudobulbar palsy

40. The following are true of the axillary plexus:

- ❑ A the radial nerve comes from the posterior cord
- ❑ B the median nerve comes from the medial cord alone
- ❑ C the ulnar nerve comes from the medial cord alone
- ❑ D a lesion of the axillary nerve causes sensory loss over the trapezius muscle
- ❑ E coracobrachialis is innervated by the musculocutaneous nerve

41. Chorea is a recognised complication of

- ❑ A prochlorperazine
- ❑ B metoclopramide
- ❑ C amitriptyline
- ❑ D selegiline
- ❑ E tetrabenazine

42. The following are true of Duchenne muscular dystrophy:

❑ A it is inherited as an X-linked recessive disorder
❑ B limb weakness usually affects distal musculature
❑ C limb contractures are an early clinical manifestation
❑ D eyes, face and bulbar musculature are usually spared
❑ E EMGs show a typically neuropathic appearance

43. In multiple sclerosis

❑ A there is reduced MHC class II expression in the CNS
❑ B helper T cells are found in acute lesions
❑ C saltatory conduction is normal
❑ D oligodendrocytes proliferate
❑ E the blood brain barrier is impaired

44. Huntington's disease

❑ A neuronal degeneration results from apoptosis
❑ B is X-linked
❑ C is caused by an expansion of a polyglutamine trinucleotide repeat in the Huntington's gene
❑ D degeneration is primarily in the olive and Purkinje neurones
❑ E characteristically presents by age 40

45. *Listeria monocytogenes*

❑ A is a Gram-positive anaerobe
❑ B infection rates are increased in pregnancy
❑ C induces host-cell actin assembly
❑ D is resistant to phagocytosis
❑ E requires listerolysis O for pathogenecity

46. *Helicobacter pylori*

❑ A do not predispose to an increased risk of gastric lymphoma
❑ B produce ammonia
❑ C are Gram-positive rods
❑ D infection is frequently asymptomatic
❑ E should be irradicated in reflux oesophagitis

47. Beta-haemolytic streptococci

❑ A may cause neonatal septicaemia and meningitis
❑ B all possess the Lancefield group A cell-wall antigen
❑ C may have an M-protein in the outer coat which is the main determinant of virulence
❑ D may cause epidermal necrolysis
❑ E are more frequently responsible for glomerulonephritis in the tropics than in temperate climates

48. Proliferative diabetic retinopathy

❑ A is treated with laser to the new vessels
❑ B is common at presentation of IDDM
❑ C improves in pregnancy
❑ D is associated with rubeosis iridis
❑ E precludes driving a car

49. Delusions of persecution can occur in

❑ A paraphrenia
❑ B paranoid personality disorder
❑ C reactive depression
❑ D myxoedema
❑ E amphetamine abuse

50. The following occur in anorexia nervosa:

❑ A amenorrhoea
❑ B osteoporosis
❑ C hyperkalaemia
❑ D raised plasma cortisol
❑ E depressed mood

51. Grief reaction

❑ A is typically self-limiting
❑ B characteristically includes denial
❑ C is best treated with tricyclic antidepressants
❑ D typically includes suicidal ideas
❑ E is a form of psychosis

52. In a tuberculous lesion

- ❑ A initially infiltration with lymphocytes occurs
- ❑ B there is progressive destruction of the organisms by macrophages
- ❑ C caseation consists of dead polymorphs
- ❑ D the presence of numerous giant cells is evidence of healing
- ❑ E the presence of caseation, macrophages and epithelioid cells is diagnostic

53. In non small cell lung cancer

- ❑ A over expression of the ras oncogene is associated with poor progress
- ❑ B proliferating cell nuclear antigen expression is inversely correlated with survival
- ❑ C outcome is independent of the Karnowsky Scale
- ❑ D adjuvant chemotherapy is superior if histology is non-squamous
- ❑ E the relative risks of combined exposure to asbestos and cigarette smoking are not additive

54. The physiological adaptations to high altitude living include

- ❑ A development of a mild systemic acidosis
- ❑ B reduced renal excretion of bicarbonate
- ❑ C reduced red cell 2,3 diphosphoglycerate (2,3 DPG)
- ❑ D no change in circulating blood volume
- ❑ E pulmonary hypertension

55. In cystic fibrosis

- ❑ A the sweat chloride concentration is characteristically elevated
- ❑ B rectal prolapse may be a presenting feature
- ❑ C it may present with bile stained vomiting in the neonatal period
- ❑ D the affected males are usually infertile
- ❑ E the gene is located in chromosome number 5

56. Concerning type I and type II pneumocytes

- ❑ A type I pneumocytes are more numerous than type II cells
- ❑ B type I pneumocytes predominantly provide the epithelial lining of the alveoli
- ❑ C type II pneumocytes produce surfactant
- ❑ D type II pneumocytes have phagocyte capacity
- ❑ E only type I pneumocytes are ciliated

57. The following are recognised features of rheumatoid arthritis:

- ❑ A ankle oedema
- ❑ B iritis
- ❑ C mouth ulcers
- ❑ D upper motor neurone signs
- ❑ E splenomegaly

58. In rheumatoid arthritis

- ❑ A there is an association with HLA DR3
- ❑ B activated T cells are present in the synovium
- ❑ C anti-tumour necrosis factor beta antibody can suppress disease activity
- ❑ D concordance in twin surveys is greater than 80%
- ❑ E chondrocytes express HLA class II antigens

59. Reiter's disease

- ❑ A is associated with HLA B27
- ❑ B antibodies to extractable nuclear antigen Jo1 develop
- ❑ C can follow infection with shigella
- ❑ D is more frequent in males
- ❑ E complicates gonococcal urethritis

60. The diastolic blood pressure readings of 1000 8-year-old children were found to have a statistically normal distribution with a mean value of 61 mmHg and a standard deviation of 8 mmHg:

- ❑ A the mean and standard deviation completely define the distribution of diastolic blood pressures for this age group
- ❑ B the mean diastolic blood pressure for this sample is equal to that for the whole population
- ❑ C 95% of the sample data lie within an interval defined by the mean ± 2 standard deviations (i.e. the range 45–77 mmHg)
- ❑ D the median is 53 (i.e. 1 standard deviation below the mean)
- ❑ E the variance is 64 (i.e. the square of the standard deviation)

PRACTICE PAPER 1: ANSWERS

1. Systemic blood pressure **Answers: B D E**

The blood pressure may be calculated by the following equation:

Blood pressure = Cardiac Output x Peripheral Resistance

Therefore, it rises when peripheral resistance increases on exposure to cold – this is sometimes used as a 'cold pressor' test. It falls when venous return and hence cardiac output falls, and a transient drop of blood pressure on rising may be seen in normal subjects but this should not persist. It does not necessarily increase when the heart rate increases, as an increased heart rate does not necessarily produce an increase in cardiac output. Stimulation of the peripheral chemoreceptors and hypoxia itself act on the pressor area in the medulla to give an increase in blood pressure.

2. Narrow complex tachycardia **Answers: B C**

Intravenous adenosine slows conduction across the AV node, therefore in re-entrant supraventricular tachycardias involving the AV node adenosine may cardiovert the patient to sinus rhythm. In atrial fibrillation and atrial flutter adenosine slows conduction and therefore the heart rate, and may assist in diagnosis. Vagal manoeuvres such as carotid sinus massage, the Valsalva manoeuvre and cold water immersion of the face may convert re-entrant arrhythmias to sinus rhythm. Disopyramide is negatively inotropic and cannot be used in heart failure, however cardioversion may be performed in the presence of heart failure and indeed may be essential. Overdrive pacing is effective in atrial flutter but is ineffective in atrial fibrillation.

3. Aortic valve disease **Answers: A D E**

Severe aortic stenosis accompanied by left ventricular failure is associated with a very poor long-term prognosis. With syncope the median survival is 3 years and with angina 5 years. In the presence of significant LV impairment the echo gradient may greatly underestimate the valve gradient, the systolic blood pressure is also an unreliable guide. Paradoxically the risk of endocarditis is greater in young people with mild aortic valve disease e.g. bicuspid aortic valve. Nifedipine is the only agent shown to improve long-term outcome in aortic regurgitation.

4. Chronic ischaemic heart disease **Answers: A C E**

Exercise-induced hypotension has a predictive value of 50% for triple vessel or left main coronary artery disease. Exercise-induced hypertension is associated with a better long-term prognosis. Other factors associated with a poor prognosis are: inability to exercise beyond stage 1 of the Bruce protocol, ST segment depression > 2 mm in multiple leads extending into the recovery phase and high grade ventricular ectopy. The presence of symptoms does not affect the prognostic value of ST depression in known ischaemic heart disease. Claudication is associated with a high risk of cardiac events in patients with ischaemic heart disease.

5. Acute massive pulmonary embolism **Answers: All false**

The treatment of choice is intravenous thrombolysis and heparin; the subcutaneous route is only appropriate for prophylaxis. The arterial pCO_2 and pO_2 are characteristically reduced. The chest X-ray is normal more often than not but may show areas of radiolucency due to oligaemia. There may also be vessel 'cut off' and later, even without infarction, evidence of atelectasis. Diagnosis is best made by perfusion scanning, which also may be useful to monitor the effects of therapy.

6. Cardiovascular changes **Answers: B C D**

In pregnancy, peripheral and pulmonary vascular resistance fall and blood volume increases by about 40% at 30 weeks. There is an increase in the volume of plasma and in the number of red cells but the disproportionate increase in plasma leads to haemodilution. Cardiac output increases to about 45% above normal levels at 20 weeks. The increase in cardiac output is due to an increased heart rate and to larger stroke volume.

7. Calcium channel blockers **Answers: B E**

These drugs inhibit calcium influx during stage 2. The negatively inotropic effect of verapamil may be fatal if given to a patient in ventricular tachycardia.

8. Cannabis abuse **Answers: C D**

Chronic cannabis abuse produces reversible intellectual impairment. Initial reports of cerebral atrophy have not been confirmed. Cannabis smoke may be carcinogenic.

9. Enzyme inducers and inhibitors **Answers: A B D**

Some drugs act as pure enzyme inducers, while others act as enzyme inhibitors. Occasionally, a drug can possess both properties: the same or different (iso)enzymes may be affected by the drug. Thus, alcohol taken acutely acts as an enzyme inhibitor while during chronic usage, it acts as an enzyme inducer. With alcohol, the same enzyme (cytochrome P450 2E1) is affected. Isoniazid similarly can act as both inducer and inhibitor of CYP2E1. In contrast, omeprazole inhibits one particular P450 isoform (P450 2C9), while inducing a different isoform (P450 1A2). Cimetidine and erythromycin act as enzyme inhibitors.

10. Cyclosporin A **Answer: B E**

Cyclosporin A exerts its immunosuppressive action by interference with interleukin-2 gene transcription by inhibition of calcineurin phosphatase. Vasoconstriction of the renal afferent arterioles reduces glomerular filtration rate and is a major side-effect often necessitating dose reduction. Allopurinol blocks xanthine oxidase and increases azathioprine toxicity but does not interact with cyclosporin. Cyclosporin A has been used to treat early autoimmune type I diabetes to prolong the honeymoon period – it does not cause glucose intolerance (unlike FK506). It does cause gingival hyperplasia, particularly when used in combination with calcium antagonists.

11. Octreotide **Answers: A B**

Octreotide delays gastric emptying and decreases splanchnic arterial blood flow thereby reducing portal venous blood loss by limiting mesenteric blood flow. It also decreases small intestinal secretions and prolongs transit and may be given subcutaneously to control high stoma output in patients with an ileostomy. Unlike its predecessors, vasopressin and glypressin, it has no effect on coronary arterioles.

12. Crohn's colitis **Answers: C D E**

Plane xanthomas (any site, yellow palmar creases) are pathognomonic of type III dysbetalipoproteinaemia. They also occur in secondary hyperlipidaemias associated with conditions of chronic biliary obstruction or prolonged cholestasis such as primary biliary cirrhosis. If generalized search for a myeloma.

Localised cutaneous amyloid may be primary or secondary with a variety of cutaneous tumours. Signs of skin involvement in systemic amyloidosis include petechiae, waxy-translucent or purpuric papules, nodules, plaques, pigmentory changes, bullous lesions, alopecia, nail dystrophy and macroglossia.

13. In insulin dependent diabetes **Answers: B E**

Despite the fact that insulin resistance is a major problem in the obese non-insulin dependent diabetic, patients presenting with hyper-osmolar coma are typically very sensitive to insulin. Small doses of insulin are therefore used initially to bring about slow changes in the disordered metabolic state. Although the half-life of glibenclamide is relatively short, it has active metabolities with a long half-life. Glipizide and its metabolites have a short duration of action and is therefore much safer in the elderly. Metformin does not normally induce clinical hypoglycaemia, even in overdose. Facial flushing with alcohol is an autosomal dominant determined condition present in 15–20% of patients treated with chlorpropamide.

14. Phaeochromocytoma **Answer: D**

Phaeochromocytoma is the ten percent tumour (10% bilateral, 10% malignant and 10% extra-adrenal). Constipation is common, as are the more usual hypertension, sweating and tachycardia. Tumour localisation with modern CT scanning is usually adequate although 131-Iodine labelled MIBG may be required for extra-adrenal tumours. Associated medullary thyroid carcinoma may be a feature of MEN type 2 syndrome. Alpha blockade is the most important initial treatment and only when this has been achieved is it safe to undertake beta blockade.

15. Hirsutism **Answers: A D E**

Hirsutism (increased androgen dependent hair growth) affects up to 20% of women. In over 95% of cases it is due to increased ovarian androgen production with mildly raised free testosterone levels, often associated with oligomenorrhoea, polycystic ovaries, obesity and a degree of insulin-resistance (polycystic ovary syndrome, PCOS). Cliteromegaly is rare, indicates true virilisation (along with breast atrophy and voice change) and should prompt a search for other causes such as an ovarian or adrenal tumour, or congenital adrenal hyperplasia (CAH). So-called 'late-onset CAH' usually results from relatively conservative mutations in the 21-hydroxylase gene and produces a phenotype indistinguishable from PCOS.

16. Chronic pancreatitis **Answers: A B E**

Portal hypertension may result from peripancreatic fibrosis. Endoscopic retrograde pancreatography is the gold standard for making the diagnosis. Steatorrhoea results only when 90% of exocrine function is lost. The high incidence of peripheral vascular disease is not solely a reflection of the tendency to develop diabetes secondary to endocrine failure.

17. Crohn's disease — Answers: B E

Nearly 75% of patients with Crohn's disease require surgery at some time in their lives. The earlier the surgery is in the history the more likely is the need for repeated surgery. Corticosteroid usage is predominantly short term to induce remissions. A small number (5–10%) of patients become steroid dependent. The major metabolic problem with this latter group is osteoporosis, and azathioprine has a useful steroid-sparing role in these patients. Acute phase protein responses are higher in large bowel disease.

18. Irritable bowel syndrome — Answers: A C D E

The irritable bowel syndrome is well recognised following *Salmonella* gastro-enteritis. Although previously thought to represent abnormal neuromuscular coordination of the colon, no characteristic abnormality of large bowel motility has yet been defined. An increased awareness of colonic action is characteristic of the syndrome and may be secondary to a lowered threshold of activity in colonic afferent neurons. Dysuria, headache, low back pain and non-ulcer dyspepsia are all associated and may represent a similar underlying pathophysiology of other organs.

19. Autosomal dominant — Answers: B C D

A condition is dominant if the disease is expressed despite normal copies of the gene being present on one chromosome; i.e. heterozygotes have the disease as well as homozygotes. A condition is recessive if the genes on both of the chromosomes have to be abnormal for the disease to be expressed. Wilson's disease and Erb's muscular dystrophy are recessive, while arachnodactyly, familial polyposis coli and tuberous sclerosis are dominantly inherited.

20. Syphilis — Answers: A B C

During the primary stage of syphilis all serological tests are initially negative with the exception of the FTA which is then followed by the TPHA and lastly by the VDRL. In the secondary stage of syphilis all serological tests are positive but in tertiary late syphilis, 5–25% of non-specific tests (VDRL) are negative in the absence of past treatment. Following effective treatment the specific tests (TPHA) remain positive whereas the non-specific tests become negative. The non-specific tests (VDRL) may be falsely positive in many infectious diseases whereas the specific tests (TPHA) are not.

21. Thalassaemia major **Answers: B C D E**

The predominant haemoglobin is type F in all neonates: the thalassaemic state appears later as the child converts from HbF to HbA. Widespread marrow hyperplasia results in bony overgrowth. The prognosis is grave and many children fail to survive into adult life.

22. In multiple myeloma **Answers: B C D E**

Radiotherapy is only useful for bone pain in myeloma. Poor renal function is closely correlated with a poor prognosis. Hyperviscosity occurs in IgA myeloma due to polymerisation of paraprotein molecules. Polyneuropathy occurs due to amyloidosis, or it may be of unknown aetiology as with carcinoma.

23. Polycythaemia rubra vera **Answer: D**

In the classical case, evidence of increased production of all the marrow elements and splenomegaly distinguishes polycythaemia rubra vera from secondary and relative ('stress') polycythaemia. The serum iron tends to be low and the serum B12 high due to an increase in the vitamin B12 binding proteins.

24. Paroxysmal nocturnal haemoglobinuria **Answers: B D E**

Paroxysmal nocturnal haemoglobinuria (PNH) is an acquired genetic disorder of the glycosyl-phosphatidyl-inositol anchor that binds the complement neutralising protein decay accelerating factor to the red cell membrane. The result is increased red cell sensitivity to complement lysis. This is exacerbated by acidosis – explaining the nocturnal nature of haemolysis – and is the basis for Ham's acid lysis test. PNH results in thrombotic events such as hepatic vein thrombosis and is associated with aplastic anaemia and a number of leukaemias.

25. Secretory IgA antibody **Answer: A C E**

Secretory IgA is dimeric. IgE (not IgA) binds to mast cells and basophils.

26. Humoral immunity **Answer: A C D**

Impaired humoral immunity is present in disorders of the B-cell lineage, hypogammaglobuliaemias and the combined immunodeficiencies (SCID, ataxia telangiectasia, Wiskott-Aldrich). Chediak-Higashi and the similar chronic granulomatous disease are disorders of innate immunity. CLL is a cause of hypogammaglobulinaemia. Sarcoidosis impairs cell mediated immunity.

27. di George syndrome **Answer: B**

The di George syndrome is a primary T-cell deficiency and therefore produces severely impaired cell mediated immunity. Though common bacterial infections can be dealt with, infections with vaccinia, measles or BCG can prove fatal. The syndrome, which is not familial, is due to a defect in the development of the thymus and 3rd and 4th branchial arches. The parathyroids are absent, causing severe hypocalcaemia and convulsions. Cardiovascular anomalies occur.

28. Hepatitis C **Answers: C E**

Hepatitis C is an RNA flavivirus. It is less likely to produce jaundice than hepatitis B but a greater percentage of those infected will have a chronic active hepatitis that will progress to cirrhosis, perhaps taking 20 years or more. Hepatocellular carcinoma is well recognised. Hepatitis D only complicates hepatitis B infection.

29. *Plasmodium falciparum* malaria **Answers: B C**

Pyrimidine and G6PD synthesis can occur *de novo*; purines are exogenous. *Plasmodium vivax* and *ovate*, but not *Plasmodium falciparum*, have a persisting hepatic cycle, from which late relapse can occur. The normal incubation period is 7–14 days, but this may be affected by concomitant antimalarial therapies. Regarding Falciparum malaria, 90% of patients present within one month and 99% within six months of leaving an endogenous area.

30. *Escherichia coli* 0157:H7 **Answers: A D E**

Escherichia coli 0157:H7 has emerged as a major cause of bloody diarrhoea and it is a causative organism of the haemolytic-uraemic syndrome. The organism adheres to the colonic mucosal surfaces and produces one or more shigella-like toxins that induce a haemorrhage colitis, pseudo membranes may be present. The toxin can initiate the haemolytic-uraemic syndrome if it gains access to the circulation. The majority of infection arises from transmission of the organism through the consumption of undercooked infected ground beef. The incubation period is typically 3 to 4 days.

31. Botulism **Answers: C D**

Ophthalmoparesis, facial weakness and bulbar palsy are the most frequent initial symptoms of botulism. Limb weakness and respiratory compromise may follow. The disease is caused by a toxin synthesised by *Clostridium botulinum,* a Gram-positive rod. The toxin impedes the formation of functioning acetylcholine vesicles thereby producing a presynaptic neuromuscular block. Post-tetanic potentiation of the compound muscle action potential, due to increased calcium mediated acetylcholine release, is a hallmark of presynaptic lesions. In affected patients only 35% have detectable toxin in their serum, stool specimens are more likely to be diagnostic.

32. The human parvovirus (B19) **Answers: C D**

Roseola infantum or the 'sixth disease' is caused by the human herpes virus 6. The human parvovirus (B19) causes erythema infectiosum or the 'fifth disease' which is characterised by a mild febrile illness, erythematous rash on the cheeks (slapped cheek appearance) and a fine reticular rash over the extremities. It is also known to cause aplastic crisis in haemolytic disease, and polyarthralgia. The epidemic form of HUS is thought to be caused by verotoxin-producing *E. coli.*

33. Serum bicarbonate concentration **Answers: A C**

Carbon dioxide retention in chronic respiratory disease leads to renal conservation of bicarbonate to maintain plasma pH. Carpopedal spasm may be a feature of hypocalcaemia and both metabolic and respiratory alkalosis. 21-hydroxylase deficiency leads to a mild metabolic acidosis in the untreated state (low plasma bicarbonate) and this will also be observed in primary hyperparathyroidism and ureterosigmoidostomy.

34. Secondary hyperlipidaemia **Answers: All true**

The aetiology of the hypercholesterolaemia associated with anorexia is not clearly defined. Chronic renal failure, particularly where there is nephrotic syndrome may be associated with very high levels of circulating lipids. Hypothyroidism classically produces an elevation of cholesterol (type II). Therapeutic doses of steroids may produce a mixed picture and alcohol excess typically causes a high serum triglyceride level.

35. Hyperuricaemia **Answers: A B C E**

Hypercalcaemia giving renal failure or due to hyperparathyroidism is associated with hyperuricaemia. Polycythaemia and other myelo-and lymphoproliferative diseases give overproduction of uric acid, and this may also be seen in secondary polycythaemia (which will accompany cyanotic heart disease). Deficiency of HGPRT is the cause of the Lesch-Nyhan syndrome in which gross overproduction of uric acid is associated with choreoathetosis, spasticity, variable mental deficiency and self-mutilation. Children with type I glycogen storage disease develop gout as a consequence of impaired uric acid excretion secondary to lactic acidosis and ketonaemia, and increased *de novo* purine synthesis. Xanthine oxidase inhibitors such as allopurinol lower blood urate levels.

36. Osteoporosis **Answers: A C D**

Osteoporosis is most commonly age-related and/or post-menopausal. Other causes include hypogonadism, thyrotoxicosis, steroid excess, immobility, myeloma, rheumatoid arthritis, phenytoin and heparin. Bone density is reduced to less than 2.5 standard deviation units below that of healthy young subjects. There are no biochemical markers which fall outside the normal range, although bone formation (indicated by serum osteocalcin, alkaline phosphatase and urinary procollagen peptides) must be lower than the rate of bone resorption (indicated by urinary hydroxyproline or pyridinium–collagen crosslinks). Treatment with bisphosphonates, either cyclical etidronate or alendronate (continuously), have been shown to increase bone density and reduce vertebral fractures. Bone density is best measured by dual energy X-ray absorptiometry (DEXA) but the inaccuracy is such that significant changes can usually only be detected over 1–2 years.

37. Endothelin–I **Answers: A C D E**

Endothelin–I is an endothelium-derived vasoconstrictor and pressor peptide with mitogenic properties that is generated from a precursor, 'big' endothelin–I, through the action of endothelin converting enzyme (that is distinct from angiotensin converting enzyme). Endothelin–I is present in plasma but it is mainly released towards smooth muscle and acts in a paracrine fashion. It is elevated in heart failure, vasospasm and acute renal failure. Endothelin–I acts on type A receptors in smooth muscle to cause vasoconstriction. Type B receptors are on endothelial cells and modulate vasoconstriction by generation of the vasodilators, nitric oxide and prostacyclin.

38. Adhesion molecule interactions **Answers: A B D**

Adhesion molecules include the integrins, immunoglobulin superfamily, cadherins and selectins. They orchestrate cell–cell and cell–matrix interactions and as such are involved in a wide range of processes including embryogenesis, inflammatory reactions and wound repair. Several adhesion molecules (including cadherins and platelet-endothelial cell adhesion molecule – PECAM) can bind to an identical molecule on another cell (homophilic adhesion). Cadherins establish molecular links between adjacent cells at adherens junctions. The integrins recognise the amino acid sequence arginine–glycerine– aspartic acid (RGD) motif present in the extracellular matrix. Signal transduction follows adhesion molecule interaction and affects many processes inside the cell including proliferation, secretion and apoptosis. Beta 2 microglobulin is not an adhesion molecule – it is part of the HLA system.

39. Diabetic microalbuminuria **Answers: B E**

Microalbuminuria is the first manifestation of diabetic nephropathy, but it may not occur until the second to third decades after the diagnosis of diabetes. It is best assessed by examination of early morning urine specimens, as albumin excretion can vary diurnally. Albuminuria can be reduced by optimising glycaemic control and blood pressure; ACE inhibitor agents have been shown to be of particular benefit in the treatment of hypertension.

40. Nephrotic syndrome **Answers: B C D E**

Cholesterol emboli complicate atheromatous aorto-renovascular disease and are not associated with the hypercholesterolaemia of the nephrotic syndrome. Hypocomplementaemia and hypoglobulinaemia predispose to most bacterial infections, especially pneumococcal disease. Acute renal failure, due to ATN, may complicate the nephrotic syndrome if intravascular volume is severely depleted; hypokalaemia often accompanies loop diuretic therapy.

41. Adult polycystic kidney disease **Answers: B C**

Polycystic kidney disease is associated with hepatic cysts (in about 70% of cases) and also pancreatic cysts, although failure of the respective organs is rare. Berry aneurysms in the cerebral circulation occur in 25% of patients. Large or infected kidneys may need to be removed prior to transplantation.

42. Dialysis patients **Answers: A B C D**

Significant cardiovascular events occur at least 20 times more frequently in dialysis patients than in the general population; cardiac arrest due to hyperkalaemia, transient systemic vasodilation and coronary disease is also well recognised during haemodialysis. Haemodialysis with cuprophane allows accumulation of beta-2-microglobulin, and development of dialysis-related amyloid. Aluminium toxicity, once common with aluminium-containing phosphate binders and with previously untreated water, is now rare due to reverse osmosis water treatment and frequent assessment of aluminium concentration.

43. Lewy body dementia **Answers: B C E**

Lewy body dementia may cause up to 25% of dementia in patients over 70 years and is associated with Lewy bodies (an inclusion body typically detected in the brains of patients with Parkinson's disease) throughout the cerebral cortex as well as in the substantia nigra. Patients may present with typical idiopathic Parkinson's disease or with cognitive change alone. Hallucinations and a fluctuating mental state are characteristic clinical features. Lewy bodies have been more easily recognised in recent years because of the development of staining for ubiquitin, a degradation protein found within all inclusion bodies.

44. Diplopia **Answers: A C**

When assessing the cause of diplopia the first task is to determine which eye is involved. The cover test is the simplest method. Each eye is covered in turn while the patient is looking in the direction which causes most marked diplopia. When the paretic eye is covered, the most peripheral of the two images will disappear. The diplopia will be maximal in the direction of gaze produced by the paretic muscle. The main action of the superior oblique muscle is to depress the adducted eye. Adduction is not possible with a third nerve palsy and the eye is usually deviated down and out by the effect of the still intact muscles lateral rectus (sixth cranial nerve) and superior oblique (fourth cranial nerve). In a third nerve palsy, the action of the intact superior oblique can be seen by its secondary action of intorsion of the eye (watch a conjunctival blood vessel whilst the patient tries to look at the tip of his nose).

45. Pseudobulbar palsy **Answers: C E**

The gag reflex is usually present or pathologically brisk. Wasting of the tongue indicates lower motor neurone involvement and together with the upper motor neurone signs of pseudobulbar palsy suggests motor neurone disease (progressive bulbar palsy). Syringobulbia causes a 'true' bulbar palsy due to involvement of the IXth, Xth, and XIIth cranial nerve nuclei from below. Pseudobulbar palsy is due to bilateral lesions above the IXth, Xth, XIIth cranial nuclei and may be due to cerebrovascular disease, multiple sclerosis or motor neurone disease.

46. Lower limbs **Answers: A B C E**

In the lower limb the sciatic nerve supplies motor to the hamstrings and short head of biceps as well as forming the tibial and common peroneal nerves. Sensory supply is purely below the knee. The tibial nerve supplies gastrocnemius, popliteus, plantaris and soleus, tibialis posterior, flexor digitorum longus and flexor hallucis longus before becoming the medial and lateral plantar nerves (small muscles of the foot). The common peroneal nerve: superficial branch – peroneus longus and brevis; deep branch – tibialis anterior, extensor digitorum longus and brevis, extensor hallucis longus and peroneus.

47. Parkinson's disease **Answers: All false**

The onset of Parkinson's disease is usually between the ages of 55 and 70. Tremor is most pronounced at rest and rigidity is equally pronounced in limb flexion and extension. Broad-based gait disturbance and early urinary incontinence are features of normal pressure hydrocephalus.

48. Dystrophia myotonica **Answers: C D E**

Dystrophia myotonica is an autosomal dominant disorder. The abnormal gene is a trinucleotide repeat on chromosome 19. The clinical manifestations are more pronounced in succeeding generations (anticipation), particularly if the affected parent is female. Cataracts, gonadal atrophy, cardiomyopathy and dementia may occur.

49. Foramen magnum **Answers: D E**

The two vertebral arteries pass through the foramen magnum, only becoming the basilar artery on the pons lying superiorly. The hypoglossal nerves have their own canal (anterior condylar canal) lying just anterolaterally. The foramen magnum does, however, transmit all the cervical rootlets which ascend into the skull from upper cervical nerves, forming the spinal branch of the accessory nerve XI. All layers of the meninges, including contents of the extradural space, pass through the foramen.

50. Schneiderian 'first rank' symptoms — Answers: A B E

Schneider considered symptoms of 'first rank' to be pathognomonic of schizophrenia in the absence of brain disease. They include specific auditory hallucinations (voices repeating or anticipating thoughts out loud, referring to the subject in the third person or maintaining a running commentary on the subjects thoughts or behaviour), thought interference (thought insertion, withdrawal and broadcasting), delusional perception (a form of primary delusion) and passivity phenomenon (the subject's feelings, impulses, acts and sensations appear under alien control). Schneider's 'second rank' symptoms included perplexity, emotional blunting and other kinds of hallucination and delusion. Bleuler, who coined the term 'schizophrenia' felt that loosening of associations, characterised by Knight's move thinking, was central to this disorder.

51. Puerperal psychosis — Answer: E

Puerperal psychosis usually begins within the first one or two weeks, but rarely in the first two days. There are three main types of clinical picture: acute organic, affective (depressive or manic) and schizophrenic. The most common presentation is depressive. The onset is usually acute and the prognosis good. The risk of recurrence in subsequent pregnancies is between 1:3 and 1:7.

52. Suicide — Answers: A B C D

The most obvious warning sign of suicide is a direct statement of intent by the patient. There is no truth in the theory that people who talk about killing themselves actually do not do it. The presence of a feeling of hopelessness is a predictor of both immediate and subsequent suicide. Of the social factors, positive family history of suicide, prolonged physical illness and living alone indicate a higher risk. Paranoid delusions can occur in depressive illness, but do not have any special significance in assessing suicide risk.

53. Dementia — Answers: A C E

It is important to look for treatable causes of dementia. Treatable causes include B12, folic acid or thiamine deficiency, normal pressure hydrocephalus, Wilson's disease, cerebral syphilis and cerebral neoplasms.

54. Oxygen debt **Answers: A D E**

This indicates that the subject is capable of six times the exertion that would have been possible without it. Trained athletes are able to increase the oxygen consumption of their muscles to a greater degree than untrained individuals. Consequently, they are capable of greater exertion without increasing lactic acid production and hence contract smaller oxygen debts for a given amount of exertion. The production of lactic acid, which is inevitable with the anaerobic pathway in action, results in a lowering of the pH due to an accumulation of acid. Thus the use of the anaerobic pathway is self-limiting.

55. Sarcoidosis **Answers: A D E**

Sarcoidosis is a multisystem disorder of unknown aetiology characterised by accumulation of T cells, monocytes and non- caseating granulomas in involved tissues. Bronchopulmonary lavage usually reveals lymphocytic pleocytosis with a predominance of CD4 +ve T cells. In comparison to the BAL findings, the peripheral blood of patients with pulmonary sarcoidosis shows a T cell lymphopenia due to reduced CD4 +ve T cells. There is also generalised B cell hyperactivity with hypergammaglobulinaemia. The hypercalcaemia of sarcoidosis is secondary to elevated calcitriol secreted by activated pulmonary macrophages.

56. Respiratory function tests **Answer: B**

In chronic bronchitis the vital capacity and total lung capacity fall, but residual volume is increased because of chest overexpansion. In interstitial lung diseases such as cryptogenic fibrosing alveolitis, extrinsic allergic alveolitis (e.g. farmer's lung) and lymphangitis carcinomatosis the major features are significantly reduced lung volumes and impaired transfer factor. Flow volume loops can distinguish intra from extra-thoracic obstruction because large airway intrathoracic obstruction affects expiration more than inspiration. In neuromuscular disease, such as Guillain–Barré syndrome, arterial pO_2 is a poor predictor of subsequent respiratory failure – a falling PEFR is a much better predictor.

57. Antiphospholipid syndrome **Answers: A B C E**

Antiphospholipid and anticardiolipin antibodies are found in 5% of the general population and in association with several connective tissue vasculitides, infection and malignancy. Arterial and venous thrombosis and spontaneous abortion are classic features but skin disorders and CNS abnormalities are increasingly described. A 'catastrophic' variant leads to multiple organ failure with widespread thrombosis. The treatment of recurrent disease is high dose warfarin at an INR of 3–4.

58. Rheumatoid arthritis **Answers: A B**

The occipital artery may be involved as well as the temporal in temporal arteritis. The loss of the corneal reflex is due to compression of the spinal tract of the Vth cranial nerve which reaches to the level of the atlanto-axial joint of the neck. Nail-fold vasculitis is benign and self-limiting. Iron therapy is ineffective, and may make inflammation worse. Gold is given intramuscularly.

59. Inflammatory myopathies **Answers: A B D**

Polymyositis and dermatomyositis are very similar. Muscles are often painful although onset of weakness may be painless. Dermatomyositis is usually more acute and severe. It is associated with malignancy, the percentage with underlying malignancy being about the same as the patient's age (age 50, 50%, age 70, 70% etc.). Extraocular muscles are typically spared.

60. Clinical trial of a new drug **Answer: C**

The difference in the efficacies of the two treatments (improvement rates of 77% for the active drug and 57% for the placebo) is reasonably impressive numerically. However, a formal statistical test is needed to estimate the probability of the difference occurring by chance under the null hypothesis that the two treatments are equipotent (this probability is actually approximately 1%, so the difference is statistically significant). The appropriate test of significance for comparing frequencies/proportions is the chi-squared test; Pearson's coefficient is a measure of correlation. Student's t-test is used for continuous data. Sequential analysis requires the patients to be paired and for a direct comparison of each pair to be made as the study progresses.

PRACTICE PAPER 2: ANSWERS

1. ECG **Answers: A B C E**

The development of tall R waves in the anterior chest leads in posterior infarction can be considered the 'mirror image' of Q waves looked at from the other side of the heart. Tricuspid atresia is associated with a very small right ventricle producing little voltage. WPW syndrome type A is associated with a tall R wave in lead V1 but type B is not. Perhaps a majority of patients with acute pulmonary embolism show no ECG changes apart from sinus tachycardia and T-wave inversion over the right-sided precordial leads. $S_1Q_3T_3$ pattern, P pulmonale, right axis deviation and right bundle branch block occur, but a dominant R wave in V1 is not a feature of an acute load on the right side of the heart. This occurs, however, with right ventricular hypertrophy due to many causes.

2. Sick sinus syndrome **Answers: A E**

Sick sinus syndrome may be associated with both tachy- and bradyarrhythmias; a degree of AV block is common. Pacing is indicated in those with documented bradycardia associated with symptoms on ambulatory ECG monitoring. Pauses of 2 seconds are not uncommon in the normal population. Pacing does not improve life expectancy (unlike complete heart block). Sinus node disease occurs in up to 5% of cases of myocardial infarction and is associated with occlusion of the circumflex or right coronary arteries which supply the SA node in the majority of cases. A prolonged sinus node recovery time may give rise to periods of asystole after restoration of sinus rhythm in patients with atrial fibrillation.

3. Atrial septal defect **Answers: B C E**

In a patient with an atrial septal defect, right axis deviation suggests a secundum defect (the most common type) and left axis deviation suggests a primum defect (less common). Sinus venosus defects are the least common type of defect and are frequently associated with anomalous right pulmonary venous drainage. Sinus arrhythmia is only present in patients with small defects and a tricuspid flow murmur suggests a large shunt. Pulmonary hypertension is a late feature of atrial septal defects and symptoms may only develop in middle age.

4. Streptokinase **Answers: All false**

The use of streptokinase in the treatment of myocardial infarction is associated with a reduction in mortality of about 25%. Older patients derive a greater benefit than young patients. No thrombolytic agent has been shown to reduce mortality in unstable angina, treatment with heparin and aspirin is indicated. Streptokinase antibodies develop 3 days or more after treatment and last up to 4 years. Within a three day window streptokinase may be used without loss of efficacy. Patients presenting with left bundle branch block and pain should be treated with thrombolysis if myocardial infarction is suspected.

5. Pericarditis **Answers: A B D**

Pericarditis is a late finding in patients with severe renal impairment. In hypothyroidism, other cardiological abnormalities include low ECG voltage, bradycardia and ischaemic heart disease. Carditis, including pericarditis is one of the major diagnostic criteria of acute rheumatic fever. Subarachnoid haemorrhage may cause widespread ST segment changes in the ECG but this is due to pericarditis.

6. Sulphasalazine **Answers: A B E**

Sulphasalazine comprises sulphapryidine and 5-aminosalicylic acid. The former produces nausea, rashes, headaches, oxidative haemolysis and a reversible reduction in sperm count. The latter has been associated with diarrhoea and renal impairment.

7. Benzodiazepines **Answers: A B C D**

Benzodiazepines are anxiolytic, sedative, anticonvulsants and act as a muscle relaxant. They enhance GABA neurotransmission. Benzodiazepines are well tolerated and side-effects tend to be a result of overdosage which leads to ataxia, drowsiness and confused thinking especially in the elderly. They potentiate the effects of central nervous system depressants such as alcohol. Dosage should be reduced in patients with impaired renal and liver function.

8. Digoxin toxicity **Answers: A B D E**

The side-effects of digoxin are protean and often affect elderly patients who have reduced tolerance to the drug. Gastrointestinal symptoms are prominent with anorexia, vomiting, abdominal pain, diarrhoea and weight loss. Confusion, delirium and seizures may occur. Visual symptoms include alterations in colour vision and even blindness. A wide variety of ventricular and supraventricular rhythms may occur and can be difficult to treat.

9. Beta interferon in multiple sclerosis **Answers: B C D E**

Beta interferon may influence the activity of multiple sclerosis (MS) through several mechanisms including down regulation of abnormal CNS HLA class II antigen expression, enhanced activity of suppressor T cells and inhibition of gamma interferon. In relapsing MS, beta interferon reduces the clinical relapse rate by approximately 30%. Magnetic resonance scanning can document blood–brain barrier leakage in active disease and this has been shown to improve following beta interferon treatment. However, short term use (for less than 6 months) may exacerbate disease.

10. Omeprazole **Answers: A B C**

Gynaecomastia occurs rarely with omeprazole and is more commonly seen with H2-antagonist treatment. Severe headache is probably the commonest reason for discontinuing omeprazole therapy. Bradycardia, occasionally due to atrioventricular block, and pancreatitis have not yet been reported with omeprazole but both are recognised side-effects of H2-antagonist treatment.

11. Systemic disease **Answers: A C E**

Pityriasis rosea: scaly erythematous patches on trunk and proximal limbs, may be confused with secondary syphilis.

Pompholyx: vesicular rash on hands and feet associated with atopy and psoriasis.

Severe seborrhoic dermatitis is seen in some HIV positive patients, who may also have dry skin, worsening or new-onset psoriasis, diffuse alopecia and atypical or more severe signs of cutaneous infection.

Kerion: severe inflammatory pattern of scalp-ringworm infection. Alopecia areata is associated with other auto-immune conditions, most commonly vitiligo and thyroid disease.

12. Graves' disease **Answers: A B C E**

Some degree of asymmetry of exophthalmos is a relatively common finding, and occasionally, it may be unilateral, especially at the outset. Loss of vision (malignant exophthalmos) may be due to increasing pressure in the eye causing optic neuritis and atrophy or corneal ulceration and severe pain may be an associated feature. Although there is an increased incidence of high titre thyroid stimulating immunoglobulins (formerly known as LATS) in patients with severe ophthalmic Graves' disease, there is no evidence that these are responsible for the ocular complications.

13. Cranial diabetes insipidus **Answers: All true**

Diabetes insipidus normally follows destruction of the posterior lobe of the pituitary or part of the hypothalamus. This may occur with space occupying or granulomatous lesions. Severe head injury may cause transient or rarely permanent cranial diabetes insipidus, probably as a consequence of damage to the pituitary stalk.

14. *Helicobacter pylori* **Answer: B**

H. pylori is a Gram-negative organism that survives in the mucous layer of the gastric mucosa. It most often produces non-erosive antral gastritis and can be found in 90% of duodenal ulcer sufferers. The urease breath test is used to confirm the presence of the organism.

15. Ulcerative colitis **Answers: B D E**

Ulcerative colitis classically involves the colon and rectum causing mucosal ulceration which, if severe enough, has a pseudopolypoid appearance. It represents islands of remaining mucosa. Diarrhoea and rectal bleeding are classical presenting symptoms. Fistula formation is more typical of Crohn's disease and cobblestoning describes the X-ray appearance of the mucosa in that disease.

16. Total parenteral nutrition **Answers: A B**

Chronic cholestasis rarely progressing to liver failure is a recognised complication of TPN but the underlying pathophysiology is poorly understood. Hyperlipidaemia is also recognised and is easily correctable. Aspiration pneumonia is a complication of enteral nutritional support, and severe pancreatitis is an indication for TPN.

17. Tuberose sclerosis **Answers: A C D**

The classical lesions of tuberose sclerosis are adenoma sebaceum, red-brown papules in the butterfly distribution on the face, 'ash leaf' hypopigmented patches, and 'shagreen patches', usually over the lumbosacral area. However about 10% of patients have café-au-lait patches of pigmentation. Other CNS manifestations include epilepsy in association with cerebral malformations known as tubers and mental retardation. About 5% of children with tuberose sclerosis develop cerebral gliomas. Renal malformations may occur and cardiac rhabdomyomas are present in up to one-third of patients.

18. Down's syndrome — Answers: A B E

Primary hypothyroidism and the incidence of other autoimmune disorders is increased. Atlanto-axial instability occurs in 10–20%. Hypotonia is one of the most constant signs in Down's syndrome babies. Duodenal atresia is the commonest gastrointestinal malformation. Premature senility and degenerative brain changes similar to Alzheimer's disease occur in older patients.

19. *Pneumocystis carinii* pneumonia — Answers: A C D E

The LDH is invariably raised in pneumocystis pneumonia and the arterial gases abnormal with hypoxaemia after exercise. Cavities are rarely seen in pneumocystis unless the patient has been receiving pentamidine inhalation prophylaxis. The absence of clinical signs is completely compatible with bad pneumocystis and some patients presenting early have a normal chest X-ray. Pleural effusion should suggest another cause, such as *M. tuberculosis* or Kaposi's sarcoma.

20. Chronic myeloid leukaemia — Answers: All true

The chronic leukaemias are characterised by an increased number of mature white cells in the blood, the acute leukaemias by an increased number of primitive blast cells. Basophilia is characteristic of the myeloproliferative disorders. A low NAP score is found in CML, most cases of AML and PNH. High NAP is found in infections, pregnancy and polycythaemia rubra vera. Recent MRC trials have confirmed that interferon treatment prolongs the chronic phase by a mean of about two years. Priapism, splenic infarction and stroke may be a feature of the hyperleukocytosis sometimes found in CML at presentation.

21. Multiple myeloma — Answers: A D E

The blood count will reflect the effects of chemotherapy as well as the bone marrow failure associated with marrow infiltration. The serum immunoglobulin and paraprotein levels will reflect the myeloma cell mass (except in non-secretory myeloma). The urinary protein level will also reflect the myeloma cell mass in Bence–Jones positive cases.

22. Polycythaemia rubra vera — Answers: All true

The worsening pruritus is due to histamine release. Iron deficiency is almost invariable. Gout is due to high cellular turnover. Raised leucocyte alkaline phosphatase could be due to infection or thrombosis. Splenomegaly is the only physical finding of diagnostic significance.

23. Sézary syndrome **Answer: C D**

Sézary syndrome is part of a spectrum of T cell malignancies which often involve the skin in a diffuse erythrodermic reaction. The cells are large, cleaved, mononuclear cells distinct from the small spiky (or hairy) cells of hairy cell leukaemia. Immunological markers have shown these cells to be helper T cells in origin. The prognosis is poor, most patients die within a few years, often from a non-Hodgkin's lymphoma.

24. Levels of IgE **Answer: B C E**

Atopic disease, parasitic disease, Wiskott-Aldrich syndrome, di George syndrome, selective IgA deficiency, rheumatoid arthritis, cystic fibrosis and nephrotic syndrome all cause elevated levels of IgE.

25. Class II MHC molecules **Answer: B D**

Class I MHC molecules are present on virtually all cells. They are transmembrane peptides associated with β2-microglobulin and signal to cytotoxic T-cells. Class II are heterodimers present on B cells, macrophages and some endothelial cells. They signal to T helper cells. The MHC is on chromosome 6 in humans and chromosome 2 in mice. Haplotypes are sets of allelic variants. An example would be HLA-A1,B8,DR3.

26. Hypogammaglobulinaemia **Answers: A B D E**

A number of drugs are implicated including phenytoin, gold (aurothiomalate), penicillamine and cytotoxics. Cyclosporin's action, however, is mainly on T-cells. Other causes are severe malnutrition, protein loss (enteropathy, burns, nephrotic syndrome), and lymphoproliferative disorders (myeloma, CLL). It may be hereditary.

27. Respiratory symptoms **Answers: A B C D**

All helminths that migrate through the lungs can cause transient pulmonary symptoms. Tropical pulmonary eosinophilia is generally caused by filarial species. *Paragonimus westermani* is a lung fluke causing cavitating lesions that may be mistaken for tuberculosis. *Ancylostoma braziliensis* is a dog hookworm that causes cutaneous larva migrans in man.

28. Rabies virus **Answers: A D E**

Animal bites in rabies endemic countries should be treated by thorough washing followed by rabies specific immunoglobulin and vaccination. No immune response is detectable in man and symptomatic infection is invariably fatal. The diagnosis can be confirmed by detecting rabies antigen in the dermal nerves of a full thickness skin punch biopsy taken from the hairy part of the neck.

29. Vancomycin resistant enterococci **Answers: B C**

Vancomycin-resistant enterococci (VRE) make a set of enzymes that modify the peptidoglycan binding site that vancomycin normally binds to blocking cell wall synthesis, thereby inhibiting its binding and action. They do not rapidly metabolise vancomycin. Risk factors for VRE include length of hospital stay, immunosuppression, severity of illness, treatment with multiple antibiotics and renal failure. The organisms are spread by the faecal–oral route and frequently colonise patients without causing disease. They are, however, also highly resistant to penicillin and to aminoglycosides.

30. Pneumococci **Answers: A C D**

Pneumococci are a major cause of pneumonia, empyema, otitis media, septicaemia and meningitis. The mucosal epithelium of the nasopharynx is the primary site of colonisation and subsequently pneumococci gain access to the lung by aspiration where they adhere to type II pneumocytes. The capsular polysaccharide protects pneumococci from phagocytosis and is the basis of serotyping, cell wall components induce the production of cytokines, including TNF, and initiate the inflammatory response by enhancing leucocyte recruitment. Resolution of pneumococcal infection begins when anticapsular antibodies opsonise the pneumococci and facilitate phagocytosis by polymorphonuclear cells.

31. Syndrome of inappropriate antidiuretic hormone **Answers: A D E**

SIADH can be caused by a number of pathologies, including pituitary/intracranial disease, pulmonary lesions, Guillain–Barré syndrome and acute intermittent porphyria. Lithium is a cause of nephrogenic diabetes insipidus not SIADH. The urine osmolality is inappropriately high in relation to serum (which is usually less than 270 mosmol/l) and typically is in the range of 350–400 mosmol/l. Oedema does not occur because aldosterone secretion is suppressed, which in turn causes increased urinary sodium excretion. Demeclocycline is effective for chronic SIADH and acts by blocking the renal tubular effect of ADH.

32. Hypophosphataemic rickets Answers: B C D

Hypophosphatemic rickets is characterised by an X-linked dominant inheritance and affects both males and females. Whereas an excessive tubular loss of phosphate is considered to be the fundamental cause of the condition, it is possible that there is an increased gastro-intestinal loss. Treatment is based on giving large doses of vitamin D together with phosphate supplements, but even with treatment from an early age, it is not thought that normal stature will be obtained. Some cases present in adult life. Calcification of interspinous ligaments occurs, sometimes confused with ankylosing spondylitis or hyperostosis

33. Acute intermittent porphyria Answers: A B

Despite the fact that it is an autosomal dominant condition, more women than men are affected in AIP, probably as a result of the effect of oestrogens. Increased urinary porphobilinogen is characteristic as a result of reduced activity of the enzyme porphobilinogen deaminase. Photosensitive metabolites are not produced in this condition. Characteristic clinical features include peripheral neuropathy, tachycardia, hypertension, abdominal pain. Mononeuropathies are not characteristic although a radial nerve palsy may be seen in the related condition of lead poisoning (some similar clinical and biochemical features). Acute attacks of AIP may be characterised by hyponatraemia due to inappropriate ADH secretion.

34. Idiopathic infantile hypercalcaemia Answers: C D E

Hypercalcaemia in idiopathic infantile hypercalcaemia (IH) is caused by increased gastrointestinal calcium absorption. Urinary calcium excretion in IH is usually increased and can lead to nephrocalcinosis. The hypercalcaemia is treated with a calcium and vitamin D deficient diet, until it resolves, unusually in the first few years of life. Patients with William's syndrome have 'elfin-like' facial features, mental retardation and aortic stenosis. Not all the patients with William's syndrome are hypercalcaemic. The reason for elevated plasma cholesterol concentrations in some infants with IH/William's syndrome is not known.

35. Constitutive nitric oxide synthase **Answer: A**

Constitutive nitric oxide synthase is present in endothelial cells and requires a rise in cytosolic free calcium for activation. Stimulation of the constitutive nitric oxide synthase generates nitric oxide of picomolar concentrations, while the amount of nitric oxide produced by the inducible enzyme, after exposure to endotoxin and cytokines is much greater. The inducible nitric oxide synthase is calcium independent. Inhibition of constitutive nitric oxide synthase causes a rise in blood pressure demonstrating that basal nitric oxide production by endothelial cells is physiologically important in blood flow regulation. Nitric oxide is produced from arginine not citrulline.

36. *p53* **Answers: A C E**

p53 is a tumour suppressor gene present on chromosome 17. It is not a viral protein. It encodes a nuclear phosphoprotein that acts as a transcription factor; it delays entry into S phase of the cell division cycle thus allowing time for DNA repair to occur before cell replication. Mutation of *p53* promotes tumour formation. Somatic mutation of the *p53* gene occurs at both alleles in 50–80% of spontaneous human cancers. *p53* is not required for normal development, but is a necessary cofactor for programmed cell death (apoptosis).

37. Hypokalaemia **Answers: A B D**

All the factors listed cause hypokalaemia and total body potassium depletion which may be profound and symptomatic. The important differential diagnosis is from Conn's syndrome, in which primary adrenal overproduction of aldosterone increases sodium–potassium exchange in the distal tubule, causing sodium retention (leading to hypertension) and excessive urinary potassium losses. In primary hyperaldosteronism, plasma renin activity is suppressed by sodium and water overload, as is also the case with carbenoxolone, a steroidal compound with similar sodium-retaining and potassium-losing effects. The membrane bound enzyme 11-betahydroxysteroid dehydrogenase metabolises cortisol but not aldosterone and hence normally protects the mineralocorticoid receptor from stimulation by cortisol. Deficiency of this enzyme activity causes the syndrome of apparent mineralocorticoid excess. Although hypokalaemia occurs in this syndrome the renin-angiotensin-aldosterone system is suppressed. In conditions such as excess vomiting, diuretic or laxative abuse, sodium and water losses and the resulting intravascular volume depletion stimulate plasma renin activity.

38. Rapidly progressive glomerulonephritis **Answers: A C D E**

There is an increased incidence of prior exposure to volatile hydrocarbons in patients developing rapidly progressive glomerulonephritis. More than half of the patients have systemic vasculitis with or without anti-neutrophil cytoplasmic antibody (ANCA), and the remainder have anti-glomerular basement membrane disease, or other systemic disease such as cryoglobulinaemia, SLE or malignancy. Goodpasture's syndrome is more common in smokers. An acute nephritic onset is usual. Response to treatment is variable but less likely in anuric patients and those with anti-glomerular basement membrane disease.

39. Chronic renal disease **Answers: C E**

It can sometimes be difficult to distinguish acute renal failure and an acute presentation of end-stage renal disease, although a full history often provides the necessary clues. Other evidence of longstanding renal failure includes the presence of renal osteodystrophy, neuropathy, anaemia and small kidneys. Pericarditis may occur in both acute and chronic renal failure.

40. Low plasma sodium **Answers: A B C E**

ADH released by blood volume contraction contributes to the hyponatraemia of salt depletion and hyperglycaemia. Also, in dehydration, increased proximal tubular reabsorption limits the volume of fluid reaching the diluting segment of the distal tubule and hence water excretion. Oat cell lung cancers may secrete ADH. In hyperglycaemia, osmotically active solute in the blood also contributes to hyponatraemia. ADH is also released inappropriately in cirrhosis of the liver where hypoproteinaemia will also contribute to the redistribution of salt and water as interstitial oedema. In hyperlipidaemia, hyponatraemia is more apparent than real, due to plasma water being replaced by sodium-free lipid.

41. Alzheimer's disease **Answers: All false**

Alzheimer's disease is the most common cause of dementia and the majority (90%) of cases occur sporadically. Amnesia and spatial dysfunction are typical early clinical features and social graces are usually maintained until late in the disease. The underlying pathology predominantly affects the temporal and parietal cortices. Extrapyramidal rigidity, long tract signs and myoclonus are all late clinical manifestations. The EEG is typically abnormal.

42. Internuclear ophthalmoplegia **Answers: A B D**

INO is caused by a lesion in the medial longitudinal bundle, which prevents messages from the pontine centre for lateral gaze reaching the contralateral medial rectus part of the IIIrd nerve nucleus. Messages reach the ipsilateral VIth nerve nucleus normally. Hence, with a lesion of the left medial longitudinal bundle, causing a left INO, there will, on right lateral gaze, be normal abduction of the right eye but slow or restricted adduction of the left eye. Ataxic nystagmus, greatest in the abducting eye is often an associated feature. Bilateral INO is typical but not diagnostic of MS and may be detected in myasthenia gravis. Retraction nystagmus is a sign of a lesion in the dorsal midbrain.

43. Nerve supply **Answers: B C**

The median nerve supplies the first and second lumbricals. The ulnar nerve (C7, 8, T1) supplies the majority of the intrinsic muscles of the hand including the dorsal interossei, adductor pollicis and the third and fourth lumbricals.

44. Carpal tunnel syndrome **Answers: A E**

The pain of median nerve compression can radiate to the forearm and may even present as a painful shoulder. Fasciculation is not a feature especially not of the small muscles of the hand as they are innervated by the ulnar nerve. Exacerbation by raising CSF pressure on coughing suggests nerve root compression in the neck. An underlying condition is rarely present in practice: most cases occurring in middle-aged people are a combination of hardening of the flexor retinaculum plus a congenitally small tunnel.

45. Myasthenia gravis **Answers: A E**

Myasthenia gravis causes fatiguable weakness of ocular, facial, bulbar and proximal limb musculature. Dysarthria and dysphagia are due to bulbar involvement whereas dysphasia is indicative of a cerebral cortical lesion. Tendon reflexes are typically preserved.

46. In the leg **Answers: A B E**

In the arm, spasticity in a patient with hemiplegia is most pronounced in the flexor muscles and weakness in the extensor muscles. The converse is true in the leg. The peroneal nerve supplies skin over the lateral aspect of the lower leg. The saphenous branch of the femoral nerve supplies skin over the medial aspect of the lower leg. A sciatic nerve palsy causes weakness of hip extension, knee flexion and foot dorsiflexion, plantar flexion, inversion and eversion. A femoral nerve palsy causes weakness of knee extensions.

47. Progressive supranuclear palsy **Answers: C D**

Progressive supranuclear palsy presents with postural instability and falls, a levodopa-unresponsive Parkinsonian-like syndrome, vertical supranuclear palsy, dysarthria, dysphagia and frontal lobe abnormalities. It is not linked with apolipoprotein E (unlike Alzheimer's disease) or a mitochondrial DNA lesion. It is characterised by abundant neurofibrillar tangles in the basal ganglia and brain stem.

48. Radial nerve lesion **Answers: B C**

Brachialis is supplied by the musculocutaneous nerve (C5,6). The radial nerve (C5,6,7,8) supplies brachioradialis. Abductor pollicis brevis and first lumbrical are supplied by median nerve (C6,7,8, 1). Sensory loss due to a radial nerve lesion affects skin over the lateral aspect of the dorsal hand surface.

49. Eaton–Lambert syndrome **Answers: A B**

Eaton–Lambert myasthenic syndrome is an autoimmune paraneoplastic phenomenon secondary to antibodies against voltage-gated calcium channels (VGCC) expressed by the tumour (typically small cell lung cancer) that react with VGCC at the presynaptic level of neuromuscular cholinergic synapses. The syndrome usually responds to treatment of the underlying malignancy. It does not cause ventricular arrthymias or cerebellar degeneration.

50. Scleritis **Answers: A C E**

Scleritis in rheumatoid disease can lead to thinning of the cornea and subsequent perforation, so called scleromalacia perforans. Conjunctivitis may occur in lupus but scleritis is not seen. Scleritis is a typical feature of Wegener's granulomatosis. Iritis is prominent in ankylosing spondylitis and scleritis does not occur.

51. Schizophrenia **Answers: B D**

The patient with early onset schizophrenia usually suffers more chronic personality deterioration. The presence of affective change, depression or mania seems to indicate preservation of personality and better prognosis. There is no evidence that any individual symptom such as visual, rather than auditory, hallucinations, influences prognosis. Echolalia is usually a symptom of organic brain damage.

52. Obsessive-compulsive neurosis **Answers: A C E**

The key feature of an obsessional symptom is that the patient feels compelled to think or act in a certain way (compulsion) he recognises as absurd and attempts to resist (resistance). Ruminations are repetitive internal arguments about simple actions. Rituals are repeated irrational patterns of behaviour. There is probably a hereditary component in the aetiology of the condition but this is probably very small. The superficial similarity of obsessional symptoms and some of the features of schizophrenia is deceptive: there is no association between these two conditions.

53. Deliberate self-harm **Answers: A B E**

The most typical pattern of deliberate self harm is an impulsive drug overdose taken with mixed motives in a state of mental turmoil often by a young single girl after a quarrel or rejection. Important associations include recent life events, marital conflict, unemployment (in men), recent alcohol consumption (especially in men), personality disorder and epilepsy. In the year following an overdose, risk of suicide is 1–2% (100 times that of the general population).

54. Korsakov's syndrome **Answer: A**

Korsakov's syndrome is characterised by relatively circumscribed memory deficit where new information is registered but quickly forgotten. This results in disorientation in time. Patients usually have little awareness of their problem and make up stories (confabulate) to cover gaps in their memory. Associations include irritability, peripheral neuropathy and the Wernicke syndrome (ataxia, ophthalmoplegia and impaired consciousness). Common aetiologies are thiamine deficiency (due to alcohol abuse or gastrointestinal disease) and lesions of the mammillary bodies and medial thalamus. Echopraxia (automatic imitation of another's movements) is a symptom of catatonia.

55. Extrinsic allergic alveolitis **Answer: A**

Precipitating antibodies may give support to the diagnosis but can occur in the absence of disease. Symptoms occur in a few hours after exposure and the onset is over seeks or months. Rheumatoid factor is not a feature of extrinsic allergic alveolitis.

56. Calcified extra cardiac lesions **Answers: A C D E**

Asbestosis can cause calcified pleural plaques. Chickenpox causes fine nodular calcification. Silicosis causes 'eggshell' calcification in lymph nodes. Collections of haemosiderin containing macrophages can enlarge and calcify in the lung fields in mitral stenosis. The infiltrates in farmers' lung do not calcify.

57. Community acquired pneumonia **Answers: A C D**

Mycoplasma occurs in 3 to 4 yearly cycles. Adverse prognostic indicators include an admission serum urea greater than 7 mmol/l, diastolic blood pressure of less than 60 mmHg and increasing age. Hypoxia is quite common in acute pneumonia but usually with a normal carbon dioxide (type I respiratory failure).

58. Systemic lupus erythematosus **Answers: C D**

Autoantibodies can cause a haemolytic anaemia, neutropenia, lymphopenia, or thrombocytopenia; the bone marrow is usually hypercellular but may be aplastic as a consequence of treatment. The CRP is usually normal and if raised may suggest sepsis. Other investigations show raised levels of immunoglobulins and a reduced complement. Antiphospholipid/anticardiolipin antibodies are found in some cases of SLE and are prothrombotic.

59. Scleroderma **Answers: A B D E**

The vascular fibrogenic response that characterises scleroderma is mediated by transforming growth factor-beta (TGF-b) in conjunction with platelet derived growth factor and basic fibroblast growth factor. Scleroderma renal crisis is frequent in patients with anti-RNA polymerase antibodies (24%) in contrast to those with anti-topoisomerase 1 antibodies (10%). Females are affected three times more frequently than males. The hypertension of scleroderma is mediated by activation of the renin-angiotensin system and should be treated by ACE inhibition. Diuretics which activate the renin-angiotensin system should be avoided as they can precipitate renal crisis.

60. Study **Answer: C**

r is simply the correlation coefficient and there is a positive association between the two variables. A statistically significant correlation does not necessarily imply a causal relationship. The small value of p implies that the mathematical relationship present has been established as statistically significant, so more than sufficient infants were studied.

PRACTICE PAPER 3: ANSWERS

1. Complete heart block **Answers: A B**

Complete and lesser degrees of A-V block are more common with inferior myocardial infarcts and characteristically resolve. This is probably related to the fact that the A-V node and bundle of His are supplied by the right coronary artery in about 90% of cases. When complete heart block occurs with anterior infarcts it usually indicates massive necrosis; hence the poor prognosis, which is mainly related to the poor left ventricular function and severe coronary disease. However, if residual complete or incomplete atrio-ventricular block or peripheral blocks persist, consideration should be given to a permanent pacemaker. An echo usually elucidates the cause of mitral reflux and is useful to distinguish it from an acute VSD in infarction. Chronic complete heart block is often due to conduction tissue fibrosis, either idiopathic sclerosis (Lenegre's disease) or fibrocalcific degeneration (Lev's disease), without clinically important ischaemic disease.

2. Mitral regurgitation **Answer: A**

The murmur of mitral regurgitation (MR) is pansystolic and extends to and fractionally beyond the second sound. Surgery is indicated in patients who are symptomatic or in those where the left ventricular function is impaired as a consequence of severe MR. Mitral leaflet prolapse (MLP) occurs in about 3% of the population and may be associated with severe MR. By the age of 75, 5.5% of men with MLP will require mitral valve repair or replacement. Vasodilators are useful in MR and are not contraindicated by pulmonary hypertension. Balloon valvuloplasty is used in the treatment of mitral stenosis.

3. Infective endocarditis **Answers: A E**

Infective endocarditis may result in an immune-complex nephritis. Combined benzylpenicillin and gentamicin is the treatment of choice in *Streptococcus faecalis* endocarditis. Invasive procedures such as sigmoidoscopy and cytoscopy result in bacteraemia and increase the risk of endocarditis in susceptible subjects. Atrial septal defect does not predispose to infective endocarditis. Echocardiography cannot be used to rule out endocarditis.

4. Hypertrophic cardiomyopathy **Answers: B C D**

55% of cases of hypertrophic cardiomyopathy are familial. Presentation with syncope in childhood or adolescence or a family history of sudden death indicates a poor prognosis. Non-sustained VT on Holter monitoring is associated with a 7-fold increase in mortality. Treatment with beta blockade, verapamil and dual chamber pacing may help with symptoms.

5. Vincristine therapy **Answers: B C E**

Vincristine can cause neuropathy, joint pain, alopecia, paralytic ileus and inappropriate ADH secretion. Pulmonary fibrosis is seen with busulphan and bleomycin and skin pigmentation also occurs with busulphan. Vincristine (Oncovin) is part of the MOPP regime for Hodgkin's disease and is used in acute lymphoblastic leukaemia and other lymphomas.

6. Paracetamol poisoning **Answers: A B D**

The major pathway of paracetamol metabolism is saturable. Glutathione helps to inactivate the toxic intermediate metabolite but cells are damaged as supplies become exhausted. Plasma paracetamol concentrations above a critical threshold 4–12 hours after ingestion indicate risks of liver cell damage. The first direct evidence of damage is a slow decay of paracetamol concentration or prolongation of the prothrombin time. Acetylcysteine at adequate concentration reactivates oxidised glutathione but once hepatic coma is established response to any therapy is poor.

7. Warfarin **Answers: A D E**

The main interactions with warfarin are due either to hepatic enzyme inhibition e.g. cimetidine, cotrimoxazole, or to enzyme induction e.g. anticoagulants, rifampicin, phenytoin. Non-steroidal anti-inflammatory drugs may predispose to gastric erosion and ulceration, with consequent risk of G.I. bleeding.

8. Side-effects of NSAIDs **Answers: A D E**

Nephrotic syndrome with or without interstitial nephritis is a rare side effect of NSAIDs - particularly propionic acid derivatives. NSAIDs inhibit prostaglandin-mediated renin release resulting in hypoaldosteronism and consequent hyperkalaemia. NSAID-induced ulcers are not related to *H. pylori* infection, serological markers and biopsy evidence of gastric colonisation are no greater than in normal controls. NSAIDs antagonise the effects of arginine vasopressin which can result in either hyponatraemia or fluid retention which can precipitate heart failure.

9. Tricyclic antidepressants **Answer: C**

Tricyclic antidepressants take at least ten days to have their effect. They have no interaction with food as do the monoamineoxidase inhibitors, and do not induce sensitivity to sunlight as do the phenothiazines. They have no direct effect on weight, except that as the depression resolves, the appetite should improve. Initial side-effects include dry mouth, but this usually clears up after a few days. Patients should be given this information so that they are encouraged to persist with treatment.

10. Ototoxic drugs Answers: A B D E

Aminoglycosides have long been known to be ototoxic, with some affecting the cochlear system (amikacin, neomycin, kanamycin), while others affect the vestibular system (streptomycin, gentamicin and tobramycin). The mechanism of toxicity is still unclear, and therapeutic drug monitoring is important in preventing toxicity. Minocycline affects the vestibular system and can cause severe vertigo; the incidence has been quoted to be between 30% and 76%. Vancomycin affects the cochlear system rather than the vestibular system. Loop diuretics such as frusemide and ethacrynic acid can lead to deafness especially when administered by rapid intravenous infusion (vestibular damage is rare). Salicylate ototoxicity is generally dose-dependent and is reversible provided the drug is withdrawn.

11. Skin and gut lesions Answer: D

Fabry disease: x-rec. Angiokeratomas initially umbilicus, buttocks, genital area, then generalised. Lack of a-galactosidase leads to accumulation of glycolipids in cells. Mainly cardiac, CNS and renal problems.

Albright's hereditary osteodystrophy: Pseudohypoparathyroidism, cutaneous osteomas, short stature, bradydactyly.

Refsum's disease: rare ichthyosis associated with lipid abnormalities and neurological problems. Loss of vision from retinitis pigmentosa, cardiac arrhythmias, bilateral sensorineural deafness, cerebellar ataxia and peripheral polyneuropathy.

Peutz-Jeghers syndrome: aut. dom., multiple freckles lips, buccal mucosa, sometimes periorbital, acral as well as conjunctival. Hamartomatous polyps anywhere in the GI tract. Risk of GI carcinoma and also pancreatic carcinoma, genital and mammary tumours.

Tungiasis: impregnated *Tunga penetrans* (Sand flea) burrows into feet of large mammals to produce eggs.

12. Hyperprolactinaemia Answers: B C E

The predominant influence on prolactin secretion is an inhibitory one through dopamine secretion by the hypothalamus and transport of this through the pituitary portal vessels. Clozapine is a modern antipsychotic which like all centrally acting antidopaminergic agents may inhibit the action of dopamine. Growth hormone secreting tumours may also secrete prolactin or cause hyperprolactinaemia through pituitary stalk disruption. True seizures may be distinguished from pseudoseizures by the elevation of prolactin which occurs in the former. Hypothyroidism (but not thyrotoxicosis) may lead to elevated serum prolactin as a consequence of reflex increase in thyrotrophin releasing hormone which has a weak prolactin stimulating effect.

13. Gluten sensitivity **Answers: A C D**

Howell-Jolly bodies represent blood cells which are usually removed in the spleen and their appearance in the blood film is in keeping with splenic atrophy. Oral aphthous ulceration and osteoporosis are recognised although atypical presenting features of gluten sensitivity. Focal biliary cirrhosis is the pathognomic liver lesion in cystic fibrosis.

14. Pseudomembranous colitis **Answer: D**

The presence of the bacteria is not sufficient to produce the effects; there must be *Cl. difficile* toxin. Rectal biopsy is often helpful although the condition can be right-sided. Toxic dilatation is an important complication. Treatment is with oral vancomycin or oral metronidazole. The recurrence rate is high.

15. Primary sclerosing cholangitis **Answers: A D**

Primary sclerosing cholangitis is a chronic progressive cholestatic liver disease characterised by continuing inflammation, necrosis and obliteration of intrahepatic and extrahepatic ducts. Approximately 75% of patients have inflammatory bowel disease (87% ulcerative colitis; 13% Crohn's disease) and two-thirds are male. It is associated with perinuclear antineutrophil cytoplasmic antibodies in a minority of cases. Ursodeoxycholic acid significantly improves the results of biochemical tests but does not improve symptoms, histological findings or prognosis. The disease usually progresses and results in cirrhosis, portal hypertension, and liver failure, ultimately necessitating liver transplantation. Sclerosing cholangitis does not recur post-transplant.

16. Gastric secretion **Answers: A C E**

Gastric secretion is stimulated by the vagus nerve, gastrin and histamine (therefore reduced by H2 blockade); it is inhibited by sympathetic nervous activation, low gastric pH and small intestine inhibitory peptides (cholecystokinine-pancreazimin, GIP). Approximately 3 litres of gastric secretions are produced per day with a concentration profile of approximately hydrogen 100 mmol/l, sodium 50 mmol/l potassium 15 mmol/l, chloride 140 mmol/l and bicarbonate 15 mmol/l.

17. Neurofibromatosis **Answers: A C D E**

Neurofibromatosis is the commonest autosomal dominantly inherited neurocutaneous disorder. The hallmark of the disease is a combination of multiple pigmented 'café-au-lait' spots, cutaneous neurofibromas and plexiform neuromas. There is a tendency to develop schwannomas and neurofibromas on peripheral and cranial nerves. There may be bilateral acoustic neuromas and a tendency to develop cerebral astrocytomas, particularly optic gliomas. In children cerebrovascular occlusive disease including carotid occlusion may occur and hydrocephalus due to aqueduct stenosis is frequent. More than five 'café-au-lait' spots measuring 1.5 cm or more are suggestive of the diagnosis and axillary freckling is a characteristic feature. Further complications include phaeochromocytoma, Wilms' tumour and non-lymphocytic leukaemia.

18. Treatment of HIV and opportunistic infection **Answers: B C D**

AZT, DDI D4T, ddc and 3TC (lamivudine) are nucleoside reverse-transcriptase inhibitors. Saquinavir, ritonavir and indinavir are proteinase inhibitors. Ganciclovir competitively blocks the incorporation of deoxyguanosine triphosphate, acting as a chain terminator. Side-effects of ganciclovir include azoospermia, granulocytopenia, thrombocytopenia, anaemia and a raised serum creatinine. Toxoplasmosis should be treated with sulphdiazine and pyrimethamine, clindamycin being reserved for patients who react to sulphonamides. There is no suitable prophylaxis or treatment for cryptosporidia.

19. Chronic granulocytic leukaemia **Answers: B C E**

Approximately 5% of cases lack the characteristic Philadelphia chromosome: many of these cases do have the associated bor:abl hybrid gene if investigated by PCR. Most cases transform into a blast crisis though a few do become myelofibrotic. Patients under the age of 45 should receive transplants if they have an HLA matched suitable sibling donor. If aged under 25 then a matched unrelated donor should be sought from the national panels such as the Anthony Nolan.

20. Idiopathic thrombocytopenic purpura **Answer: D**

Most cases resolve spontaneously in childhood, and the patients usually do not have splenomegaly. Even though the mother may be clinically 'cured' by splenectomy, circulating antibodies may still be present and can affect the baby at the time of delivery. In ITP, megakaryocytes are normal or increased in the marrow.

21. Cold autoimmune haemolytic anaemia **Answers: A C D**
Cold autoimmune haemolytic anaemia is a disorder of the elderly. Secondary cases occasionally occur in association with non-Hodgkin's lymphoma, Mycoplasma pneumoniae or infectious mononucleosis. The red cells become coated with IgM antibodies to the I-antigen in the patient's cold extremities. As the blood warms, complement is activated and intravascular haemolysis occurs. Cryoglobulins are immunoglobulins which form precipitates in the cold – they are distinct from cold agglutinins.

22. Anaphylaxis **Answers: A B D E**

23. Immunodeficiency **Answers: A B D**
CLL and nephrosis mainly affect humoral immunity. In sarcoid and di George's syndrome the defect lies in cell mediated immunity.

24. HLA B_{27} antigen **Answers: B C D**
The B_{27} antigen is associated with various members of the seronegative arthropathy group and uveitis. Its strongest association is with reactive arthritis.

25. Cryptococcal meningitis **Answers: B D E**
Cryptococcus neoformans is a fungus found throughout the world. Meningitis is typically of insidious onset with headache, neck stiffness, fever, nausea and vomiting. Only 5% of patients have negative CSF cryptococcal antigen tests. Standard treatment is with intravenous amphotericin B and oral flucytosine. Relapses occur in 10-20% of patients.

26. Neutrophil leucocytosis **Answer: B**
A neutrophil leucocytosis is in general suggestive of bacterial, rickettsial and spirochaetal infections. In dengue (flavivirus), brucellosis and typhoid fever the neutrophil count is usually normal or low.

27. Fever and pulmonary infiltrate **Answers: All true**
Other atypicals include *Mycoplasma, Mycobacterium*, cytomegalovirus, aspergillosis and pneumocystis.

28. *Legionella pneumophila* **Answers: C D**

Although the natural habitat of *L. pneumophila* is water, moist soil and mud it has not been isolated from sea-water as it is inhibited by sodium chloride; it grows well in warm water but only slowly multiplies where temperatures are below 20ºC. Confirmation of the diagnosis in Legionnaire's disease is usually serological, but the organism can be cultured on selective charcoal yeast extract (CYE) media and also after inoculation into guinea pigs. Infection is environmental/nosocomial rather than transmitted from infected patients. Pontiac fever describes a short febrile illness unaccompanied by physical signs or pneumonia and caused by *L. pneumophila*.

29. Phosphate metabolism **Answers: B C D E**

Dietary phosphate is absorbed (both active and passive) throughout the small bowel, mostly from the jejunum. The kidney responds immediately to changes in serum phosphate levels and normally over 90% of the filtered load is reabsorbed from the proximal tubules. Chronic renal failure is the most common cause of hyperphosphataemia; raised levels are also found in hypoparathyroidism, hyperthyroidism, acromegaly, tumoral calcinosis and with bisphosphonate therapy. An increased phosphate load may be a feature of vitamin D toxicity, cytotoxic therapy and rhabdomyolysis. Renal phosphate wasting is seen in Fanconi's syndrome and ketoacidosis; other causes of hypophosphataemia include alcoholism and the administration of glucose and insulin. High levels of phosphate lead to hypocalcaemia and tetany; very low levels result in 2,3 DPG and tissue ATP deficiency and associated haemolytic anaemia and muscle weakness.

30. Osteopenia **Answers: A B C D**

Osteopenia is defined as reduced bone mineral content. Factors which increase the risk of osteopenia and which may increase the risk of fracture include low weight, oestrogen deficiency (and testosterone deficiency in men), smoking, thyrotoxicosis, primary hyperparathyroidism, cortico-steroid treatment and Cushing's syndrome, chronic liver disease, alcohol excess, immobility and transplant recipients. Reflex sympathetic dystrophy (Sudeck's atrophy or algodystrophy) is characterised by osteopenia, sweating and pain, usually following fracture.

31. Hypothermia **Answer: D**

This is generally defined as a core (rectal) temperature less than 35°C. Inability to shiver is one of the causative mechanisms. ECG changes include sinus bradycardia, atrial fibrillation and ventricular fibrillation (particularly below 28°C). The J wave is seen in hypothermic patients as a small positive wave after the R wave; the delta wave is a feature of Wolff-Parkinson-White syndrome. Alcoholism is a common precipitant (remember pancreatitis), as are myocardial infarction, stroke and debilitating infection in the elderly. Hypothyroidism is a rare though important cause. Metabolic acidosis, due in part to tissue hypoxia, is a characteristic finding.

32. Tumour necrosis factor **Answers: A D**

Tumour necrosis factor is a proinflammatory cytokine released primarily from macrophages in response to bacterial toxins, inflammatory products and other invasive stimuli. It is present in the circulation in free form and complexed to binding proteins derived from cleavage fragments of TNF receptors. The cellular effects of TNF include cytotoxicity against tumour cells, suppression of adipocyte lipoprotein lipase and reduction of myocyte resting membrane potential. Acute exposure to high doses of TNF causes shock, fever, vascular leak syndrome and widespread tissue injury. At low doses chronic exposure leads to cachexia and protein catabolism but tachyphylaxis to TNF actions occur.

33. Acute inflammation **Answers: A B C**

Diapedesis is the passive movement of red cells out of vessels, complement activation will result in production of chemotactic factors which can induce a directional movement of inflammatory cells. Both occur in acute inflammation, but do not contribute to the fluid exudate.

34. Impairment of renal function **Answers: A D E**

ACE inhibitors, such as captopril, may cause renal failure. The risk is increased in the presence of renal artery stenosis, peripheral vascular disease and cardiac failure. Renal function must be regularly monitored. Gentamicin is a well-recognised cause of renal failure. The risk is reduced by once daily dosing. NSAIDs are among the most common drugs to impair renal function, especially in elderly patients.

35. Renal vasculitis **Answer: D**

Renal vasculitis usually involves small vessel inflammation as in microvascular polyarteritis. Wegener's and SLE; infarction is uncommon. A crescentic GN is the most common lesion, and urinary red cells and casts may point to the diagnosis. Systemic ill health with pyrexia, weight loss, myalgia and arthralgia often precede the renal presentation; eosinophilia occurs in polyarteritis nodosa and Churg-Strauss syndrome and is therefore uncommon. With prompt diagnosis and immunosuppressive therapy progression of the disease can be prevented in the majority of cases.

36. von Hippel–Lindau disease **Answers: A C D**

Von Hippel–Lindau (VHL) disease is an autosomal dominant disorder characterised by CNS haemangioblastoma formation, phaeochromocytoma, renal tumours and pancreatic tumours and cysts. The VHL gene is on the short arm of chromosome 3 and normally functions as a tumour suppressor gene. In VHL disease the gene is mutated or deleted. Retinoblastomas are due to the loss of a different tumour suppressor gene on chromosome 13.

37. Acute renal failure **Answers: A B D**

Haemodialysis is more haemodynamically stressful to patients than PD and should be avoided, generally, when the circulatory state is at particular risk, after a myocardial infarct, in the elderly and in the hypotensive, PD, splinting the diaphragms, can lead to respiratory problems even with 1 litre exchanges. It may also not provide adequate urea clearance to correct the uraemia if urea production is especially high. The optimal urea clearance with PD is about 25–30 ml/min compared with 100 ml/min or more for haemodialysis.

38. Ptosis **Answers: B E**

A lateral medullary, dorsolateral pontine and dorsolateral midbrain lesion may produce an ipsilateral Horner's syndrome. In addition, a basal and paramedian midbrain lesion may produce an ipsilateral third cranial nerve palsy. Myotonic dystrophy may be associated with bilateral partial ptosis.

39. Unilateral lesion in the midbrain **Answers: B C D**

The unilateral paramedian midbrain lesion will produce an ipsilateral third cranial nerve palsy and contralateral ataxia (Benedikt's syndrome) due to involvement of the red nucleus which interrupts the dentato-rubro-thalamic tract. A unilateral basal midbrain lesion will produce an ipsilateral third cranial nerve palsy and contralateral hemiplegia (Weber's syndrome). A unilateral dorsolateral midbrain lesion will produce an ipsilateral Horner's syndrome, contralateral total sensory loss and ipsilateral ataxia due to involvement of the superior cerebellar peduncle. The sixth cranial nerve nucleus is located in the pons. Bilateral lesions are require to produce a pseudobulbar palsy.

40. Axillary plexus **Answers: A C E**

Posterior cord – Radial nerve (PR). Medial cord – Ulnar nerve (MU). Medial and Lateral cords – Median nerve (MLM). The axillary nerve (posterior cord C5–6) supplies deltoid and teres minor. A lesion causes weakness of shoulder abduction between 15 and 90 degrees and sensory loss over the anterior aspect of the shoulder. The musculocutaneous nerve (lateral cord C5–6) innervates biceps, brachialis and coracobrachialis (BBC) and skin over the outer border of the upper arm.

41. Chorea **Answers: A B C D**

Chorea may be caused by drugs which increase striatal dopamine activity (L-dopa, selegiline, tricyclic antidepressants) or stimulate striatal dopamine receptors (bromocriptine). Tardive chorea is caused by dopamine blocking agents (including the commonly used metoclopramide and prochlorperazine) and is thought to be caused by receptor hypersensitivity. Tetrabenazine is used in the treatment of Huntington's chorea.

42. Duchenne muscular dystrophy **Answers: A D**

Limb weakness affects proximal limb musculature whereas pseudohypertrophy affects more distal musculature of the calves and forearms. Limb contractures may be a late clinical manifestation of Duchenne muscular dystrophy but are an early feature of Emery-Dreifuss muscular dystrophy (X-linked recessive). EMGs show a typically myopathic appearance.

43. Multiple sclerosis **Answers: B E**

In MS, breakdown of the blood brain barrier precedes both symptoms and MRI signs of demyelination. Perivascular helper T cells are found in acute MS lesions and there is abnormal MHC class II expression on macrophages and astrocytes resulting in antigen presentation. The resulting T cell proliferation and activation of B cells with macrophages leads to demyelination by killing of oligodendrocytes which have little, if any, proliferative capacity. The loss of myelin prevents saltatory conduction between the nodes of Ranvier.

44. Huntington's disease **Answers: A C**

Huntington's disease is an autosomal dominant neurodegenerative disorder characterised by variable age at onset (typically 45–65), uncontrolled movements, altered behaviour and cognitive decline. It is caused by expansion of a polyglutamine trinucleotide repeat in the coding region of the gene – the size of the expansion predicts age of onset. Neurodegeneration is primarily in the caudate and putamen by apoptosis. The spinocerebellar ataxias (which cause Purkinje and olive degeneration) are due to similar polyglutamine trinucleotide repeats in their respective genes. Trinucleotide repeat diseases are characteristically worse in each subsequent generation.

45. *Listeria monocytogenes* **Answers: B C E**

Listeria monocytogenes is an aerobic Gram-positive bacillus that is ubiquitous in the environment. Infection with this micro-organism is increased in the elderly, immunocompromised and pregnant (x 17 relative risk). Listeria monocytogenes is readily phagocytosed but has an enzyme – listerolysis O – an exotoxin that lyses the cell membrane of the phagolysosome and allows the organism to escape into the cytoplasm. Listeria exploit the host-cell contractile system for locomotion and cell-to-cell spread by promoting actin assembly that propels the micro-organism.

46. *Helicobacter pylori* **Answers: B D**

Helicobacter pylori is a microaerophilic Gram-negative rod. *H. pylori* colonise the stomach in at least a third of the world's human population. These organisms are urease positive and can therefore produce ammonia which is thought to result in epithelial damage. *H. pylori* infection is often asymptomatic but can result in peptic ulcer disease, gastritis, gastric carcinoma and gastric lymphoma. Helicobacter irradication is not recommended for reflux oesophagitis.

47. Beta-haemolytic streptococci **Answers: A C E**

Several strains of streptococci are characterised by their ability to lyse red blood cells; these include organisms with the Lancefield group A antigen (*Str. pyogenes*), group B (*Str. agalactiae*, which can cause serious neonatal infections), and also C and G. Group A streptococci are the most frequently pathogenic in man; the presence of the M-protein in their cellular wall is important for virulence. These organisms may cause skin infections such as erysipelas and impetigo, the latter occurring in epidemic proportions in some tropical countries such that post-infective glomerulonephritis is a frequent complication.

48. Proliferative diabetic retinopathy **Answer: D**

Proliferative diabetic retinopathy is treated initially by pan-retinal photocoagulation, not directed at the abnormal vessels. Rubeosis iridis is a feature of new vessels on the iris. All microvascular complications are exceptionally rare in presentation in IDDM. Unfortunately, pregnancy may lead to a deterioration in pre-existing retinopathy. Patients may continue to drive provided that they fulfil the requirements for visual fields and acuity.

49. Delusions of persecution **Answers: A D E**

Persecutory delusions are the leading feature of paraphrenia, a psychosis typically of elderly deaf, socially isolated women with premorbid schizoid or paranoid traits. Myxoedema can produce a variety of serious mental disorders, including paranoid psychosis. Amphetamine abuse frequently produces a psychotic disorder with paranoid delusions and hallucinations, which may remit rapidly with abstinence. Patients with paranoid personalities have a pervasive sense of being slighted or tricked which does not reach delusional intensity. Persecutory delusions occur in endogenous (psychotic) depression rather than reactive depression.

50. Anorexia nervosa **Answers: A B D E**

The central clinical features of anorexia nervosa are low body weight (15% below normal weight), distorted body image and amenorrhoea. Vomiting and laxative abuse may lead to hypokalaemia. Several hormonal abnormalities may occur: raised growth hormone, raised plasma cortisol with loss of diurnal variation, low gonadotrophins and low triiodothyronine. There are numerous medical complications such as bradycardia, hypotension, cardiac arrhythmias, oedema, osteoporosis, hypothermia, salivary gland enlargement, pancreatitis, hypoglycaemia and erosion of tooth enamel. Depressed mood is common.

51. Grief reaction **Answers: A B D**

The initial stages of a grief reaction is a period of numbness with little or no emotional reaction. This is the period of denial. Subsequent stages follow to a state of depression, and suicidal ideas are often expressed. These may reflect feelings of guilt or identification with the dead person. The reaction is self-limiting although there may be delays up to several years. The treatment of choice would be some form of psychotherapy or counselling. The reaction is neurotic rather than psychotic.

52. Tuberculous lesion **Answer: B**

There is initial transient acute inflammation with polymorphs. Caseation consists of altered macrophages and dead tissue cells. Fibroblasts, not giant cells, provide evidence of healing. Although the combination of caseation, macrophages and epithelioid cells is very suggestive of tuberculosis, it is not diagnostic.

53. Non small cell lung cancer **Answers: A B**

Molecular genetic markers of prognosis in non small cell lung cancer include the ras oncogene and p21 expression. The ras oncogenes modulate cell growth via regulation of the signal transduction pathway. ras genes are expressed in virtually all cells, but mutations can lead to over expression and increased production of p21, the protein product of ras – this is associated with poor outcome. Proliferating cell nuclear antigen, a nuclear protein that binds to DNA polymerase and can be used as a marker of cell proliferation, is also associated with poor outcome. Karnowsky performance status, extent of disease and weight loss are the most powerful determinants of survival. Histological type does not affect response to adjuvant chemotherapy. The risks of smoking (relative risk increased by 11) and asbestos (relative risk increased by 6) exposure are multiplicative (relative risk increased by 59).

54. Physiological adaptations to high altitude **Answer: E**

The response to chronic hypoxia (e.g. high altitude acclimatisation) includes increased ventilation which reduces carbon dioxide levels and causes a mild alkalosis that is corrected by increased renal bicarbonate excretion. Red cell 2,3 DPG is increased facilitating shift of the Hb-O_2 dissociation curve to the right. Haemoglobin concentration and circulating blood volume increase and there is pulmonary hypertension due to pulmonary vasoconstriction caused by chronic hypoxia.

55. Cystic fibrosis **Answers: A B C D**

Sweat sodium and chloride concentrations are characteristically elevated. Rectal prolapse is a recognised clinical feature of cystic fibrosis in infancy. Approximately 10% of cases present in the neonatal period with intestinal obstruction due to meconium ileus. Aspermia is a uniform finding in males, resulting from obliteration of the vas deferens. The gene is located on chromosome number 7.

56. Type I and type II pneumocytes **Answers: B C D**

Type II pneumocytes are slightly more numerous than type I cells, but cover less of the epithelial lining. The type I cells have an extremely attenuated cytoplasm and thus only provide a thin barrier to gas exchange across the alveolar membrane. They are derived from type II pneumocytes. In contrast, type II pneumocytes are more cuboidal in shape and cover a more limited surface area. The principal physiological activity of type II pneumocytes is production of surfactant but they also have limited phagocytic ability. Surfactant is an insoluble liproprotein largely consisting of dipalmitoyl lecithin which lowers the surface tension in the alveoli. Cilia only extend to the respiratory bronchiole; neither pneumocyte is ciliated.

57. Rheumatoid arthritis **Answers: A C D E**

Ankle oedema may be a feature of cardiac failure, constrictive pericarditis or amyloid and nephrotic syndrome. Mouth ulcers may be associated with sicca syndrome, drugs or neutropenia. Splenomegaly is a feature of Felty's syndrome. Cervical cord compression may occur with sub-luxation leading to upper motor neurone neuropathy; mono-neuritis multiplex and peripheral nerve entrapment are also common. Iritis is no more common than in the general population.

58. Rheumatoid arthritis **Answers: B E**

Rheumatoid arthritis is associated with HLA DR1and HLA DR4, but twin surveys reveal a concordance of less than 30%, suggesting a polygenic rather than single gene effect. There is evidence of B cell overactivity (rheumatoid factor, autoantibodies) and increased activated T cells in the peripheral blood and joints. Interleukin-I and tumour necrosis factor alpha are elevated in the joints and blockade of TNF-alpha with monoclonal antibody therapy reduces disease activity. Abnormal HLA class II expression or chondrocytes, fibroblasts and endothelial cells occur and are likely to be involved in antigen presentation to the T cell receptor.

59. Reiter's disease **Answers: A C D**

Reiter's disease is a reactive arthritis secondary to infection – frequently dysentery or non-specific urethritis (not gonococcal). The disease is thought to be due to immune complex deposition but antibodies to nuclear antigens are not a feature. The disease usually affects males aged 16 to 35 years and is strongly associated with HLA B27. Other features of Reiter's disease include plantar fascitis, keratoderma blennorrhagica and circinate balinitis.

60. Diastolic blood pressure readings study **Answers: A C E**

It is hoped that the sample mean will be equal to the population mean, but in reality they are rarely exactly equal. The median is equal to the mean when the data are normally distributed.

REVISION CHECKLIST FOR THE MRCP 1 EXAM

Numbers in brackets indicate relative frequency of topics.

BASIC SCIENCES

Physiology

- Changes in pregnancy (2)
- Haemoglobin function
- Physiology of bone
- Aetiology of oedema

Pathology

- Amyloid plaques
- Apoptosis

Hormone and mediator biochemistry

- Atrial natriuretic peptides (4)
- Insulin/insulin resistance (3)
- Nitric oxide (3)
- Angiotensin (2)
- Neurotransmitters (2)
- Prostacyclin (2)
- Adenosine
- ADH
- Aldosterone
- H2 receptors
- Somatostatin
- Steroid receptors

Miscellaneous

- Organelles with DNA (2)
- Apolipoproteins
- Alpha$_1$-antitrypsin
- Oncogenes

CARDIOLOGY

Valvular heart disease

- Heart sounds (4)
- Mitral stenosis (3)
- Valve lesions/murmurs (3)
- Antibiotic prophylaxis
- Catheterisation data
- Mitral valve prolapse

Arrhythmias

- Wolff-Parkinson-White/SVT (6)
- Atrial fibrillation (3)
- Ventricular tachycardia (3)
- LBBB (2)
- Prolonged Q-T (2)
- Torsades des pointes

Pericardial disease

- Constrictive pericarditis (7)
- Cardiac tamponade (1)
- Pericardial effusion
- *IHD/heart muscle disease*
- Myocardial infarction (6)
- Cardiomyopathy (3)
- Left ventricular failure (2)
- Unstable angina (2)
- Coronary bypass surgery
- Left ventricular hypertrophy
- Signs underlying heart disease

Congenital heart disease

- Cyanotic heart disease/ Eisenmenger's (4)
- ASD (3)
- Patent ductus arteriosus
- VSD

Large vessel disease

- Pulmonary embolus (4)
- Aortic dissection (3)
- Pulmonary hypertension (3)

Miscellaneous

- Cannon "a" waves in JVP (4)
- Alcohol and the heart (3)
- Carotid body/cardiac sympathetics (2)
- Coronary circulation
- Left atrial myxoma

DERMATOLOGY

Specific skin lesions

- Erythema multiforme (2)
- Psoriasis (2)
- Alopecia areata
- Erythema nodosum
- Papular rash
- Purpura

Systemic manifestations

- Pruritus (3)
- Photosensitivity (2)
- Skin manifestations of systemic disease

Miscellaneous
- ➢ Foot ulcers
- ➢ Lesions on limbs

ENDOCRINOLOGY
Diabetes and glycaemic control
- ➢ Diabetes (11)
- ➢ Hypoglycaemia (4)
- ➢ Glycosylated haemoglobin
- ➢ Hepatic gluconeogenesis
- ➢ Insulinoma

Adrenal disease
- ➢ Cushing's syndrome (8)
- ➢ Addison's disease (4)
- ➢ Congenital adrenal hyperplasia (4)
- ➢ ACTH action

Thyroid disease
- ➢ Thyroxine action/metabolism TFTs (6)
- ➢ Thyroid cancer/nodule (3)
- ➢ Graves'disease/exophthalmos (2)
- ➢ Hypothyroidism (2)

Parathyroid disease
- ➢ PTH/hyperparathyroidism (4)
- ➢ Calcitonin (2)

Pituitary disease
- ➢ Acromegaly (5)
- ➢ Chromophobe adenoma (2)
- ➢ Hyperprolactinaemia (2)
- ➢ Hypopituitarism
- ➢ Pituitary hormones

Miscellaneous
- ➢ Polycystic ovary syndrome/infertility (4)
- ➢ SIADH (3)
- ➢ Short stature
- ➢ Weight gain/Prader-Willi Syndrome (2)
- ➢ Endocrine changes in anorexia
- ➢ Hirsutism
- ➢ Hormone physiology (including pregnancy)
- ➢ Sweating

GASTROENTEROLOGY
Liver disease
- ➢ Chronic liver disease (2)
- ➢ Jaundice (4)
- ➢ Primary biliary cirrhosis (4)
- ➢ Gilbert's syndrome (2)
- ➢ Hepatic mass/sub-phrenic abscess (2)
- ➢ Alcohol & liver
- ➢ Portal vein thrombosis

Small bowel disease/Malabsorption
- ➢ Coeliac disease (7)
- ➢ Malabsorption/protein-losing enteropathy (4)
- ➢ Cholera toxin/gastroenteritis (3)
- ➢ Carcinoid syndrome
- ➢ Whipple's disease

(see also 'Crohn's disease' below)

Large bowel disorders
- ➢ Crohn's disease (6)
- ➢ Ulcerative colitis/colonic carcinoma (6)
- ➢ Irritable bowel syndrome (3)
- ➢ Diarrhoea (2)
- ➢ Inflammatory bowel disease – general (2)
- ➢ Pseudomembranous colitis

Oesophageal disease
- ➢ Gastro-oesophageal reflux/tests (4)
- ➢ Achalasia (3)
- ➢ Dysphagia/oesophageal tumour (2)
- ➢ Oesophageal chest pain

Stomach and pancreas
- ➢ Acute pancreatitis (4)
- ➢ Gastric acid secretion (2)
- ➢ Persistent vomiting
- ➢ Stomach cancer

Miscellaneous
- ➢ GI tract bleeding (4)
- ➢ Abdominal X-ray
- ➢ GI hormones
- ➢ Physiology of absorption
- ➢ Recurrent abdominal pain

GENETICS

Syndromes

- ➢ Klinefelter's syndrome (4)
- ➢ Turner's syndrome (2)
- ➢ Down's syndrome (2)

Modes of inheritance

- ➢ X-linked conditions (2)
- ➢ Autosomal recessive (2)
- ➢ Autosomal dominant
- ➢ Genetic anticipation
- ➢ Inheritance patterns (various)

Miscellaneous

- ➢ Abnormal karyotype (4)
- ➢ Chorionic villous sampling
- ➢ Chorionic defects

HAEMATOLOGY

Red cell physiology and anaemias

- ➢ Iron deficiency/metabolism/ therapy (4)
- ➢ Macrocytosis/pernicious anaemia (4)
- ➢ Folate deficiency (3)
- ➢ Basophilia (2)
- ➢ Erythropoiesis/Hb physiology (2)
- ➢ Haem biosynthesis (2)
- ➢ Sideroblastic anaemia (2)
- ➢ Aplastic anaemia
- ➢ Investigation of anaemia
- ➢ Vitamin B12 metabolism

Haemolytic anaemia

- ➢ Haemolytic anaemia (7)
- ➢ Sickle cell/Haemoglobinopathy (7)
- ➢ Hereditary spherocytosis (2)
- ➢ Reticulocytosis (2)
- ➢ G-6-PD deficiency
- ➢ Haemolytic-uraemic syndrome
- ➢ Intravascular haemolysis

Bleeding disorders

- ➢ Thrombocytopaenia (2)
- ➢ Haemophilia (2)
- ➢ Bleeding time
- ➢ Fresh frozen plasma
- ➢ Von Willebrand's disease

Haematological malignancy

- ➢ Hodgkin's/Non-Hodgkin's lymphoma (5)
- ➢ Leukaemia (2)
- ➢ Pancytopenia/splenomegaly (5)
- ➢ Polycythaemia (2)

Miscellaneous

- ➢ Hyposplenism (2)
- ➢ Methaemoglobinaemia (2)
- ➢ Neutropaenia (2)
- ➢ Thrombocytosis (2)
- ➢ Bone infarction
- ➢ Bone marrow test
- ➢ Eosinophilia
- ➢ Hyperuricaemia and haematological disease

(see also Metabolic Disease)

- ➢ Paroxysmal nocturnal haemoglobinuria

IMMUNOLOGY

Cytokines

- ➢ Tumour necrosis factor (3)
- ➢ Interferon (2)
- ➢ Inflammatory mediators (general)
- ➢ Leukotrienes

Cellular immunity

- ➢ T lymphocytes/deficiency (5)
- ➢ Cell-mediated immunity (2)

Immunoglobulins/autoimmunity

- ➢ IgA/IgE/IgG (4)
- ➢ Autoimmune disease/ANCA (2)
- ➢ Hypogammaglobulinaemia (2)
- ➢ Monoclonal gammopathy (2)
- ➢ Tissue receptor antibodies (2)
- ➢ Circulating immune complexes
- ➢ Precipitating antibodies in diagnosis

Miscellaneous

- ➢ Complement/CH_{50} (2)
- ➢ Angioneurotic oedema (2)
- ➢ Hypersensitivity reactions (2)
- ➢ Mast cells
- ➢ Polymerase chain reaction
- ➢ Post-splenectomy
- ➢ Transplant rejection

INFECTIOUS DISEASES

Viral Infections

- Hepatitis (6)
- Infectious mononucleosis (6)
- Chickenpox/measles/mumps (5)
- AIDS/HIV (4)
- Adenovirus
- Genital herpes
- Parvovirus

Bacterial Infections

- Venereal disease (8)
- Brucellosis (4)
- TB/BCG (4)
- Tetanus (4)
- Toxoplasmosis (4)
- Typhoid/cholera (4)
- Bacteroides
- *Haemophilus influenza*
- *Helicobacter pylori*
- Lyme disease
- Meningitis
- Pneumonia
- Staphylococcus

Routes of infection

- Transmission by insect bite (3)
- Faecal-oral transmission (2)

Tropical and protozoal infections

- Malaria (9)
- Tropical fever/splenomegaly (2)
- Giardiasis
- *Pneumocystis carinii*
- Schistosomiasis

Miscellaneous

- *Chlamydia trachomatis* (2)
- Other infections/diarrhoea (2)
- Chronic infection and anaemia
- Infections and eosinophilia
- Prion disease

METABOLIC DISEASE

Overdose and poisoning

- Carbon monoxide/other poisoning (5)
- Salicylate/paracetamol overdose (4)
- Tricyclic/theophylline overdose (4)
- Excess alcohol (2)
- Iron toxicity

Disorders of bone

- Osteoporosis (4)
- Vitamin D metabolism (4)
- Achondroplasia
- Calcium homeostasis
- Increased alkaline phosphatase
- Increased prostate-specific antigen
- Paget's disease

Disorders of acid/base and electrolytes

- Hyper/hypokalaemia (4)
- Alkalosis/vomiting (3)
- Hypomagnesaemia (3)
- Hyponatraemia/chloride depletion (2)
- Hypophosphataemia (2)
- Hypercalcaemia
- Hypernatraemia
- Polydipsia

Inherited metabolic disorders

- Hypercholesterolaemia (2)
- Wilson's disease (2)
- Alpha$_1$-antitrypsin deficiency (*see also Basic Science*)
- Homocystinuria
- Malignant neuroleptic syndrome

Miscellaneous

- Hypothermia (2)
- Hypercarotenemia
- Hyperuricaemia
- Kwashiorkor
- Marfan's syndrome
- Obesity
- Thiamine deficiency

NEPHROLOGY

Nephrotic syndrome/related glomerulonephritis

- Nephrotic syndrome (9)
- Membranous glomerulonephritis (4)
- Minimal Change disease (4)
- Hypocomplementaemia & glomerulonephritis (2)
- Renal vein thrombosis (2)
- Acute glomerulonephritis
- SLE nephritis

Renal failure
- ➢ Acute renal failure (4)
- ➢ Acute versus chronic (3)
- ➢ Chronic renal failure (3)
- ➢ Haemolytic-uraemic syndrome (2)
- ➢ Rhabdomyolysis (2)
- ➢ Anaemia in renal failure
- ➢ Contrast nephropathy

Urinary abnormalities
- ➢ Macroscopic haematuria (2)
- ➢ Discolouration of the urine
- ➢ Nocturia
- ➢ Polyuria

Basic renal physiology
- ➢ Normal renal physiology/ function (6)
- ➢ Water excretion/urinary concentration (2)
- ➢ Serum creatinine

Miscellaneous
- ➢ Distal renal tubular acidosis (5)
- ➢ Renal papillary necrosis (4)
- ➢ Diabetic nephropathy (3)
- ➢ Analgesic nephropathy
- ➢ Polycystic kidney disease
- ➢ Renal calculi
- ➢ Renal osteodystrophy
- ➢ Retroperitoneal fibrosis
- ➢ Steroid therapy in renal disease

NEUROLOGY

Abnormalities of brain & cerebral circulation
- ➢ Dementia/Alzheimer's (5)
- ➢ Transient ischaemic attacks (4)
- ➢ Benign intracranial hypertension/brain tumour (3)
- ➢ Head injury (3)
- ➢ Lateral medullary/circulatory syndromes (3)
- ➢ Subdural haematoma (3)
- ➢ Encephalitis (2)
- ➢ Parietal lobe/frontal cortical lesions (2)
- ➢ Temporal lobe epilepsy (2)
- ➢ Amnesia
- ➢ Central pontine myelinolysis
- ➢ Cerebral abscess
- ➢ Creutzfeldt-Jakob disease
- ➢ EEG
- ➢ Intracranial calcification
- ➢ Midbrain (Parinaud's) syndrome
- ➢ Normal pressure hydrocephalus
- ➢ Wernicke's encephalopathy

Spinal cord and peripheral nerve anatomy & lesions
- ➢ Innervation of specific muscles (4)
- ➢ Median nerve/brachial plexus (3)
- ➢ Posterior nerve root/spinal ganglia lesions (3)
- ➢ Dorsal interosseous nerve (2)
- ➢ Guillain-Barré (2)
- ➢ Pyramidal tracts/posterior column pathways (2)
- ➢ Sciatic nerve lesion (2)
- ➢ Autonomic spondylosis
- ➢ Cervical spondylosis
- ➢ Motor neuron disease
- ➢ Paraesthesia
- ➢ Spinal cord lesions

Cranial nerve anatomy & lesions
- ➢ Facial nerve (6)
- ➢ Cranial nerve lesions (5)
- ➢ Third nerve palsy/pupillary reflex (3)
- ➢ Bulbar palsy
- ➢ Internuclear ophthalmoplegia
- ➢ 4th nerve palsy

Dyskinesias
- ➢ Ataxia (2)
- ➢ Benign essential tremor (2)
- ➢ Dyskinesia
- ➢ Parkinson's disease

Muscular disorders
- ➢ Duchenne muscular dystrophy (4)
- ➢ Myotonic dystrophy (2)
- ➢ Myaesthenia gravis

Miscellaneous
- ➢ Multiple sclerosis (5)
- ➢ Headache/migraine (4)
- ➢ Lumbar puncture/CSF (3)
- ➢ Nystagmus (3)
- ➢ Pseudofits (2)

- Vertigo/dysarthria (2)
- CNS involvement in AIDS

PHARMACOLOGY

Interactions/dose adjustment

- Drug interactions (10)
- Pregnancy/breast feeding (7)
- Adverse effects - general (4)
- Dose adjustment in renal failure (3)
- Drugs in porphyria
- Polymorphism of drug metabolism

Specific side-effects of drugs

- Asthma exacerbation (2)
- Causing hypothyroidism (2)
- Gynaecomastia/ hyperprolactinaemia (2)
- Hepatic enzyme inducers
- Hypokalaemia
- Aggravation of skin disorders
- Convulsions
- Haemolytic anaemia

Fundamental pharmacology

- Mechanisms of drug/antibiotic action (2)

Most frequently considered individual agents

- Antipsychotics/depressants (5)
- ACE inhibitors (4)
- Amiodarone (4)
- Thiazides (4)
- Anti-convulsants (3)
- Digoxin (3)
- Lithium (3)
- Sulphasalazine (2)
- Metronidazole
- Radio-iodine

Other 'topical' agents

- Azidothymidine (AZT)
- Cimetidine
- Gentamicin
- Griseofulvin
- HMG Co-A reductase inhibitor
- L-dopa
- Metronidazole
- Penicillamine
- Retinoic acid
- Warfarin

PSYCHIATRY

Psychotic disorders

- Schizophrenia (8)
- Depression (7)
- Mania (6)
- Hallucinations/delusions (3)

Anxiety states/compulsive disorders

- Neurosis/psychogenic/ conversion disorders (5)
- Obsessional/compulsive disorders (5)
- Panic attack

Eating disorders

- Anorexia nervosa (9)
- Bulimia (2)

Other cognitive disorders

- Differentiation of dementia and depression (3)
- Acute confusional state (2)

Miscellaneous

- Psychiatric manifestations of organic disease (6)
- Alcohol dependency (3)
- Insomnia (2)
- Narcolepsy (2)
- Endocrine causes of psychiatric disease
- Psychiatric manifestations in adolescence

RESPIRATORY DISEASE

Respiratory infections

- Pneumonia (7)
- Broncho-pulmonary aspergillosis (3)
- Acute bronchiolitis
- Psittacosis
- Viral infections

Lung cancer

- Bronchial carcinoma (5)
- Surgery for cancer (3)
- Pancoast's tumour
- Small cell cancer

Pulmonary physiology
- Lung function tests (4)
- Normal physiology (3)
- Transfer factor (2)
- Forced hyperventilation

End-stage lung disease
- Respiratory failure (4)
- Long-term oxygen

Interstitial lung disease/fibrosis
- Extrinsic allergic alveolitis (6)
- Bronchiectasis (4)
- ARDS (3)
- Sarcoidosis (3)
- Emphysema (2)
- Fibrosing alveolitis (2)
- Pulmonary fibrosis (2)
- Asbestosis
- Cystic fibrosis

Miscellaneous
- Asthma (5)
- Sleep-apnoea syndrome (5)
- Autoimmune disease and lung (3)
- Abnormal chest X-ray (2)
- Lung cavitation
- Pulmonary eosinophilia

RHEUMATOLOGY

Auto-immune disease
- Rheumatoid arthritis (7)
- SLE (7)
- Wegener's granulomatosis (2)

Other vasculitides
- Polymyalgia rheumatica (4)
- Cranial arteritis
- Vasculitic disease

Other arthritides
- Reiter's syndrome (3)
- Ankylosing spondylitis/HLA B27 (2)
- Arthralgia (2)
- Behçet's disease (2)
- Arthropathy (general)
- Hypertrophic osteo-arthropathy
- Osteoarthritis
- Pseudogout

Miscellaneous
- Anti-phospholipid syndrome (3)
- Digital gangrene
- Peri-articular calcification
- Systemic sclerosis

STATISTICS

Statistical populations
- Normal distribution (4)
- Standard deviation (3)
- Skewed distribution

Tests of significance
- Significance test (6)
- Chi-square test
- Type I and II errors
- Skewed distribution

Miscellaneous
- Specificity of clinical trials (2)

REVISION INDEX

The numbers in this index refer to the page the relevant question appears on.